Diffusion of Innovations in Health Service Organisations

A systematic literature review

Diffusion of Innovations in Health Service Organisations

A systematic literature review

Trisha Greenhalgh
Primary Care and Population Sciences, University College London, Highgate Hill, London N19 5LW

Glenn Robert
Centre for Health Informatics and Multiprofessional Education (CHIME), University College London, Highgate Hill, London N19 5LW

Paul Bate
Centre for Health Informatics and Multiprofessional Education (CHIME), University College London, Highgate Hill, London N19 5LW

Fraser Macfarlane
The School of Management, University of Surrey, Guildford, Surrey GU2 7XH

Olivia Kyriakidou
The School of Management, University of Surrey, Guildford, Surrey GU2 7XH

FOREWORD BY
Sir Liam Donaldson

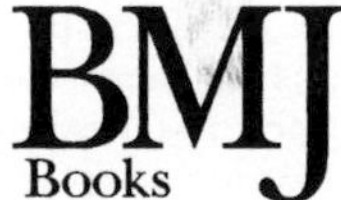

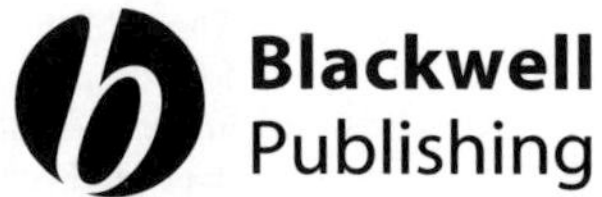

Blackwell Publishing, Inc., 350 Main Street, Malden, Massachusetts 02148-5020, USA
Blackwell Publishing Ltd, 9600 Garsington Road, Oxford OX4 2DQ, UK
Blackwell Publishing Asia Pty Ltd, 550 Swanston Street, Carlton, Victoria 3053, Australia

First published 2005

Library of-Congress Cataloging-in-Publication Data

Diffusion of innovations in health service organisations : a systematic literature review/ Trisha Greenhalgh ... [et al.]; foreword by Sir Liam Donaldson.

p. ; cm.

Includes bibliographical references and index.

ISBN-13: 978-0-7279-1869-7 (alk. paper)

ISBN-10: 0-7279-1869-9 (alk. paper)

1. Medical care—Quality control. 2. Health services administration—Quality control. 3. Diffusion of innovations. 4. Medical care—Research—Methodology.

[DNLM: 1. Delivery of Health Care—trends. 2. Diffusion of Innovation. 3. Health Services Administration—trends. W 84.1 D569 2005] I. Greenhalgh, Trisha.

RA399.A1D54 2005

362.1′068′5–dc22 2005004104

ISBN-13: 978-0-7279-1-8697
ISBN-10: 0-7279-1869-9

A catalogue record for this title is available from the British Library

Set in 9.5/12pt Sabon by Kolam Information Services Pvt. Ltd, Pondicherry, India
Printed and bound by Replika Press Pvt. Ltd, India

Commissioning Editor: Mary Banks
Development Editor: Nick Morgan
Production Controller: Debbie Wyer

For further information on Blackwell Publishing, visit our website:
http://www.blackwellpublishing.com

The publisher's policy is to use permanent paper from mills that operate a sustainable forestry policy, and which has been manufactured from pulp processed using acid-free and elementary chlorine-free practices. Furthermore, the publisher ensures that the text paper and cover board used have met acceptable environmental accreditation standards.

Contents

Acknowledgements, viii
Foreword, ix
How to read this book, x

Summary overview, 1

Chapter 1: Introduction, 20

1.1 What is diffusion of innovations theory?, 20
1.2 Why did the UK Department of Health want to research the diffusion of innovations?, 22
1.3 Scope of this research, 25
1.4 Definitions, 26
1.5 Structure of this book, 31

Chapter 2: Method, 32

2.1 Outline of method, 32
2.2 Planning phase, 34
2.3 Search phase, 35
2.4 Mapping phase, 37
2.5 Appraisal phase, 38
2.6 Synthesis phase, 40
2.7 Meta-narrative review: philosophical origins and links with other approaches to the synthesis of complex evidence, 42

Chapter 3: The research traditions, 48

3.1 The origins of diffusion of innovations research, 49
3.2 Rural sociology, 51
3.3 Medical sociology, 53
3.4 Communication studies, 55
3.5 Marketing and economics, 56
3.6 Limitations of early diffusion research, 58
3.7 Development studies, 60
3.8 Health promotion, 62
3.9 Evidence-based medicine and guideline implementation, 64
3.10 Structural determinants of organisational innovativeness, 66
3.11 Studies of organisational process, context and culture, 68
3.12 Interorganisational studies: networks and influence, 70
3.13 Knowledge-based approaches to diffusion in organisations, 70
3.14 Narrative organisational studies, 77
3.15 Complexity and general systems theory, 79
3.16 Conclusion, 80

Chapter 4: Innovations, 83

4.1 Background literature on attributes of innovations, 83
4.2 The Tornatzky and Klein meta-analysis of innovation attributes, 87
4.3 Empirical studies of innovation attributes, 90
4.4 Limitations of conventional attribution constructs for studying adoption in organisational settings, 94
4.5 Attributes of innovations in the organisational context, 97

Chapter 5: Adopters and adoption, 100

5.1 Characteristics of adopters: background literature, 100
5.2 Adoption as a process: background literature, 103
5.3 Assimilation of innovations in organisations, 106

Chapter 6: Diffusion and dissemination, 114

6.1 Communication and influence through interpersonal networks, 114
6.2 Opinion leaders, 118
6.3 Champions and advocates, 126
6.4 Boundary spanners, 129
6.5 Change agents, 130
6.6 The process of spread, 130

Chapter 7: The inner context, 134

7.1 The inner context: background literature, 134
7.2 Organisational determinants of innovativeness: meta-analyses, 135
7.3 Organisational determinants of innovativeness: overview of primary studies in the service sector, 140
7.4 Empirical studies on organisational size, 141
7.5 Empirical studies on structural complexity, 146
7.6 Empirical studies on leadership and locus of decision-making, 148
7.7 Empirical studies on organisational climate and receptive context, 150
7.8 Empirical studies on supporting knowledge utilisation and manipulation, 154

Chapter 8: The outer context, 157

8.1 Interorganisational influence through informal social networks, 157
8.2 Interorganisational influence through intentional spread strategies, 163
8.3 Empirical studies of environmental impact on organisational innovativeness, 170
8.4 Empirical studies of impact of politics and policymaking on organisational innovativeness, 172

Chapter 9: Implementation and institutionalisation, 175

9.1 Overview of the implementation literature, 176
9.2 Measuring institutionalisation and related concepts, 178
9.3 Implementation and institutionalisation: systematic reviews and other high-quality overviews, 180
9.4 Empirical studies of interventions aimed at strengthening predisposition and capacity of the user system, 186
9.5 Empirical studies of interventions aimed at strengthening the resource system and change agency, 190
9.6 Empirical studies of linkage activities to support implementation, 191
9.7 Empirical studies that have investigated 'whole-systems' approaches to implementation, 195

Chapter 10: Case studies, 199

10.1 Developing and applying a unifying conceptual model, 199
10.2 Case study 1: integrated care pathways ('the steady success story'), 202
10.3 Case study 2: GP fundholding ('the clash'), 204
10.4 Case study 3: telemedicine ('the maverick initiative'), 206
10.5 Case study 4: the electronic health record ('the big roll-out'), 208
10.6 Conclusion, 210

Chapter 11: Discussion, 219

11.1 Overview and commentary on main findings, 219
11.2 A framework for applying the model in a service context, 220
11.3 Recommendations for further research, 225
11.4 Conclusion, 231

Appendix 1: Data extraction form, 232

Appendix 2: Critical appraisal checklists, 234

Box A.1 Quality checklist for experimental (randomised and non-randomised controlled trial) designs, 234
Box A.2 Quality checklist for quasi-experimental (interrupted time series) designs, 235
Box A.3 Quality checklist for attribution studies, 236
Box A.4 Quality checklist for questionnaire surveys, 237

Box A.5 Quality checklist for qualitative studies, 238
Box A.6 Quality checklist for mixed-methodology case studies and other in-depth complex designs, 239
Box A.7 Quality checklist for comparison of 'real-world' implementation studies, 240
Box A.8 Quality checklist for action research designs, 242

Appendix 3: Descriptive statistics on included studies, 245

Table A.1 Main sources and yield of papers, books and book chapters, 247
Table A.2 Breakdown of studies included in the book, 248
Table A.3 Yield from hand search of journals, 249
Table A.4 Yield from search of electronic databases, 252
Table A.5 Yield from electronic citation tracking, 254

Appendix 4: Tables of included studies, 255

Table A.6 Narrative overviews used as key sources in this review, 255
Table A.7 Empirical studies of attributes of health care innovations in the organisational setting, 257
Table A.8 Empirical studies that focused on the *process* of adoption in health care organisations, 260
Table A.9 Network analyses of interpersonal influence in health care organisations, 262
Table A.10 Empirical studies of opinion leadership in health care organisations, 263
Table A.11 Controlled trials of opinion leaders as an intervention in health care organisations, 265
Table A.12 Empirical studies of impact of champions in health care organisations and selected other examples, 267
Table A.13 Meta-analyses that addressed the impact of the organisational context on adoption of innovations, 269
Table A.14 Empirical studies of 'inner' context determinants of innovation in health care organisations and selected other examples, 271
Table A.15 Empirical studies from health care that looked at the organisational context for innovation from a knowledge utilisation perspective, 274
Table A.16 Empirical studies of informal inter-organisational influence amongst health care organisations and selected other examples, 276
Table A.17 Empirical studies on health care quality improvement collaboratives, 278
Table A.18 Empirical studies of impact of environmental factors on innovation in health care organisations and selected other examples, 280
Table A.19 Empirical studies of impact of political and policymaking forces on organisational innovation, 283
Table A.20 Systematic reviews relevant to the question of dissemination, implementation and sustainability of innovations in service delivery and organisation, 285
Table A.21 Surveys of perceptions about capacity or of association between capacity and implementation in health care organisations, 287
Table A.22 Empirical studies of interventions to enhance user system capacity in health care organisations, 289
Table A.23 'Whole-systems' approaches to implementation and sustainability of innovations in health care organisations and selected other examples, 291

Glossary, 293
References, 296
Index, 313

Acknowledgements

We are especially grateful to Richard Peacock for librarian input to this study.

This work would not have been possible without the support of the Department of Health Service Delivery and Organisation Programme and the input of the following colleagues, friends and peer reviewers:

Amanda Band
Lindsay Forbes
Andrew Moore
Marcia Rigby
Anna Donald
Martyn Eccles
Chris Henshall
Mary Dixon-Woods
David Patterson
Mike Dunning
Diane Ketley
Mike Kelly
Francis Maietta
Paul Plsek
Gene Feder
Ray Pawson
Helen Roberts
Sandy Oliver
Huw Davies
John Øvretveit
Jennie Popay
Sarah Fraser
Jeremy Grimshaw
Stephanie Taylor
Jos Kleijnen
Stuart Anderson
Jerome Bruner

Foreword

In the mid-1990s, long before I became Chief Medical Officer, I met Michael Peckham who had just been appointed as the first Director of Research and Development for the National Health Service (NHS). He was scoping the role of the new research and development function. I suggested that he should give priority to health services research, and also that he should find a place for a programme looking at how, why and when research can be translated into beneficial change (either in clinical practice or in the provision of health services). We spent a couple of hours talking through this concept (which had not featured in Michael Peckham's other meetings), and becoming increasingly fascinated by its potential for improving the NHS.

Subsequently, as a member of the Central Research and Development Committee, I did the preparatory work that led to the formation of the NHS Service Delivery and Organisation programme. 'The SDO', as it has come to be known, has funded numerous empirical research studies into the organisation and management of health services, as well as several systematic literature reviews. This review by Trisha Greenhalgh and her colleagues was part of a wider SDO-funded research programme on change management.

For those who are already working in a relevant field – the adoption of innovations, the implementation of best practice or the translation of research findings into service improvements – this book is of major significance. Not only does it synthesise the diverse fields of research that have a bearing on this complex issue, it genuinely breaks new ground in conceptualising and mapping a vast intellectual terrain in a way that provides insight and adds practical value. It summarises and builds on the excellent work done by Everett Rogers who wrote the original textbook *Diffusion of Innovations* in the 1960s. It focuses especially on the kind of complex and multifaceted innovations that we often need to introduce in health services, drawing extensively on the organisational and management (O&M) and knowledge management (KM) literature.

For those unfamiliar with the territory, who may be both enticed and somewhat confused by vocabulary such as the 'innovation adoption curve', 'early adopters', 'laggards', 'opinion leaders' and 'champions', this new work provides an accessible and balanced account of an immensely complex subject.

This book is a towering work of remarkable scholarship. It bathes in light what was previously a shadowland of opacity, misconception, theory-hopping and misplaced enthusiasm.

Sir Liam Donaldson
Chief Medical Officer
Department of Health
79 Whitehall
London SW1A 2NS

How to read this book

This book is a detailed write-up of an extensive systematic review of over 1000 papers on the diffusion, spread and sustainability of innovation in health service organisations. The review raised methodological questions about how to undertake systematic reviews of complex bodies of evidence. The best way to read this book is probably to study the Summary Overview (page 1) and then turn to the chapter(s) that interest you most. Table 1.1 (page 23) also provides a useful overview of the different research literatures that contributed to this review.

If you want a quick revision of classical diffusion of innovations theory as developed by Everett Rogers and colleagues, turn to Section 1.1 (page 20). If you want to read about why the UK Department of Health were keen to explore the diffusion of innovations literature in 2002 when this work was commissioned, see Section 1.2 (page 22). The scope of this study – i.e. a broad-brush summary of what we included in, and what we omitted from, our research – is set out in Section 1.3 (page 25) and the definitions we used (such as 'innovation', 'diffusion' and so on) are given in Section 1.4 (page 26).

If you are particularly interested in the methodological issues raised by this review, for example if you plan to tackle a complex area of literature, you should read Chapter 2 (page 32). Chapter 3 (page 48) gives a brief overview of each of the 13 research traditions that we explored for this review. This is a long chapter and is useful for orientating yourself around the many different contributions to the literature on diffusion of innovations. You do not need to read it all before going on to the main results chapters, but you may like to return to it periodically.

The main results of the review are set out in the subsequent six chapters, divided into innovations (Chapter 4, page 83), adopters and adoption (Chapter 5, page 100), diffusion and dissemination (Chapter 6, page 114), the inner (organisational) context (Chapter 7, page 134), the outer (environmental) context (Chapter 8, page 157) and implementation and institutionalisation (Chapter 9, page 175). Each chapter includes a summary of key points on the first page.

In Chapter 10 (page 199), we offer a unifying model of diffusion of innovations in health service organisations (see page 201 for a summary diagram), and apply this model to four case studies of organisational innovations in health services. Chapter 11 (page 219) discusses the strengths and limitations of our method, suggests how it may be applied in a service context (page 220) and makes detailed suggestions for future research (including setting out areas where we believe further research is *not* needed—see page 225 et seq.).

Finally, we have provided additional detail for reference in the appendices, including our quality criteria for evaluating empirical studies (pages 234–242); the tables of included sources (pages 247–254); and the results from secondary and primary studies (pages 257–292). For the criteria we used to grade levels of evidence, see Box 2.4 (page 42).

Summary overview

Introduction and methods

Background. This book describes a systematic review of the literature on the diffusion, spread and sustainability of innovations in the organisation and delivery of health services. It was commissioned by the UK Department of Health via the National Health Service (NHS) Service Delivery and Organisation (SDO) Programme and undertaken between October 2002 and December 2003. The brief for the project was to inform the modernisation agenda set out in the white paper the *NHS Plan*[1] and related policy documents. Although an earlier (draft) version was produced as an internal report for the SDO Programme, this book includes minor factual amendments and refinements of style and presentation but covers the same empirical material.

Scope. Our systematic review covered a very wide range of literature. It focused primarily but not exclusively on research studies in the service sector, and the health care sector in particular. In areas where this literature was sparse, or where a wider literature provided important theoretical, methodological or empirical information, we broadened the scope of the review accordingly. Given the breadth of the research question and the limitations of time and resources (funding was limited to £80 000 and the contract required a definitive report after 9 months), we did not attempt an encyclopaedic coverage of all possibly relevant literature. Throughout this book, we have indicated areas where we believe additional work should be undertaken.

Definitions. We define a systematic literature review as one undertaken according to an explicit, rigorous and reproducible methodology. Innovation in service delivery and organisation refers to a novel set of behaviours, routines and ways of working, which are directed at improving health outcomes, administrative efficiency, cost-effectiveness, or user experience, and which are implemented by means of planned and coordinated action. We distinguish between diffusion (a passive phenomenon of social influence), dissemination (active and planned efforts to persuade target groups to adopt an innovation) and implementation (active and planned efforts to mainstream an innovation). There is an ambiguity in the notion of sustainability (the more an innovation is sustained or 'routinised' in an organisation, the less the organisation will be open to new innovations). These definitions and inherent tensions are discussed in Section 1.3 (page 25).

Search strategy. We used a broad search strategy (described in detail in Section 2.3, page 35), covering 15 separate electronic databases as well as hand searching 30 journals in health care, health services research, organisation and management, and sociology literature. Despite this, our initial yield of relevant quality papers was disappointing. Searching references of references, using electronic tracking to forward track citations, and seeking advice from experts in the field added considerably to our yield. Details of included sources are given in Tables A.1–A.5 (pages 245–254).

Inclusion criteria. Our initial intention was to include studies that (a) had been undertaken in the health service sector; (b) had addressed innovation in service delivery and organisation; (c) had looked specifically at the spread or sustainability of these innovations; and (d) had met stringent criteria for methodological quality as set out in Appendix 2 (page 234). In practice, as explained above, we used a pragmatic and flexible approach to inclusion that took account of the availability of research in different topic areas. We did not approach the literature as a whole with a strict and unyielding 'hierarchy of evidence'. Rather, we used an iterative and pluralist approach to defining and evaluating evidence, as set out below.

Making sense of the literature. Our search strategy led us to scan over 6000 abstracts and identified around 1000 full-text papers and over 100 books that were possibly relevant, of which some 500 contributed to the analysis and are referenced in this book. It was initially very difficult to develop any kind of taxonomy of the literature, and indeed previous reviewers had used expressions such as 'a conceptual cartographer's nightmare' to describe its theoretical complexity. In order to aid our own exploration of the literature, we developed a new technique, which we called 'meta-narrative review', described in detail in Chapter 2 (see in particular Box 2.1, page 33). In the initial mapping phase, we divided the literature broadly into research traditions* and traced the historical development of theory and empirical work separately for each tradition. Within each tradition, we identified the seminal theoretical and overview papers using the criteria of scholarship, comprehensiveness, and contribution to subsequent work within that tradition, as described in detail in Box 2.2 (page 37). We then used these papers to identify, classify and evaluate other sources within that tradition.

*As explained on page 38, a research tradition is defined as a coherent body of theoretical knowledge and a linked set of primary studies in which successive studies are influenced by the findings of previous studies.

Data extraction and analysis. We developed a data extraction form (adapted for different research designs), to summarise the research question, research design, validity and robustness of methods, sample size and power, nature and strength of findings, and validity of conclusions for each empirical study. We adapted the critical appraisal checklists used by the Cochrane Effective Practice and Organisation of Care Group for evaluation of service innovations, and added other checklists for qualitative research, mixed-methodology case studies, action research, and realist evaluation (these checklists are reproduced in Appendix 2, pages 234–242).

Grading strength of evidence. The grading system for strength of evidence is a modified version of the WHO Health Evidence Network system for public health evidence and is explained in more detail in Box 2.4 (page 42). Briefly, we classified evidence as strong (plentiful, consistent, high-quality), moderate (consistent and good quality), or limited (inconsistent or poor quality) and as direct (from research on health service organisations) or indirect (from research on other organisations).

Data synthesis. We grouped the findings of primary studies under six broad themes: (a) the innovation itself; (b) the adoption process; (c) diffusion and dissemination (including social networks, opinion leadership, and change agents); (d) the inner (organisational) context; (e) the outer (interorganisational) context; and (f) the implementation/sustainability process. Within each of these themes, we further divided data from the primary studies into subtopics. We built up a rich picture of each subtopic by grouping together the contributions from different research traditions. Because different researchers in different traditions had generally conceptualised the topic differently, asked different questions, privileged different methods, and used different criteria to judge 'quality' and 'success', we used narrative, rather than statistical, summary techniques.[2] We highlighted the similarities and differences between the findings from different research traditions and considered reasons for any differences from both an epistemological and an empirical perspective. In this way, heterogeneity of approaches and contradictions in findings could be turned into data and analysed systematically, allowing us to draw conclusions that went beyond statements such as, 'the findings of primary studies were contradictory' or that 'more research is needed'.

Developing and testing a unifying conceptual model. We developed a unifying conceptual model based on the evidence from the primary studies. We applied this model to four case studies on the spread and sustainability of particular innovations in health service delivery and organisations. We purposively selected these case studies to represent a range of key variables: strength of evidence for the innovation, technology dependence, source of innovation (central or peripheral), setting (primary or secondary care), sector (public or private), context (UK or international), timing (historical or contemporary example), and main unit of implementation (individual, team or organisation). The case studies are described in Chapter 10 (page 199).

Outline of research traditions

We identified 13 major research traditions that had, largely independently of one another, addressed (or provided evidence relevant to) the issue of diffusion, dissemination or sustainability of innovations in health service delivery and organisation. We classified four of these as 'early diffusion research':

1 **Rural sociology**, where Rogers[3] first developed his highly influential diffusion of innovations theory. In this tradition, innovations were defined as ideas or practices perceived as new by practitioners; diffusion was conceptualised as the spread of ideas between individuals, largely by imitation. The adoption decision was perceived as centring on the imitation of respected and homophilous individuals. Interventions aimed at influencing the spread of innovations focused on harnessing the interpersonal influence of respected individuals within a social network,* especially opinion leaders and change agents. Research in this tradition mapped the social network and studied the choices of intended adopters.

2 **Medical sociology**, in which similar concepts and theoretical explanations were applied to the clinical behaviour of doctors (most notably, the classic study by Coleman *et al.*[5] on the spread of prescribing of newly introduced antibiotics). Early studies in medical sociology set the foundations for network analysis – the systematic study of 'who knows whom' and 'who copies whom' – and led to the finding that well-networked individuals are generally better educated, have higher social status, and are earlier adopters of innovations.[6]

3 **Communication studies**, in which the innovation was generally new information (often 'news') and spread was conceptualised as the transmission of this information by either mass media or interpersonal communication. Research centred on measuring the speed and direction of transmission of news and on improving key variables such as the style of message, the communication channel (spoken or written, etc.) and the nature of the exposure of the intended adopter to the message.[7]

4 **Marketing and economics**, in which the innovation was generally a product or service, and the adoption decision was conceptualised as a rational analysis of costs and benefits by the intended adopter. The spread of innovations was addressed in terms of the success of efforts to increase the perceived benefits or reduce the perceived costs of an innovation. An important stream of research in this tradition centred on developing mathematical models to quantify the influence of different approaches.[8]

Early diffusion research as addressed by these traditions produced some robust empirical findings on

*As discussed in Section 6.1 (page 114), a social network is 'the pattern of friendship, advice, communication and support that exists among members of a social system'.[4]

the attributes of innovations, the characteristics and behaviour of adopters, and the nature and extent of interpersonal and mass media influence on the adoption decision. However, the early tradition had a number of theoretical limitations, which are discussed in detail in Section 3.6 (page 58). Of particular note were the erroneous assumptions that (a) the only relevant unit of analysis is the individual innovation or the individual adopter; (b) an innovation is necessarily better than what has gone before and adoption is more worthy of study than non-adoption or rejection; (c) patterns of adoption reflect fixed personality traits; and (d) the findings of diffusion research are invariably transferable to new contexts and settings. Research traditions that emerged as developments – and sometimes as breakaways – from such conceptual models, include:

5 **Development studies**, in which a key concept was the political and ideological context of the innovation and any dissemination programme, and the different meaning and social value that particular innovations held in different societies and political contexts. Adoption of innovations was reframed as centrally to do with the appropriateness of particular technologies and ideas for particular situations at particular stages in development. Two important contributions from this tradition have been that (a) an innovation may hold a very different meaning for the agency that introduces it to that held by the intended adopters; and (b) 'innovation–system fit' (related to the interaction between the innovation and its potential context) is generally a more valid and useful construct than 'innovation attributes' (often assumed to be fixed properties of the innovation in any context).[9]

6 **Health promotion**, in which innovations were defined as good ideas for healthy behaviours and lifestyles, and the spread of such innovations was expressed as the reach and uptake of health promotion programmes in defined target groups. Health promotion research was traditionally framed around the principles of social marketing (developed from marketing theory – see above), but more recently, a more radical 'developmental' agenda has emerged in health promotion, with parallels to development studies. In the latter, positive changes are increasingly seen in terms of the development, empowerment, and emerging self-efficacy of vulnerably communities rather than in terms of individual behaviour change in line with instructions disseminated outwards from central agencies.[10]

7 **Evidence-based medicine (EBM) and guideline implementation**, in which innovations are defined as health technologies and practices supported by good scientific evidence. Spread of innovation was initially couched in terms of behaviour change in individual clinicians in line with evidence-based guidelines. It is increasingly recognised in this research tradition that the implementation of most clinical guidelines requires changes to the organisation and the delivery of services and hence change at the organisational level as well as that of the individual clinician.[11] It is also increasingly recognised by some protagonists of EBM that the evidence base for particular technologies and practices is often ambiguous or contested – and must be interpreted and reframed in the light of local context and priorities.[12] Hence, the EBM research tradition now contains an inherent tension – between the traditional, highly rationalist and linear perspective in which evidence-based recommendations are seen as context-independent and depicted as flowing 'like water through a pipe' from their research source to the practitioner in the clinic, to a much more constructivist perspective in which the acquisition, dissemination, interpretation and application of evidence is seen as a 'contact sport' in which the meaning and value of evidence is negotiated at its point of use.[13]

8 **Structural determinants of organisational innovativeness**, in which innovation was seen as a product or process likely to make an organisation more profitable. Organisational innovativeness was seen as primarily influenced by structural determinants, especially size, functional differentiation (an internal division of labour), slack resources, and specialisation (the organisation has a clear 'niche' in which it offers expertise and specialist resources). In this tradition, research centred on collecting quantitative data about the formal structures of organisations, usually by

sending questionnaires to the chief executive officer (CEO). Such studies were among the few in our review that were amenable to meta-analysis.[14–16]

9 Studies of organisational process, context and culture, in which the focus of research was the process of adoption, assimilation, and routinisation of an innovation. In this tradition, an organisation's innovativeness was explored in terms of 'softer', non-structural aspects of its make-up – especially the prevailing culture and climate, notably in relation to leadership style, power balances, social relations, and attitudes to risk-taking. This tradition used mainly qualitative (often ethnographic) methods, and centred on people and their relationships and behaviour. This stream of research has many overlaps with the mainstream change management literature, although there is also a distinct subtradition on innovation.[17,18]

10 Interorganisational studies, in which an organisation's innovativeness was explored in relation to the influence of other organisations – in particular by interorganisational communication, collaboration, competition, and norm-setting. This tradition applied social network theory (the notion that people are 'networked' to friends and colleagues and that these networks form channels of communication and influence[19]) to the level of the organisation (e.g. the concept of the opinion-leading organisation was introduced and explored). Interorganisational norms ('fads and fashions') were seen as a key mechanism for the spread of ideas between organisations.[20,21]

11 Knowledge-based approaches to innovation in organisations, in which both innovation and diffusion were radically re-couched in terms of the construction and distribution of knowledge.[22] A critical new concept was the absorptive capacity of the organisation for new knowledge. Absorptive capacity is a complex construct incorporating the organisation's existing knowledge base, 'learning organisation' values and goals (i.e. those that are explicitly directed towards capturing, sharing and creating new knowledge), technological infrastructure, leadership and enablement of knowledge sharing, and effective boundary-spanning roles with other organisations.[23]

12 Narrative organisational studies, in which one key dimension of organisational innovativeness – the generation of ideas – was couched in terms of the creative imagination of individuals in the organisation. An innovative organisation, according to this tradition, is one in which new stories can be told and which has the capacity to capture and circulate these stories.[24,25] This research tradition emphasises the rule-bound, inherently conservative nature of large professional bureaucracies and celebrates stories for their inherent subversiveness. Because key constructions in stories are surprise, tension, dissent, and 'twists in the plot', and because characters can be imbued with positive virtues such as honesty, courage, or determination, stories can effectively embody 'permission to break the rules'.[26] In the narrative tradition, the diffusion of innovations within organisations is about constructing and bringing into action a shared story with a new ending. Hence, interventions to support innovation are directed towards supporting 'communities of practice' with a positive story to tell.

13 Complexity studies, derived from general systems theory, in which innovation is viewed as the emergent continuity and transformation of patterns of interaction, understood as ongoing, complex responsive processes of humans relating in local situations. Diffusion of innovations is seen as a highly organic and adaptive process by which the organisation adapts to the innovation and the innovation is adapted to the organisation.[27] This organic, adaptive process is not easily – and perhaps not at all – controllable by external change agencies.[28]

These different research traditions vary considerably in how they conceptualise innovation and its spread. The dimension of controllability (from 'make it happen' to 'let it happen', with 'help it happen' lying somewhere in between) is one key dimension but not the only difference between these traditions. Figure 3.5 (page 82) illustrates where the 13 traditions lie on this dimension of controllability. One relevant tradition within organisation and management literature is organisational psychology, in which innovativeness is seen as critically dependent on good leadership, sound decision-making, and effective human resource management (especially motivation, training and support of staff). We did not explore this literature in detail as it was the subject of several other projects funded by the Department of Health Service Delivery and Organisation Programme (see www.sdo.lshtm.ac.uk/changemanagement.htm).

A model of diffusion in service organisations

Figure 0.1 shows the unifying conceptual model that we derived from our synthesis of theoretical and empirical findings; the full-annotated model (which includes additional details of the key determinants of successful diffusion, dissemination and implementation) is shown in Fig. 10.1 (page 201). As noted in Chapter 11 (page 219), the model is intended mainly as an *aide memoire* for considering the different aspects of a complex situation and their many interactions. It should not be viewed as a prescriptive formula. The next section presents key empirical findings from across the different research traditions, organised broadly around the main components of the model.

Empirical findings from primary studies

On the basis of the combined evidence from all the above traditions, we addressed the seven key topic areas as set out below:

Innovations (Chapter 4, page 83)

Different innovations are adopted by individuals, and spread to other individuals, at different rates. Some are never adopted at all; others are subsequently abandoned. A very extensive evidence base from sociology (including medical sociology) supports the notion of key *attributes* of innovations (as perceived by prospective adopters), which explain a high proportion of the variance in adoption rates between innovations. Rogers'[3] authoritative review and the conclusions given below are based on a number of more recent empirical studies of service innovations in the health care field (see Chapter 4 for full references):

1a. *Relative advantage*: Innovations that have a clear, unambiguous advantage in terms of either effectiveness or cost-effectiveness will be more easily adopted and implemented (strong indirect and moderate direct evidence[3,29–31]). If a potential user sees no relative advantage in the innovation,

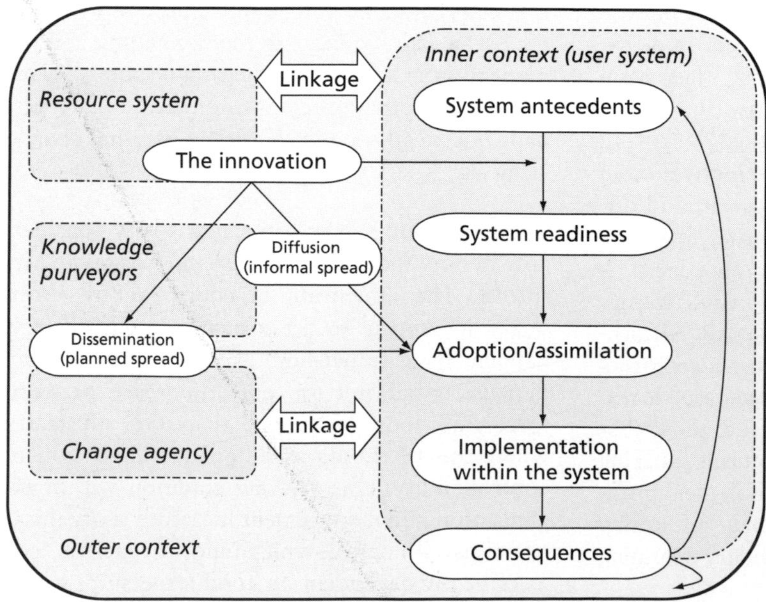

Fig. 0.1 Conceptual model for considering the determinants of diffusion of innovations in the organisation and delivery of health services.

he or she does not generally consider it further: in other words, relative advantage is a sine qua non for adoption (strong direct and moderate indirect evidence[3]). Nevertheless, relative advantage alone does not guarantee widespread adoption (strong direct evidence[11,32,33]). Even so-called 'evidence-based' innovations go through a lengthy period of negotiation amongst potential adopters, in which their meaning is discussed, contested and reframed; such discourse can increase or decrease the perceived relative advantage of the innovation (moderate direct evidence[12]).

1b. *Compatibility*: Innovations that are compatible with the values, norms and perceived needs of intended adopters will be more readily adopted (strong direct evidence[3,12,33–35]). Compatibility with organisational or professional norms, values and ways of working is an additional determinant of successful assimilation (strong direct evidence[12,12,33,36]).

1c. *Complexity*: Innovations that are perceived by key players as simple to use will be more easily adopted (strong direct evidence[3,30,31,33,37,38]). Perceived complexity can be reduced by practical experience and demonstration (moderate direct evidence[28]). If the innovation can be broken down into more manageable parts and adopted on an incremental basis, it will be more easily adopted (strong indirect and moderate direct evidence[3,28]). In the organisational setting, if the innovation has few response barriers that must be overcome, it will be more easily assimilated (strong indirect and moderate direct evidence[3]). Interventions to reduce the number and extent of such response barriers improve the chances of successful adoption (limited evidence).

1d. *Trialabililty*: Innovations that intended users can experiment with on a limited basis will be more easily adopted and assimilated (strong direct evidence[3,28,37,39]). Such experimentation can be encouraged through provision of 'trialability space' (strong indirect and moderate direct evidence[3,28,40]).

1e. *Observability*: If the benefits of an innovation are visible to intended adopters, it will be more easily adopted (strong direct evidence[33,37,38,40]). Initiatives to make the benefits of an innovation more visible (e.g. through demonstrations) increase assimilation (limited evidence).

1f. *Reinvention*: If a potential adopter can adapt, refine or otherwise modify the innovation to suit his or her own needs, it will be more easily adopted (strong direct evidence[3,31]). Reinvention is especially critical for innovations that arise spontaneously as 'good ideas in practice' and spread through informal, decentralised, horizontal social networks (moderate indirect evidence[3]). See also point 1g.

These 'standard' attributes (which, apart from reinvention, are extensively cited) are necessary but not sufficient to explain the adoption and assimilation of complex innovations in organisations. Additional key attributes are listed below (note that for clarity we have conflated some attributes that were considered separately by researchers):

1g. *Fuzzy boundaries*: Complex innovations in service organisations can be conceptualised as having a 'hard core' (the irreducible elements of the innovation itself) and a 'soft periphery' (the organisational structures and systems that are required for the full implementation of the innovation); the adaptiveness of the 'soft periphery' is a key attribute of the innovation (moderate direct evidence[33]). The concept of soft periphery links with Rogers' concept of reinvention (point 1f) and with 'innovation–system fit' as a key feature of system readiness (point 6b).

1h. *Risk*: If the innovation carries a high degree of uncertainty of outcome that the individual perceives as personally risky, it will be less likely to be adopted (strong direct evidence[31,38]). The risks and benefits of an innovation are not evenly distributed in an organisation; the more the risk–benefit balance maps to the power base of the organisation, the greater its chance of assimilation (moderate direct evidence[12,33]). Perceived risk can be reduced through familiarity and opinion leader endorsement (strong indirect evidence[41]).

1i. *Task issues*: If the innovation is relevant to the performance of the intended user's work, and if it improves task performance, it will be more easily adopted (moderate direct and strong indirect evidence[39]). Interventions to enhance task relevance improve the chances of successful adoption (limited evidence). If the innovation is feasible, workable and easy to use, it will be more easily adopted (strong direct evidence[34,38,39,42]). Interventions to improve the feasibility and workability of innovations for key staff members and teams improve the chances of successful adoption (limited evidence).

1j. *Nature of the knowledge required to use it*: If the knowledge required for the innovation's use can be codified and separated from one context so as to be transferred to a different context, it will be more easily adopted (strong indirect and moderate direct evidence[35,43,44]).

1k. *Augmentation/support*: If a technology is supplied as an 'augmented product' (e.g. with customisation, training and a helpdesk), it will be more easily assimilated (strong indirect and moderate direct evidence[35]).

In Chapter 4, we give a number of examples of studies that failed to support the importance of even the most well established innovation attributes in certain settings. This finding illustrates the important principle that the attributes are neither stable features of the innovation nor sure determinants of their adoption or assimilation. Rather, it is the *interaction* between the innovation, the intended adopter(s) and a particular context that determines the adoption rate.

Adoption by individuals (Chapter 5, page 100)

As discussed in Chapter 5, people are not passive recipients of innovations. Rather (and to a greater or lesser extent in different individuals), they seek innovations out, experiment with them, evaluate them, find (or fail to find) meaning in them, develop feelings (positive or negative) about them, challenge them, worry about them, complain about them, 'work round' them, talk to others about them, develop know-how about them, modify them to fit particular tasks, and attempt to improve or redesign them (often through dialogue with other users).

This diverse list of actions and feelings highlights the complex nature of adoption as a process, and contrasts markedly to the widely cited 'adopter categories' ('early adopter', 'laggard' and so on) that have been extensively misapplied as explanatory variables. The empirical work reviewed in Section 5.1 (page 100) suggests that the latter are stereotypical and value-laden; they fail to acknowledge the adopter as an actor who interacts purposively and creatively with the innovation; and they are rarely helpful in informing us of why adoption patterns are the way they are for particular innovations in particular circumstances.

On the basis of the empirical evidence set out in Chapter 5, we have included seven key aspects of adopters and the adoption process in our overall model:

2a. *General psychological antecedents*: We identified a large literature from cognitive psychology on individual characteristics associated with propensity to adopt innovations in general (e.g. personality traits such as tolerance of ambiguity, intellectual ability, motivation, values, learning style and so on) to try out and use innovations in general. This evidence has been largely ignored by researchers studying the diffusion of innovations, and we did not cover it in this review because of the constraints of our project. Therefore, we have not made any recommendations on general psychological antecedents, but we strongly recommend that further secondary research be undertaken to link this literature with the findings presented here.

2b. *Context-specific psychological antecedents*: An intended adopter who is motivated and capable (in terms of specific goals, specific skills and so on) to use a particular innovation is more likely to adopt it (strong direct evidence[12,39,45]). If the innovation meets an *identified need* in intended adopters, they are more likely to adopt it (strong indirect evidence[41,46]). If the adoption of the innovation accords with behaviour congruent with the individual's identity ('this is something that someone like me would do in these circumstances'), it is more likely to be adopted (moderate direct evidence[47]).

2c. *Meaning*: The meaning that the innovation holds for the intended adopter has a powerful influence on the adoption decision (strong indirect and moderate direct evidence[48,49]). If the meaning attached to the innovation by individual adopters is congruent with the meaning attached by top management, service users, and other stakeholders, assimilation is more likely (moderate indirect evidence[50]). The meaning attached to an innovation is generally not fixed but can be negotiated and reframed, e.g. through discourse within the organisation or across interorganisational networks (strong direct evidence[12]). The success of initiatives to support such reframing of meaning varies and is not easy to predict (limited evidence).

2d. *Nature of the adoption decision*: The decision by an individual within an organisation to adopt a particular innovation is rarely independent of other decisions. It may be contingent (dependent on a decision made by someone else in the organisation), collective (the individual has a 'vote' but ultimately must follow to the decision of a group) or authoritative (the individual is told whether to adopt or not).[3] Authoritative decisions (e.g. making adoption by individuals compulsory) may increase the chance of initial adoption by individuals but may also reduce the chance that the innovation is successfully implemented and routinised (moderate indirect evidence[3]).

Adoption is a process rather than an event, with different concerns dominating at different stages. The adoption process in individuals is generally presented as having five stages: awareness, persuasion, decision, implementation and confirmation (see Box 5.4, page 104).[3] However, we found that a less well-known model, the concerns-based adoption model (CBAM) developed in relation to innovation in schools (see Section 5.2, page 103), better explained the findings of empirical studies of complex service innovations in an organisational context. The CBAM suggests three key issues, which we have included in our model:

2e. *Concerns in the pre-adoption stage*: Important prerequisites for adoption are that intended adopters be *aware* of the innovation; have sufficient *information* about what it does and how to use it; and be clear about how the innovation would affect them *personally*, e.g. in terms of costs (strong indirect evidence[46]).

2f. *Concerns during early use*: Successful adoption of an innovation is more likely if the intended adopter has continuing access to *information* about what the innovation does, and to sufficient training and support on *task issues*, i.e. about fitting in the innovation with daily work (strong indirect evidence[46]).

2g. *Concerns in established users*: Successful adoption of an innovation is more likely if adequate feedback is provided to the intended adopter on the consequences of the innovation (strong indirect evidence), and if the intended adopter has sufficient opportunity, autonomy and support to adapt and refine the innovation to improve its fitness for purpose (strong indirect evidence[46]).

Assimilation by organisations (Chapter 5, page 100)

Most research into the diffusion of innovations has focused on simple, product-based innovations, for which the unit of adoption is the individual and diffusion occurs by simple imitation.[3] It is important not to overgeneralise from this literature to complex, process-based innovations in service organisations, for which the unit of adoption (more usually called *assimilation* at this level) is the team, department or organisation – in which various changes in structures or ways of working will be required. In such circumstances, there is almost invariably a formal decision-making process, an evaluation phase or phases, and planned and sustained efforts at implementation. In other words, empirical work in the organisation and management field has shown clearly that successful individual adoption is but one component of the assimilation of complex innovations in organisations. The evaluation of organisational (system) readiness (points 6a–6f) and the crucial implementation phase (points 8a–8h) are considered separately below, but one overarching concept should be borne in mind about the assimilation process as a whole:

3a. *The nature of assimilation*: Whilst one large, high-quality study[38] demonstrated an organisational parallel to the 'stages' of individual adoption, comprising 'knowledge-awareness', 'evaluation-choice', and 'adoption-implementation', the remaining empirical evidence was more consistent with an organic and often rather messy model of assimilation in which the organisation moved back and forth between initiation, development, and implementation, punctuated variously by shocks, setbacks and surprises (strong indirect and moderate direct evidence[18]).

Diffusion and dissemination (Chapter 6, page 114)

As described in Section 6.1 (page 114), the various influences that promote the spread of innovation can be thought of as lying on a continuum between pure diffusion (in which the spread of innovations is unplanned, informal, decentralised and largely horizontal or peer-mediated) and active dissemination (in which the spread of innovation is planned, formal, often centralised and tends to occur more through vertical hierarchies). Whilst mass media and other impersonal channels may create awareness of an innovation, interpersonal influence through social networks (defined as 'the pattern of friendship, advice, communication and support that exists among members of a social system'[4]) is the dominant mechanism for diffusion. On the basis of the evidence reviewed in Chapter 6, we have identified a number of key aspects of communication and influence for our overall model:

4a. *Network structure*: Adoption of innovations by individuals is powerfully influenced by the structure and quality of their social networks (strong indirect and moderate direct evidence[4,36,51]). Different groups have different types of social network. Doctors, for example, tend to operate in informal, horizontal networks while nurses more often have formal, vertical networks (moderate direct evidence).[51] Different social networks have different types of influence – e.g. horizontal networks are more effective for spreading peer influence and supporting the construction and reframing of meaning; vertical networks are more effective for cascading codified information and passing on authoritative decisions (moderate indirect evidence and limited direct evidence).[3,51]

4b. *Homophily*: Adoption of innovations by individuals is more likely if they are homophilous – i.e. similar in terms of socio-economic, educational, professional and cultural background – with current users of the innovation (strong direct evidence[32,36,51]).

4c. *Opinion leaders*: Certain individuals have particular influence on the beliefs and actions of their colleagues (strong direct evidence[5,52]).* Expert opinion leaders influence through their authority and status; peer opinion leaders influence by virtue of representativeness and credibility (moderate direct evidence[32,53]). Opinion leaders can have either a positive or a negative influence (moderate direct evidence[53]). If a project is insufficiently appealing (e.g. in terms of clarity of goals, organisation and resources) it will not attract the support of key opinion leaders (strong indirect and moderate direct evidence[3,53]).

4d. *Harnessing opinion leader influence*: Whilst the powerful impact of social influence (such as that of opinion leaders) in naturalistic settings (see above) is well established, active attempts to engage such individuals in planned change efforts have often had disappointing results. In trials where opinion leaders have been trained to influence the behaviour of their peers (e.g. to persuade fellow clinicians to follow a new guideline), the impact is generally positive in direction but small in magnitude (strong direct evidence[54]). Failure to identify the true opinion leaders, and in particular, failure to distinguish between monomorphic opinion leaders (only influential for a particular innovation) and polymorphic opinion leaders (influential across a wide range of innovations) may limit the success of such intervention strategies (strong indirect and moderate direct evidence[3,53]).

4e. *Champions*: Adoption of an innovation by individuals in an organisation is more likely if key individuals within their social networks are willing to back the innovation (strong indirect

*The distinction between opinion leaders and early adopters should be carefully noted: opinion leaders are usually *not* the initial enthusiasts behind an innovation, but generally lie in the 'late majority' of adopters.

and moderate direct evidence[38,55–57]). The different champion roles for organisational innovations include (a) the *organisational maverick*, who provides the innovators with autonomy from the rules, procedures and systems of the organisation so they can establish creative solutions to existing problems; (b) the *transformational leader*, who harnesses support from other members of the organisation; (c) the *organisational buffer*, who creates a loose monitoring system to ensure that innovators make proper use of organisational resources, while still allowing them to act creatively; and (d) the *network facilitator*, who defends develops cross-functional coalitions within the organisation (moderate indirect evidence[58]).* There is very little direct empirical evidence on how to identify, and systematically harness the energy of, organisational champions.

4f. *Boundary spanners*: An organisation is more likely to adopt an innovation if individuals who have significant social ties both within and outside the organisation,† and who are able and willing to link the organisation to the outside world in relation to this particular innovation, can be identified. Such individuals play a pivotal role in capturing the ideas that will become organisational innovations (strong indirect and moderate direct evidence[3,59]). Organisations that promote and support the development and execution of boundary-spanning roles are more likely to become aware of, and assimilate, innovations quickly (moderate direct evidence[12,60,61]).

4g. *Formal dissemination programmes*: In situations where a planned dissemination program is used for the innovation (e.g. led by an external change agency), this will be more effective if program organisers (a) take full account of potential adopters' needs and perspectives, with particular attention to the balance of costs and benefits for them; (b) tailor different strategies to the different demographic, structural and cultural features of different subgroups; (c) use a message with appropriate style, imagery, metaphors and so on; (d) identify and utilise appropriate communication channels; and (e) incorporate rigorous evaluation and monitoring against defined goals and milestones (strong indirect evidence[3]).

The diverse literature on diffusion and dissemination highlighted an important area of contestation in paradigms of diffusion. The vast majority of diffusion research has addressed proactively developed innovations (e.g. technologies or products developed in formal research programmes) for which the main mechanism of spread is centrally driven and controlled (what we have defined as dissemination). But many innovations in service delivery and organisation occur as 'good ideas' at the coalface, which spread informally and in a largely uncontrolled way (diffusion). This tension, which has received remarkably little attention in the literature we reviewed, is discussed in Section 6.6 (page 131).

The inner context: organisational antecedents for innovation (Chapter 7, page 134)

Different organisations provide widely differing contexts for innovations, and a number of features of organisations (both structural and 'cultural') have been shown to influence the likelihood that an innovation will be successfully assimilated (i.e. adopted by all relevant individuals and incorporated into 'business as usual').

5a. *Structural determinants of innovativeness*: We identified three previous meta-analyses that included both manufacturing and service organisations[14–16,62] (Table A13, page 269) and 15 additional empirical studies (17 papers) from the service sector[32,38,59,63–76]). Their findings are somewhat heterogeneous, although less so than is often claimed. They suggest that an organisation will assimilate innovations more readily if it is large, mature, functionally differentiated (i.e. divided into semi-autonomous departments and units), specialised,‡ with

*See Section 6.3 (page 126) for various alternative taxonomies.

†As explained in Section 6.4 (page 129), wide external ties are known as 'cosmopolitanism' in social network literature.

‡As Section 7.1 (page 134) explains, the term 'complexity' in organisation and management literature generally refers to a composite measure of the degree of specialisation, functional differentiation and professional knowledge.

foci of professional knowledge; if it has slack resources to channel into new projects; and if it has decentralised decision-making structures (strong direct evidence). Size is almost certainly a proxy for other determinants including slack resources and functional differentiation.

These structural determinants are significantly, positively and consistently associated with organisational innovativeness, but together they only account for less than 15% of the variation between comparable organisations. Furthermore, the relationship between structural determinants and innovativeness is moderated by, or contingent on, a number of additional factors (e.g. the radicalness of the innovation, whether it is administrative or technical, and the stage of adoption). There is little empirical evidence to support the efficacy of interventions to change an organisation's structure to make it more 'innovative', except that establishing semi-autonomous project teams is independently associated with successful implementation (see point 8a, page 14).

One important weakness of the literature on structural determinants of innovativeness is the assumption that they can be treated as variables whose impact can be isolated and independently quantified. For example, the empirical studies on organisational size implicitly assume that there is a 'size effect' that is worth measuring and that is to some extent generalisable. An alternative theoretical approach,[77] supported by a number of recent in-depth qualitative studies,[12,64] suggests that the determinants of organisational innovativeness interact in a complex, unpredictable and non-generalisable way with one another.

There is consistent empirical evidence for two other non-structural determinants of organisational innovativeness:

5b. *Absorptive capacity for new knowledge*: An organisation that is able to systematically identify, capture, interpret, share, reframe and re-codify new knowledge; to link it with its own existing knowledge base; and to put it to appropriate use will be better able to assimilate innovations – especially those that include technologies (strong direct evidence[12,61]). Prerequisites for absorptive capacity include the organisation's existing knowledge and skills base (especially its store of tacit, uncodifiable knowledge) and pre-existing related technologies, a 'learning organisation' culture and proactive leadership directed towards enabling knowledge sharing (strong direct evidence[12,23,61]). The knowledge that underpins the adoption, dissemination and implementation of a complex innovation within an organisation is not objective or given. Rather, it is socially constructed, frequently contested and must be continually negotiated between members of the organisation or system. Strong, diverse and organic (i.e. flexible, adaptable and locally grown) intraorganisational networks (especially opportunities for interprofessional teamwork, and the involvement of clinicians in management networks and vice versa) assist this process and facilitate the development of shared meanings and values in relation to the innovation (moderate direct evidence[12,61]).

A critical aspect of knowledge utilisation in health care organisations is the application of research evidence on the efficacy of health technologies. Health professionals should ensure that they and their staff are aware of new developments (and new definitions of what is obsolete) in diagnostic tests, drugs, surgical procedures and so on, and modify their practice accordingly. A major overview of high-quality qualitative studies on how research evidence is identified, circulated, evaluated and used in health care organisations[75] confirms those of mainstream knowledge utilisation literature, which suggest that before knowledge can contribute to organisational change initiatives, it must be *enacted and made social*, entering into the stock of knowledge constructed and shared by other individuals. Knowledge depends for its circulation on interpersonal networks, and will only diffuse if these social features are taken into account and barriers overcome.

5c. *Receptive context for change*: This composite construct incorporates a number of organisational features that have been independently associated with its ability to embrace new ideas and face the prospect of change.[78] An organisation with such a receptive context will be better able to assimilate innovations. In addition to absorptive capacity for new knowledge (point 5b), the components of receptive context include strong leadership, clear strategic vision, good managerial relations, visionary staff in key positions, a climate conducive to experimentation and risk-taking, and effective data capture systems (strong indirect and moderate direct evidence[18,61,69–71,75,76,78]). Leadership may be especially critical in encouraging organisational members to break out of the convergent thinking and routines that are the norm in large, well-established organisations (strong indirect evidence[18]).

The inner context: organisational readiness for innovation (Chapter 7, page 134)

An organisation may be amenable to innovation in general but not ready or willing to assimilate a particular innovation.* As shown in Fig. 0.1 (page 6) formal consideration of the innovation allows the organisation to move (or perhaps choose not to move) to a specific state of system readiness *for that innovation*. The elements of system readiness (discussed in Chapter 7, page 134, and also in Chapter 9, page 175, in relation to implementation and sustainability) are listed below.

6a. *Tension for change*: If staff perceive that the present situation is intolerable, a potential innovation is more likely to be assimilated successfully (moderate direct evidence[79]).

6b. *Innovation–system fit*: An innovation that fits with the existing values, norms, strategies, goals, skill mix, supporting technologies and ways of working of the organisation is more likely to be assimilated (strong indirect and moderate direct evidence[3,79]). See the related concept of 'fuzzy boundaries' (point 1g).

6c. *Assessment of implications*: If the implications of the innovation (including its knock-on effects) are fully assessed, anticipated and catered for, the innovation is more likely to be assimilated (strong indirect and moderate direct evidence[3,79]). Most of the implementation issues set out in points 8a–8h are amenable to advance assessment and planning.

6d. *Support and advocacy*: If supporters of the innovation outnumber, and are more strategically placed, than opponents, it is more likely to be assimilated (strong indirect and moderate direct evidence[3,64,79]). See also 'champions' (point 4e).

6e. *Dedicated time and resources*: If the innovation has a budget line from the outset, and if resource allocation is (a) adequate and (b) recurrent, it is more likely to be assimilated (strong indirect and moderate direct evidence[3,79]).

6f. *Capacity to evaluate the innovation*: If the organisation has tight systems and appropriate skills in place to monitor and evaluate the impact of the innovation (both anticipated and unanticipated), the latter is more likely to be assimilated and sustained (strong indirect and moderate direct evidence[3,28,79]).

The outer context: interorganisational networks and collaboration (Chapter 8, page 157)

An organisation's decision to adopt an innovation, and its efforts to implement and sustain it, depend on a number of external influences:

7a. *Informal interorganisational networks*: A key influence on an organisation's adoption decision is whether a threshold proportion of comparable (homophilous) organisations have done so or plan to do so (strong direct evidence[36,65,80,81]). A 'cosmopolitan' organisation (one that is externally well networked with others) will be more amenable to this influence (strong direct evidence[36,65,80,81]). Interorganisational networks will only promote adoption of an innovation once this is generally perceived as 'the norm'; until that time, networks can also serve to warn organisations of innovations that have no perceived advantages (strong indirect and moderate direct evidence[21,32,81]). Integrative organisational forms (such as the UK NHS, Health Maintenance Organisations, and professionally led networks between health care providers), which link provider organisations through common management and governance structures or explicit shared values and goals, can promote the spread of innovation between member organisations (strong indirect and moderate direct evidence[31]).

7b. *Intentional spread strategies*: Formal networking initiatives, such as quality improvement

*As discussed in Section 10.4 (page 206), GP fundholding in the UK was a good example of this.

collaboratives[40] or 'Beacon' schemes,[72] aimed at promoting sharing of ideas and knowledge construction, are sometimes but not always effective (moderate direct evidence[82–86]). Such initiatives are often expensive and the gains from them difficult to measure; evidence on their cost-effectiveness is limited. Key success factors from health care quality improvement collaboratives include (a) the nature of the topic chosen for improvement (comparable with attributes of the innovation discussed in points 1a–1k); (b) the capacity and motivation of participating teams – in particular their leadership and team dynamics; (c) the motivation and receptivity to change of the organisations they represent; (d) the quality of facilitation – in particular the provision of opportunities to learn from others in informal space; and (e) the quality of support provided to teams during the implementation phase (moderate direct evidence[40]).

7c. *Wider environment*: The evidence base for the impact of environmental variables on organisational innovativeness in the service sector is sparse and heterogeneous, with each group of researchers exploring somewhat different aspects of the 'environment' or 'changes in the environment'. Environmental uncertainty has either a small positive impact or no impact on innovativeness (moderate direct evidence[38,59,63]), and there may be small positive effects from interorganisational competition and higher socio-economic status of patients/clients (limited evidence).

7d. *Political directives*: Whist this review was not designed to tap centrally into the literature on policymaking and its impact, some empirical studies on innovation formally measured the effect of the policy context on the adoption of a particular innovation. A policy 'push' occurring at the early stage of implementation of an innovation initiative can increase its chances of success, perhaps most crucially by making a dedicated funding stream available (strong direct evidence[32,87–89]). External mandates (political 'must-dos') increase the predisposition (i.e. the motivation), but not the capacity, of an organisation to adopt an innovation (moderate direct evidence[90]); such mandates (or the fear of them) may divert activity away from innovations as organisations seek to second-guess what they will be required to do next rather than focus on locally generated ideas and priorities (strong indirect and moderate direct evidence[88,91]).

Implementation and routinisation (Chapter 9, page 175)

Implementation has been defined as 'the early usage activities that often follow the adoption decision'.[91] The evidence on implementation of innovations was particularly complex and relatively sparse; it was difficult to disentangle from that on change management and organisational development. Implementation depends on many of the factors already covered above in relation to the initial adoption decision and the early stages of assimilation. At the organisational level, the move from considering an innovation to successfully routinising it is generally a non-linear process characterised by multiple shocks, setbacks and unanticipated events,[18] as discussed in point 3a. The key components of system readiness for an innovation have been discussed above (points 6a–6f) and are highly relevant to the early stages of implementation. In addition, a number of additional elements are specifically associated with successful routinisation:

8a. *Organisational structure*: An adaptive and flexible organisational structure, and structures and processes that support devolved decision-making in the organisation (e.g. strategic decision-making devolved to departments; operational decision-making devolved to teams on the ground), will enhance the success of implementation and the chances of routinisation (strong indirect evidence[18,91]).

8b. *Leadership and management*: Top management support, advocacy of the implementation process and continued commitment to it will enhance the success of implementation and routinisation (strong indirect and moderate direct evidence[79,91,92]). If the innovation aligns with the prior goals of both top and middle management, and if leaders are actively involved and frequently consulted, it is more likely to be routinised (moderate direct evidence[79]). See also 'champions' (point 4e).

8c. *Human resource issues*: Successful routinisation of an innovation in an organisation depends on the motivation, capacity and competence of individual practitioners (strong direct evidence[79]). Early and widespread involvement of staff at all levels, perhaps through formal facilitation initiatives, enhance the success of implementation and routinisation (strong indirect and moderate direct evidence[91,93]). Where job changes are few and clear, high-quality training materials are available and timely on-the-job training is provided, successful and sustained implementation is more likely (strong indirect and moderate direct evidence[79,91,92,94]). Team-based training may be more effective than individual training where the learning involves implementing a complex technology (moderate direct evidence[95]).

8d. *Funding*: If there is dedicated and ongoing funding for implementation, the innovation is more likely to be implemented and routinised (strong direct evidence[32,79,87,92,96]).

8e. *Intraorganisational communication*: Effective communication across structural (e.g. departmental) boundaries within the organisation will enhance the success of implementation and the chances of routinisation (strong indirect and moderate direct evidence[91]). A narrative approach (i.e. the purposive construction of a shared and emergent organisational story of 'what we are doing with this innovation') can serve as a powerful cue to action (moderate indirect and limited direct evidence[25,97]).

8f. *Extraorganisational networks*: The greater the complexity of the implementation needed for a particular innovation, the greater the significance of the interorganisational network for implementation success (moderate indirect evidence[91,98]).

8g. *Feedback*: Accurate and timely information on the impact of implementation process (through efficient data collection and review systems) increases the chance of successful routinisation (strong indirect and moderate direct evidence[11,92]).

8h. *Adaptation/reinvention*: If an innovation is adapted to the local context, it is more likely to be successfully implemented and routinised (strong indirect and moderate direct evidence[3,40,79]). See also 'reinvention' (point 1f) and 'fuzzy boundaries' (point 1g).

Linkage between components of the model

As explained in Chapters 4–9, there is some empirical evidence (and also robust theoretical arguments) for building strong links between different parts of the system depicted in Fig. 0.1 (page 6). Specific success factors included in our model (which are covered in the various individual results chapters) are:

9a. *Linkage at development stage*: An innovation that is centrally developed (e.g. in a research centre) is more likely to be widely and successfully adopted if the developers or their agents are linked with potential users *at the development stage* in order to capture and incorporate the user perspective (strong indirect evidence[3]). Such linkage should aim not merely for 'specification' but for a shared and organic (developing, adaptive) understanding of the meaning and value of the innovation-in-use, and should also work towards shared language for describing the innovation and its impact.

9b. *Role of the change agency*: If a change agency is involved with a dissemination programme, the nature and quality of any linkage with intended adopter organisations will influence the likelihood of adoption and the success of implementation (strong indirect and moderate direct evidence). In particular, human relations should be positive and supportive; the two systems should share a common language, meanings and value systems; there should be sharing of resources in both directions; the change agency should enable and facilitate networking and collaboration between organisations; and there should be joint evaluation of the consequences of innovations. The change agency should possess the capacity, commitment, technical capability, communication skills and project management skills to assist with operational issues. This is particularly important in relation to technology-based innovations, which should be disseminated as augmented products with tools, resources, technical help and so on (moderate direct evidence[3,99]).

9c. *External change agents*: Change agents employed by external agencies will be more effective if they are (a) selected for their homophily and credibility with the potential users of the innovation; (b) trained and supported to develop strong interpersonal relationships with potential users and to explore and empathise with the user's perspective; (c) encouraged to communicate the user's needs and perspective to the developers of the innovation; and (d) able to empower the user to make independent evaluative decisions about the innovation (strong indirect and limited direct evidence[3]).

Testing the model by applying it to case studies

The case studies we selected for analysis were: integrated care pathways (ICPs), general practitioner (GP) fundholding, telemedicine, and the electronic health record (ECR) in the UK.

ICPs ('the steady success story', page 202) are an example of an innovation that has shown some – but not overwhelming – success. This innovation has high relative advantage and potentially reduces the complexity of a service; it is trialable and its results are observable. It has been adopted widely but has certainly not reached niche saturation. Furthermore, many poor quality ICPs are in circulation, and organisations may 'reinvent the wheel' because they are unaware of existing models that could be adapted. All this highlights the relative absence of interprofessional collaboration on ICPs, and suggests that were such collaborations to be developed and strengthened, further spread and greater sustainability might be achieved.

GP fundholding ('the clash', page 204) is an excellent example of an innovation whose relative advantage was perceived very differently by different players, which proved incompatible with certain value systems, for which some potential adopters had a good existing knowledge and skills base (e.g. in accounting) while others did not, and whose knock-on consequences were difficult to isolate or measure. It is also a good example of a centrally driven innovation that rose and fell with the prevailing political climate. The lack of a formal pilot phase or rigorous evaluation programme means that this historical example will always remain controversial.

Telemedicine ('the maverick initiative', page 206) tends to be introduced by individual enthusiasts rather than organisation-wide, and hence raises particular issues around sustainability. Innovators who introduce telemedicine projects (often on a research grant or short-term project funding) generally lack the skills or interest to 'mainstream' the initiative within their organisation. Costs have traditionally been high and technical ease of use low. But several factors have recently come together to swing the risk–benefit equation much more in telemedicine's favour – user-friendly technology, a fall in price–performance ratio, and better linkage between information technology (IT) companies and clients during software development and implementation. Telemedicine is thus entering an interesting phase, and it is possible that its fortunes thus far (relatively poor spread and low sustainability) may at some stage be reversed.

The ECR in the UK ('the big roll-out', page 208) has a strong external mandate for its roll-out. According to our model, this will create *predisposition* in user organisations but will not in itself increase their capacity to deliver. The very high complexity of the innovation (which requires simultaneous adoption across multiple organisations and sectors) and its low ease of use will, theoretically at least, conspire against adoption, especially since its relative advantage is not unanimously accepted. This does not, of course, mean that the innovation will fail, but it does raise challenges for the change agencies involved.

On the basis of these case studies, we believe that the model depicted above provides a helpful conceptual framework for considering the diffusion of the innovations in the first three (historical) case studies and for constructing hypotheses about the likely success of the final example – a controversial contemporary innovation that is in the early stages of dissemination and implementation. However, we emphasise that our model has yet to be tested prospectively and we make no firm claims for its predictive value at this stage.

Applying the model in a service context

As explained in Section 11.2 (page 220), because of the highly contextual and contingent nature of the diffusion process, it was not possible for us to make formulaic, universally applicable recommendations for practice and policy. Indeed, we strongly caution against any approach that seeks to produce such recommendations. Rather, we recommend a structured, two-stage framework to guide context-dependent reflection and action in the service and policymaking environment. In the first stage, the components of the model shown in Fig. 0.1 (attributes of the innovation, characteristics of intended adopters, potential agents of informal social influence, characteristics of the organisation, characteristics of the environment, nature of dissemination programme, nature of implementation programme) should be considered against the empirical evidence base presented in this book.

In the second stage, we recommend a more pragmatic approach in which the potential interaction between these variables is considered in relation to a specific local context and setting, perhaps using the realistic evaluation framework discussed in Section 11.3 (page 225). We have modified the realist framework specifically for the context-sensitive evaluation of innovations in health service delivery and organisation (see Box A.7, page 240).

Recommendations for further research

Research into diffusion of innovations in service delivery and organisation (covered in detail in Section 11.3, page 225) can be divided – somewhat arbitrarily – into research that focuses on particular components of the model and research that takes a 'whole-systems' approach and explores the interaction between components. We take these different approaches in turn.

Innovations. The main gap in the research literature on complex service innovations in health care organisations is an understanding of how they arise, especially since this process is largely decentralised, informal and hidden from official scrutiny. An additional key question is how such innovations are reinvented as they diffuse within and between organisations.

Adopters and adoption. In relation to the adoption of innovations, transferable lessons might be gleaned from a secondary study of the cognitive psychology literature on the ability and tendency of individuals to adopt particular innovations in particular circumstances; and also from a study of the social psychology literature on the impact of group and organisational categorisations and identifications on the way individuals interpret and make sense of innovations.

Diffusion and dissemination. 'Intervention trials' of opinion leadership seem to be of limited value, and the general messages from such trials are already available. However, further in-depth qualitative research is recommended on the *nature* of social influence and of the operation of different social networks in different professional and other groups in the health services. We also recommend additional qualitative studies into the different roles of champions, boundary spanners and change agents in different organisational contexts and settings.

The inner context. At the organisational level, we recommend that research be commissioned into the challenge of how organisations might create and sustain an absorptive capacity for new knowledge and how they might achieve what are now established as the key components of a receptive context for change. An additional important research question is: What steps must be taken by organisations when moving towards a stage of 'readiness' (i.e. with all players on board and with protected time and funding), and how might this overall process be supported and enhanced?

The outer context. Research at the interorganisational level might fruitfully explore the process of informal interorganisational networking and more formal interorganisational collaboration, with an emphasis on the role of the change agency (and how this might be enhanced). An explicit study of the process and effectiveness of interorganisational knowledge transfer activities through boundary spanners (such as the appointment, training and support of knowledge workers) might provide generalisable lessons for organisations seeking to develop their capacity in this area.

The implementation/sustainability process. The empirical literature on the implementation of service innovations in health care is currently extremely sparse. We recommend two areas of additional research: First, further secondary research into the extensive wider literature on change management, from which lessons about implementation and sustainability of innovations could be gleaned. Second, a wide range of in-depth qualitative or mixed-methodology studies into the process of implementation in organisations should be commissioned, perhaps ideally as responsive funding to capture innovative ideas as they emerge and spread.

Limitations of 'component'-oriented research. A consistent theme in high-quality overviews and commentaries on the diffusion of innovations in health service organisations is that empirical research has generally been restricted to a single level of analysis (individual *or* team *or* organisation *or* interorganisational); has explicitly or implicitly assumed simple causal relationships between variables; has failed to address important interactions between different levels (e.g. how different organisational settings moderate individual behaviour and decision-making) and between both measured and unmeasured variables within these levels; and has failed to take due account of contingent and contextual issues. A growing methodological literature in both organisational studies and health promotion (two traditions that are particularly focused on implementation and sustainability) criticises previous research for being too 'interventional' (conceptualised in an experimental paradigm) and insufficiently cognisant of context. These critics call for more research that is properly immersed in the practical, contextual, whole-systems world rather than the artificial and controlled world of the experimenter.

Whole-systems approaches. As depicted in Box 11.1 (page 229), a whole-systems approach to implementation research would be: (a) Theory-driven (i.e. it would explore an explicit hypothecated link between the determinants of a particular problem, the specific mechanism of the programme, and expected changes in the original situation); (b) process-rather than 'package'-oriented (it should eschew questions of the general format 'Does programme X work?' in favour of those framed as 'What features account for the success of programme X in this context and the failure of a comparable programme in a different context?'); (c) participatory (i.e. it would engage practitioners as partners in the research process); (d) collaborative and coordinated (i.e. aim to prioritise and study key research questions across multiple programmes in a variety of contexts); (e) addressed using common definitions, measures and tools to enable valid comparisons across studies; (f) multi-disciplinary and multi-method, with a primary emphasis on interpretive approaches; (g) meticulously detailed (so as to document the unique aspects of different programmes and their respective contexts to allow future research teams to interpret idiosyncratic findings and test rival hypotheses about mechanisms); and (h) ecological (i.e. it should recognise the critical reciprocal interaction between the programme and the wider setting in which it takes place).

There are many potential approaches to whole-systems research. We identified two as particularly promising for researching innovation in health service delivery and organisation, and we specifically recommend that the following methods be supported in future commissioning exercises:

Participatory action research. This approach (a) focuses on change and improvement; (b) explicitly and proactively involves participants in the research process; (c) is educational for all involved; (d) looks at questions that arise from practice; (e) involves a cyclical process of collecting, feeding back, and reflecting on data; and (f) is a process that generates knowledge.

Realistic evaluation. This is an approach linked to secondary research (realist review) developed by Pawson *et al.* and is discussed further in Section 11.3 (page 225). Briefly, the realist approach addresses the innovation–context interaction and asks 'what works, for whom, and under what circumstances?'. When evaluating any particular programme, open-ended questions (known as the 'would it work here' framework, which we have adapted and reproduced in Box A.7, page 240) are asked about the innovation, the organisation, the people, the resources and so on in order to tease out and illuminate the mechanisms of success or failure. When comparing two or more comparable programmes, each dimension of the programme is compared in relation to contextual factors using a general question format: 'What is the desirability or feasibility of changing practice, procedures and context of system B (in which the programme was successful) to match those of system A (in which it was less successful)?'

In order to produce meaningful comparisons from a realist perspective, future research studies must follow the criteria for whole-systems research set out previously. In particular, they must aim for a detailed, multidimensional picture of the experience of implementing the programme, and (therefore) must prospectively set out to capture high-quality data on a range of agreed and standardised process measures. A first step towards addressing the remaining unanswered questions in spread and sustainability is to develop, adapt and disseminate the 'would it work here?' matrix, or a similar conceptual framework, and encourage research teams to align with its recommendations.

Chapter 1
Introduction

Key points

1. This systematic review of the diffusion, spread and sustainability of innovations in health service delivery and organisation was commissioned in late 2002 by the UK Department of Health as part of a programme of research aimed at supplying the evidence base for the modernisation of the NHS. It should be interpreted with this policy context in mind.

2. We have defined innovation in service delivery and organisation as a novel set of behaviours, routines and ways of working, which are directed at improving health outcomes, administrative efficiency, cost-effectiveness or the user experience, and which are implemented by means of planned and coordinated action.

3. The mechanisms by which innovations spread include both diffusion (a passive phenomenon of adoption by individuals and organisations) and dissemination (the active attempt to influence the rate and success of adoption).

4. Sustainability of organisational innovations can be thought of as the point at which new ways of working become the norm and the underlying systems and ways of working become transformed in support. Whereas the diffusion and adoption of innovations has been widely researched at both an individual and an organisational level, their implementation and sustainability are relatively under-researched areas.

5. The study, which entailed exploring and organising a complex and diverse body of literature, raised important questions about the methodology of systematic review, which are discussed in Chapter 2.

1.1 What is diffusion of innovations theory?

'Diffusion of innovations' is a term that means different things to different groups of scholars. Classical diffusion of innovations research, as set out by Rogers,[3] is a body of knowledge built around empirical work that demonstrated a consistent *pattern* of adoption of new ideas over time by people in a social system. Its central tenet is that the adoption of new ideas by a population follows a predictable pattern. There is a slow initial (lag) phase, followed by an acceleration (take-off) in the number of people adopting in each time period, then a corresponding deceleration, and finally a tail as the last few individuals who are going to adopt finally do so (Fig. 1.1).

Underpinning diffusion theory is a simple law about the nature of growth in a closed system, observable across the biological sciences from cell division to epidemiology: one cell divides into two (or one person infects two others), two becomes four and so on, doubling with each unit of time until a point of saturation is approached when each new convert has fewer potential converts to influence, after which the process slows and tails off. Mathematically, the point of diminishing growth (or spread) is the point where an exponential function becomes a logistic function.*

*Enthusiasts for the mathematical small print are encouraged to see Henrich's[100] excellent article, based on complex mathematical modelling, on why the S-shaped adoption curve supports the hypothesis that adoption occurs via a mimetic (copying) phenomenon between

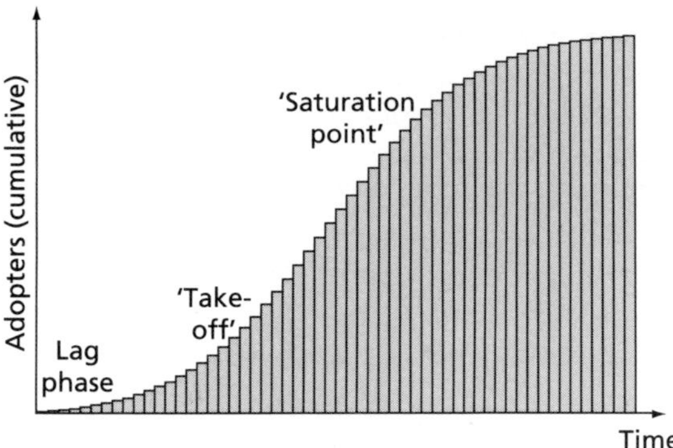

Fig. 1.1 The S-curve – cumulative distribution of adopters over time.

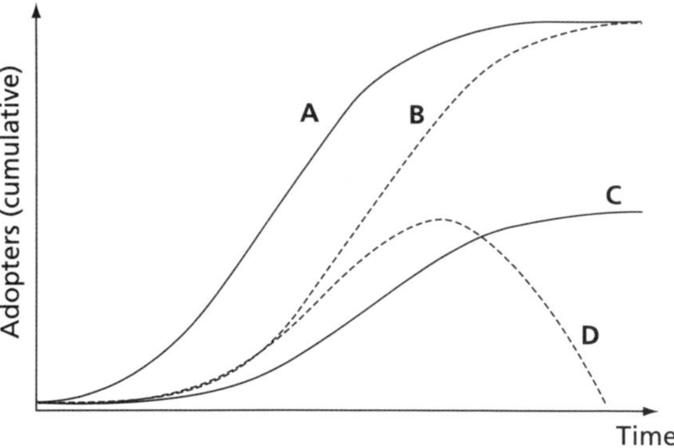

Fig. 1.2 S-curves for different innovations and populations. A = rapid and complete adoption by a population; B = similar pattern following a longer lag phase; C = slower adoption and incomplete coverage; D = adoption followed by discontinuance.

For an excellent account of these mathematics from an epidemiological perspective, see Bailey's classic text.[101]

This pattern only occurs if the population is fixed and the influence of the innovation (e.g. the value attached to it) stays constant over time. If there is rapid population turnover, infusion of new people, loss of former members or a change in the market (or other) value of the innovation, the curve will cease to be S-shaped.[102]

Within a particular population, there may be several distinct subpopulations with different adopter characteristics. If these subpopulations were separated, each would have its respective S-shaped diffusion curve with a longer or shorter lag phase and a greater or lesser proportion that ultimately adopts; the combined population will also show an S-shaped diffusion curve, which is the sum of the curves of the subpopulations. Different innovations introduced into different populations produce a cumulative adoption curve of the same basic shape as shown in Fig. 1.1, but with different slopes (rates of adoption) and intercepts (proportion of people adopting), as shown in Fig. 1.2. The explanatory challenge for diffusion of innovations theory is to account for the differences in slope and intercept of curves A, B and C – and (crucially) account for curve D (discontinuance), which is probably the commonest diffusion curve of all.

Whilst the simple law of natural growth is sufficient to *describe* the shape of the adoption curve, it does not tell us why some people adopt an innovation early while others do so much later – or why they never adopt it at all. Furthermore, classical diffusion of innovations theory takes little or no account of the complex process of adoption (or, strictly, assimilation) of innovations at the organisational level.

As Chapter 3 (page 48) describes, a wide range of conceptual and theoretical models for the adoption, diffusion, dissemination, implementation and sustainability of innovations have been proposed and empirically tested in fields as diverse as sociology, anthropology, psychology, communication studies, economics, development studies, epidemiology, organisation and management, and complexity science. Whilst we knew from the outset that the research literature crossed many disciplinary boundaries, we did not initially anticipate the wide diversity of theoretical perspectives and research designs adopted by different groups of scientists, nor that one of our central tasks would be to develop a preliminary taxonomy of the contribution, strengths and limitations of these

individuals rather than via the rational weighing up of costs and benefits by potential adopters. Henrich points out that a small proportion of adoption curves are in fact r-shaped rather than S-shaped, and discusses the underlying mechanisms for these oddities.

different research traditions. The disciplinary origins of these traditions are summarised in Table 1.1 (pages 23–24). It should be noted that the construction of Table 1.1 was a major intellectual effort that we only completed towards the end of this systematic review. As Chapter 2 (page 32) describes, we did not – and, we believe, *could* not – construct this table before the main synthesis work began. We have, however, included it in this chapter to orient readers towards the framework set out in Chapters 4–9.

1.2 Why did the UK Department of Health want to research the diffusion of innovations?

The UK NHS was set up in 1948 by the post-war labour government under the staunchly socialist Minister of Health Anyerin Bevan, who promised a Welfare State that would provide health and social care for every citizen 'from the cradle to the grave'.[499] The NHS was an explicit product of the ideology and social structure of UK in the 1950s – an era in which the solidarity of the war effort had focused communities on mutual support rather than individual gain; rationing of food and fuel was still in place; and a large proportion of medical problems comprised acute conditions requiring a straightforward package of initial treatment followed by convalescence. At that time, both science and technology were advancing at a steady but manageable pace; no-frills care was an accepted goal of politicians and public alike; the expectations of service users were relatively modest; and changes in technologies and service needs were barely discernible year on year.

This socio-political context produced the built environment of the NHS (hospitals designed for lengthy inpatient stays, general practices designed as one-man businesses for reactive care), its administrative structure (centralised, hierarchical and standardised), its values (unlimited care according to need, free at the point of delivery) and its conventions and ways of working (e.g. separate hierarchies, management structures and information systems for different professional groups).

Like any large public-sector bureaucracy, today's NHS constantly struggles against the past that shaped it. Its leaders have, arguably, been somewhat trigger-happy in the past in introducing well-intentioned changes intended to 'modernise' outdated structures and systems. In the early 2000s, the Department of Health recognised that the modernisation of the NHS should move beyond centrally driven, standardised and unpopular restructuring initiatives and begin to celebrate and support decentralised, creative change at a local level. It also recognised, perhaps in response to the growing ideology of consumerism and accountability in health care, that the service must be designed much more closely around the needs and experience of the user. The detailed vision and strategy to achieve this was set out in the 2001 white paper, the *NHS Plan*.[1] A key element of the strategy was the establishment of a new statutory body, the NHS Modernisation Agency, charged with driving through a range of organisational and cultural reforms. In the words of its chief executive:

> The NHS has embarked upon a decade of improvement. Over the next ten years the delivery of care will be transformed as the *NHS Plan* is implemented. Care will be designed around the needs of patients and their carers. Diagnosis and treatment that previously took weeks or months will be completed in days or even hours. The NHS Modernisation Agency has been created to help local staff across the service make these radical and sustainable changes.
>
> David Fillingham; Modernisation Agency website (www.modernnhs.nhs.uk/ ; accessed 31 December 2003)

Between 2001 and 2005, the Modernisation Agency worked with more than 3000 local clinical teams as part of 30 national programmes established in accordance with the *NHS Plan* in priority development areas such as primary care, cancer, heart disease and emergency care. These modernisation initiatives had mixed fortunes and few independent, in-depth evaluations have been published, but many positive outcomes were described.[103–106] One early finding from these

Table 1.1 Research traditions that have produced findings relevant to the diffusion of innovations in health service organisations, showing disciplinary roots, scope and key concepts.

Research tradition	*Academic discipline*	*Definition and scope*	*'Diffusion of innovations' conceptualised as*
Rural sociology	Sociology	The study of rural society and the relationships between its members, especially the influence of social structures and norms on behaviours and practices	Influence of social norms and values on adoption decisions. Networks of social influence.
Medical sociology	Sociology	As above for medical society	As above. Specifically, the norms, relationships and shared values that drive clinician behaviour (e.g. adoption of guidelines).
Communication studies	Psychology	The study of human communication, including both interpersonal and mass media	Structure and operation of communication channels and networks. Interpersonal influence (e.g. impact of 'experts' vs 'peers' on decision-making).
Marketing	Interdisciplinary (psychology and economics)	The study of the production, distribution and consumption of goods and services	Affordability, profitability, discretionary income, market penetration, media advertising, supply and demand.
Development studies	Interdisciplinary (anthropology, sociology, economics, political science, information and communications technology)	The study of the adoption, adaptation and use of technology, especially in a development context	Barriers to the uptake of more advanced technologies (e.g. labour-saving machinery, computers).
Health promotion	Interdisciplinary (epidemiology, social psychology, marketing)	The study of strategies and practices aimed at improving the health and well-being of populations (draws on, and overlaps with, communication studies)	'Reach' and 'uptake' of positive lifestyle choices in populations targeted by health promotion campaigns
Evidence-based medicine	Clinical epidemiology	The study of the spread of best [research] evidence on managing diseases and symptoms	Filling a 'knowledge gap' or 'behaviour gap' in targeted clinicians

Continued

Table 1.1 continued: Research traditions that have produced findings relevant to the diffusion of innovations in health service organisations, showing disciplinary roots, scope and key concepts.

Research tradition	*Academic discipline*	*Definition and scope*	*'Diffusion of innovations' conceptualised as*
Structural determinants of organisational innovativeness	Organisation and management	The study of how the structure of an organisation influences its function in relation to uptake of new ideas and practices	Organisational attributes influencing 'innovativeness' – e.g. size, slack resources, hierarchical vs decentralised lines of management
Studies of organisational process, context and culture	Interdisciplinary (organisation and management, sociology, anthropology)	The study of the development and impact of culture (meaning systems, language, traditions, accepted ways of doing things) in organisations and professional groups	Changes in culture, values and identities
Interorganisational studies (networks and influence)	Interdisciplinary (organisation and management, sociology)	The study of interorganisational norms, fashions and influence	Interorganisational fads and fashions, spread through social networks
Knowledge utilisation	Interdisciplinary (organisation and management, information and communications technology, sociology)	The study of how individuals and teams acquire, construct, synthesise, share and apply knowledge	Transfer of knowledge – both explicit (formal and codified as in a guideline) and tacit (informal and embodied as in 'knowing the ropes')
Narrative studies	Interdisciplinary (literature, sociology, anthropology)	The study of the stories (in this context, those told in and about organisations). Use of storytelling as a tool for dissemination and change in organisations	The telling, re-telling and interpretation of stories. Innovators as characters (heroes, underdogs) in a story of change. Innovation as social drama
Complexity studies	Interdisciplinary (ecology, social psychology, systems analysis)	The study of how individuals, groups and organisations emerge, evolve and adapt to their environment	Creativity, emergence and adaptation

projects was that the intensive injection of energy, expertise and resources generally produced short-term improvements in the targeted service, but two critical questions remain unanswered:
(1) To what extent would the changes achieved through a Modernisation Agency–funded initiative be sustained after the official end of the project?
(2) How could improvements achieved in one health service organisation be effectively and reliably disseminated to a wider group of comparable organisations, thus gaining maximum impact from the original efforts?

The Modernisation Agency interpreted its agenda – perhaps somewhat naively in retrospect – as identifying and defining best practices, extracting the features that were critical to the success of such practices, adapting them to new contexts, supporting their implementation and ensuring that the improvements were sustained. It explicitly sought to produce transferable tools and models that would be of direct use to staff involved in NHS modernisation.[107] It established its own Research Into Practice Team, which produced a number of internal reports about change in general and the spread and sustainability of innovation in particular.[108–112] These reports were based largely on qualitative interviews with stakeholders regarding modernisation initiatives. They were produced impressively quickly and (hence, perhaps) had considerable face validity in policymaking circles, but they were essentially studies of the intuitive impressions of front-line staff and were not designed prospectively to test empirical hypotheses about the process of change.

Whether the Modernisation Agency (due to be disbanded in early 2005) had the 'right' approach or not, it drew considerable international interest as a model of change. Professor Don Berwick described the work of the Modernisation Agency as 'to my knowledge, the most ambitious concerted systematic improvement effort ever undertaken, anywhere, by any organisation of comparable size' (Don Berwick, personal communication, May 2003).

Our own team has previously questioned whether the approach of the Modernisation Agency, based largely on intensive short-term support for specific projects, was sufficient to achieve true transformation of the NHS, and whether the underlying – and largely taken for granted – theory of change underpinning its efforts was suited to the scale, pace and type of 'second-order' shift required for NHS modernisation.[113,114] Recognising that its capacity to conduct systematic research into such questions was limited, the Modernisation Agency approached the Department of Health Service Delivery and Organisation Programme with the initial idea for the systematic review reported in this book.

Whilst we kept in mind the policy context of our work and maintained a focus on the Modernisation Agency as our ultimate 'client', we did not make any conscious political concessions to this (or any other) body. Indeed, we took some steps to ensure that our work was academically independent of the Modernisation Agency (e.g. after an initial interview to set the scope for this work, we did not invite its members to our steering group meetings), and we tried to remain distanced from the prevailing political ideologies espoused in its publications. Nevertheless, we are aware that no research study is ideologically neutral, and in accordance with standard practice in qualitative research, we have set out our own backgrounds and perspectives in Chapter 2 (page 34).

1.3 Scope of this research

The research study, including the write-up, was intended to last 9 months. Funding was provided for approximately one full-time academic post and a part-time administrator/librarian for this period. Within the constraints of our budget and timescale, we aimed to provide a comprehensive (but not encyclopaedic) summary of the literature that would describe, evaluate and summarise the relevant theoretical approaches and empirical research studies.

As explained in Section 1.2, we sought to provide information on the work of the Modernisation Agency and the *NHS Plan* in relation to the spread and sustainability of organisational innovations and to make clear recommendations for practice, policy and further research in the UK public sector. We were interested in identifying what might be termed 'critical success factors' for the spread and sustainability of innovations in an organisational setting, though we knew from the outset that many if not all such factors would be highly context-dependent.

A secondary objective was to contribute to the emerging scientific discourse on the methodology of systematic reviews of complex evidence (which, like this one, are often undertaken in a particular policy context and under resource and time constraints).[12,40,115–120] As Table 1.1 illustrates, the wealth and breadth of relevant literature promised many important insights, but it also posed major practical problems for the systematic reviewer working on a tight budget and deadline. Our frustrations on a practical level reflected fundamental epistemological questions about the nature of knowledge and the implications for synthesising, summarising and prioritising complex, cross-disciplinary and disparate bodies of evidence. This aspect of the research is discussed further in Chapter 2 (page 32).

1.4 Definitions

It is important to bear in mind when reading this book that there is not, nor will there ever be, a consensus on terminology. Different individuals, influenced by different professional, disciplinary and sociocultural traditions, use the same words in different contexts. In our research, we found a wide range of implicit and explicit definitions of these concepts ('service delivery', 'organisation', 'innovation', 'diffusion', 'spread', 'sustainability'), and a similar range of meanings for other critical terms such as 'adoption', 'communication', 'technology' and 'implementation'.

We recognise that linguistic meaning is highly context-dependent, and do not seek to privilege the definitions that we ourselves have chosen. But for the purposes of preparing a systematic review, we felt obliged to attempt to make a firm demarcation between what would be included and what would be excluded in each of the key terms in our research question. It proved impossible to hold to these definitions, since in practice different research teams used words in particular contexts. We used our judgement to interpret the work of different authors in the light of the definitions they used rather than strictly impose 'inclusion criteria' based on our own – arbitrary – definitions. Nevertheless, we set out the linguistic 'benchmarks' against which the relevance and validity of the empirical studies covered in this chapter were judged, and in Chapters 4–9 we highlight where the definitions used by other researchers differ from these.

Innovation in service delivery and organisation

Rogers'[3] much-quoted definition of innovation is (page 11):

> An innovation is an idea, practice, or object that is perceived as new by an individual or other unit of adoption. It matters little, so far as human behaviour is concerned, whether or not an idea is objectively new as measured by the lapse of time since its first use or discovery.

This definition is helpful when considering individual behaviour (e.g. when a clinical guideline might be classified as an innovation by a doctor or nurse) but it is less useful at an organisational level (e.g. when the same clinical guideline might be classified as an *organisational* innovation on a ward or in a GP surgery). Using this example, it is clear that the guideline only becomes an organisational innovation if it precipitates some kind of planned change in the structures and systems in the organisation. People in the organisation need to do more than perceive the guideline as new; they must *do* something – adopt new roles, make different decisions, form new relationships, use new technology, develop new systems and so on. And this begs the question of how innovation differs from any other kind of organisational change.

Osborne reviewed the organisational studies literature and found over 20 different definitions of innovation, from which he extracted four core characteristics:

(1) innovation represents newness;

(2) it is not the same thing as invention (the latter is concerned with the discovery of new ideas or approaches whereas innovation is concerned with their application);

(3) it is both a process and an outcome; and
(4) it involves discontinuous change.[121]

Tushman and Anderson[122] argue that discontinuity is the essential difference between innovation and incremental organisational development, while Van de Ven[123] defines organisational innovation as the development and implementation of new ideas by people who over time engage in transactions with others within an institutional order. From a sociological perspective, innovations are novel (at least to the adopting community), making communication a necessary condition for adoption.[124]

The link between innovation and implementation is particularly crucial to the modernisation agenda in the UK NHS. For this reason, Damanpour's[125] and Euan's definition of organisational innovation is particularly pertinent:

> Innovation is the implementation of an internally generated or a borrowed idea – whether pertaining to a product, device, system, process, policy, program or service – that was new to the organisation at the time of adoption. ... Innovation is a practice, distinguished from invention by its readiness for mass consumption and from other practices by its novelty.

In their review of interorganisational transfer of innovation, Goes and Park[68] offer the following sector-specific definitions (page 674):

> [A health care innovation is] a medical technology, structure, administrative system, or service that is relatively new to the overall industry and newly adopted by hospitals in a particular market area.... [Service innovations are] innovations that incorporate changes in the technology, design, or delivery of a particular service or bundle of services.

In a review based mainly on the manufacturing sector, Damanpour[16] distinguished between 'product' and 'process' innovations – a distinction that is probably less clear (and less helpful) in the world of health service delivery where many innovations are a combination of product and process. Westphal *et al.*[81] has pointed out that whereas the notion of a technological innovation is relatively straightforward, the definition of administrative innovation is more ambiguous. Administrative innovations can potentially include many different routines that can be combined in different ways, and hence it is often more difficult to identify a discontinuous change. Ultimately, a degree of subjective judgement will usually be required.

Added to this already complex taxonomy is Osborne's[126] fourfold classification of social policy innovations, comprising developmental innovations (existing services to a particular user group are improved or enhanced), expansionary (existing services are offered to new user groups), evolutionary (new services are provided to existing users) and total (new services to new users). We have not used Osborne's taxonomy because the mainstream literature on health service innovations rarely draws on it, and we did not find it especially helpful in explaining the findings of the empirical studies presented in this book.

The essential criterion of newness for an innovation immediately excludes practices and programmes that are long established, even if they fulfil key quality criteria (such as effectiveness, efficiency, affordability and acceptability). It is a recurring protest in the NHS that 'innovations' imposed from outside are not necessarily better than existing practices and processes, and indeed that (usually by means of unintended consequences) they may represent a retrograde step.

Two additional concepts should therefore be considered here: 'best practice', defined by Zairi and Whymark[127] (page 160) as 'a task, function or behaviour which, when carried out, produces above average results'; and 'potentially better practices', defined by Horbar *et al.*[86] as practices that have been shown (or which are believed) to improve outcomes in one setting, and which can be selected, modified and applied in unique ways to fit a new situation, which takes account of the fact that 'best practice' in one setting is only *potentially* an improvement on existing practice when transferred elsewhere. Interestingly, in their study of potentially better practices, Horbar *et al.* made no attempt to verify whether the practices *actually* improved outcome – indeed, they comment that the critical impetus for quality improvement may be the process of pulling together to implement anything that improves *or is perceived to improve* outcome, not the practice itself.

Taking account of all the above, we constructed a new definition for the purposes of this review: An innovation in health service delivery and organisation is a set of behaviours, routines and ways of working, along with any associated administrative technologies and systems, which are
(1) perceived as new by a proportion of key stakeholders;
(2) linked to the provision or support of health care;
(3) discontinuous with previous practice;
(4) directed at improving health outcomes, administrative efficiency, cost-effectiveness, or user experience; and
(5) implemented by means of planned and coordinated action by individuals, teams or organisations.

Such innovations may or may not be associated with a new health technology.

This definition is by no means perfect, since it presupposes a rationalist view of innovation, i.e. it implies that innovation is an event rather than a process and that the assimilation of innovations will be through planned and transformative rather than continuous and emergent change; hence, initiatives based on developmental and collaborative models would not be strictly included in this definition. The criterion 'discontinuous with previous practice' was not therefore applied in all cases, but we did use it to distinguish initiatives to spread *new* ways of working (included) from initiatives aimed at encouraging more widespread use of a practice that is generally seen as already 'mainstream' as an idea. To give a specific example, meta-analysis of 'Interventions that *increase use of* adult immunisation and cancer screening services' (emphasis added), as defined by Stone *et al.*,[128] is excluded under this criterion.

One final caveat in relation to organisational innovation is the very different meaning of the word 'organisation' in different contexts. The bulk of research into organisational innovation has been done in the commercial sector, and a high proportion of empirical studies centre on industrial manufacturing, software production and distribution, and marketing. In these contexts, the 'organisation' is generally a firm with something to sell and shareholders to answer to. Indeed, von Hippel[129] defined innovation in terms of its potential ability to make firms more competitive, suggesting that 'innovative behaviour is a strategic activity by which organisations gain and lose competitive advantage'. In the public service sector, of course, 'organisation' is a different and fuzzier concept in terms of both structure and process,* and the literature on spreading innovation is sparse by comparison. In preparing this review, we rejected a lot of material from the commercial and manufacturing sectors – but we have also included substantial elements of this literature, and the health service practitioner must judge how relevant particular findings are to their own context.

Adoption of innovations

Rogers[3] defines adoption (in relation to the individual; page 21) as 'the decision to make full use of the innovation as the best course of action available'. Damanpour and Gopalakrishnan,[130] writing about the adoption of innovations in organisations, define it as:

> [A]n organisation's means to adapt to the environment, or to pre-empt a change in the environment, in order to increase or sustain its effectiveness or competitiveness. Managers may emphasise the rate or speed of adoption, or both, to close an actual or perceived performance gap.

Both these definitions imply that people and organisations choose rationally to adopt innovations because of some actual or perceived advantage. As we shall see, the adoption of advantageous innovations often fails to take place; likewise, adoption of disadvantageous innovations is sadly very common. We shall also see (in Chapter 5) that adoption

*Take, for example, UK general practice – is the unit of analysis in organisational innovation the practice itself, the practice plus its attached staff (e.g. district nurses), the Primary Care Organisation, the health district and so on?

(and non-adoption) is not always a rational process, nor is adoption a single decision.

In the organisational context, adoption is more usually referred to as assimilation, and this is discussed further in Section 5.3 (page 160).

Diffusion, dissemination and spread

These terms have similar meanings in common parlance, and are also used interchangeably by some researchers and policymakers. But it is generally agreed that there are subtle but important distinctions between them. We have accepted Rogers'[3] own definition of diffusion (page 5): 'Diffusion is the process by which an innovation is communicated through certain channels over time among the members of a social system.'

For Rogers, diffusion thus refers to the spread of abstract ideas and concepts, technical information, and actual practices within a social system, from a source to an adopter, typically via communication and influence. As with the chemical process from which the metaphor is taken, diffusion of ideas or practices is an essentially passive process whose key mechanism is imitation ('let it happen' rather than 'make it happen' – see Fig. 3.5, page 82).

Wejnert,[41] a political scientist and author of one of the most comprehensive overviews of diffusion of innovation from a socio-political perspective, views the task of the diffusion researcher as (page 297): 'identifying the factors that influence the spread of innovations across groups, communities, societies and countries ... an area of inquiry referred to formally as diffusion'.

Dissemination, on the other hand, is a planned and active process intended to increase the rate and level of adoption above that which might have been achieved by diffusion alone ('make it happen' rather than 'let it happen' – see Fig. 3.5, page 82). Mowatt *et al.*,[131] who undertook a systematic literature review of the diffusion and implementation of health technologies, developed a standard definition of dissemination (page 669), which we have used in this review: 'Dissemination is actively spreading a message to defined target groups.'

'Spread' – a term used extensively by the Modernisation Agency in its own reports and included on the original brief for this review – is not used extensively or consistently by scientists in the research traditions we reviewed. Only 21 sources out of over 1000 screened (apart from Modernisation Agency publications) used the term in the title or abstract, compared with 140 for diffusion and 42 for dissemination. It generally refers to the transfer of ideas and practices between (inter) organisations or within (intra) a single organisation.[43] Adler, an organisational theorist, suggests that spread refers to the adoption of innovation by others, through whatever means (including passive diffusion and active dissemination). Berwick rejects 'spread' as a concept, preferring the term 'reinvention', which is also used by Rogers.[3] Indeed, he states (page 1971) that the 'word "spread" is a misnomer'[132] (implicitly, because nothing spreads in its original form since complex innovations are always changed as they become embedded in new organisational structures and systems).

Because of the lack of consistency in the definition and use of the term by others, we have used the term 'spread' sparingly in our review, preferring terms with a more widely accepted meaning ('diffusion', 'dissemination' and 'reinvention').

Sustainability

Sustainability presupposes implementation (i.e. an innovation cannot be sustained unless it has first been implemented). Mowatt *et al.*[131] define implementation in relation to health technologies (page 669) as: 'dissemination plus action to actively encourage the adoption recommendations contained in a message'.

The term 'sustainability' is even less widely used in the diffusion of innovations literature. We found it in only two out of over 1000 sources screened for this review (perhaps because the notion of adoption, at least in individuals, implies some continuity of use). The NHS Modernisation Agency's[133] working definition of sustainability is 'when new ways of working and improved outcomes become the norm'. They go on to clarify:

> Not only have the process and outcome changed, but the thinking and attitudes behind them are fundamentally altered and the

> systems surrounding them are transformed in support. In other words it has become an integrated or mainstream way of working rather than something 'added on'. As a result, when you look at the process or outcome one year from now or longer, you can see that at a minimum it has not reverted to the old way or old level of performance. Further, it has been able to withstand challenge and variation; it has evolved alongside other changes in the context, and perhaps has actually continued to improve over time.... Sustainability means holding the gains and evolving as required, definitely not going back.

This definition is supported by the academic literature in the few places where the term is mentioned at all. Von Krogh and Roos[134] emphasise the property of 'resisting erosion' – i.e. a resilience against undermining forces that consolidates innovations and turns them into normal practice (the institutionalisation of change). Others have emphasised as the essence of sustainability the durability of the attributes that produced improvement,[135] and the notions of 'routinisation' (i.e. the innovation becomes an ongoing element in the organisation's activities and loses its distinct identity).[95,123,136]

There is a hint from some publications that the Modernisation Agency and certain writers see sustainability as an intrinsic feature of the innovation itself, whereas Rogers,[3] who does not define sustainability and mentions it only in passing, implies (page 341) that sustainability is more a function of the receiving system than of the innovation itself, though as we discuss in Chapter 8 (page 157) this is not a view that organisational theorists necessarily share.

A further issue complicating the concept of sustainability is the notion that inherent to the construct is resistance to further growth and development! If an innovation is sustained indefinitely, the organisation must become resistant to further innovation in that area. In the words of Eveland[50]:

> If we aim our efforts at routinization, we are likely to damn ourselves with success. Organisations that carefully implement state-of-the-art computer systems tend to have a great deal of difficulty taking advantage of changing technology; they have too many 'sunk costs' in the old systems. It is well to remember that every old, outdated, ossified tool or practice in any organisation was once an innovation that got 'routinized' all too well.

Eveland[50] goes on to discuss the tension between rolling out good ideas *to* organisations and developing the capacity for change and innovation *within* organisations:

> To the extent that research creates new and better ways to manipulate individuals and organisations into adopting other people's views of what is a 'good thing', it will contribute by contrast to a dissolution of social progress. I realize that this may be a difficult point to swallow for those who legitimately believe they have a 'good thing' other people really need – a group that includes most of the 'true believers' in technological and social innovation. On balance, however, we are all likely to be better off by encouraging the development of the capacity for effective and purposive internalized self-directed evolution and control than by relying on any 'diffusion system' to overcome the shortcomings of organisational and individual change processes.

Weick[137] introduced the concept 'irreversible action' to denote the gains made from an innovation but also allows further development – the gains may be held or continue to be extended. Weick also introduced the notion that sustainability is a characteristic of the social system that exists within an organisation – i.e. it is fundamentally a social phenomenon, incorporated in the binding commitments people make to each other in relation to (but extending beyond) the innovation itself. Hence, when the innovation achieves 'sustainability', the organisation has moved forward in terms of the social relationships that support both this *and other* innovations. Using this definition, sustainability has a very different – and more positive – meaning from routinisation (which for some organisational theorists has the negative overtone of entrenchment[138]). Indeed, there is some evidence that the successful assimilation and implementation of one innovation makes an organisation more rather than less receptive to the next one, because the innovation itself serves as a catalyst for developing organisational sense-making capacity.[139] However, relatively few empirical studies have used Weick's definition and most organisational research reviewed here takes a more conventional view of the term.

In summary, like the term 'spread', 'sustainability' is rarely used in the mainstream literature on diffusion of innovations, and furthermore, it is a contested theme in the contemporary discourse on innovation in organisations. For these reasons, we have tried to capture the ambiguity around the meaning of 'sustainability', and to apply the term in a flexible way that embraces the tension between routinisation of one innovation and receptivity to others.

1.5 Structure of this book

Chapter 2 sets out the methods we developed for searching, prioritising, analysing and synthesising the vast literature that was relevant to this review, and gives our search strategy and synthesis methods. Chapter 3 provides an overview of the many diverse research traditions, each with its own conceptual, theoretical, methodological and instrumental approach to the problem. We also briefly mention some other potentially relevant bodies of literature that were omitted because of resource limitations. Chapters 4–9 consider evidence from all the main traditions outlined in Chapter 3 (page 48). It is divided into six separate chapters, each of which focuses on one key question:

(1) Innnovations: What features (attributes) of innovations influence the rate and extent of adoption? (Chapter 4, page 83)
(2) Adopters and adoption: What is the nature of the adoption process – and why do some people adopt innovations more readily than others? (Chapter 5, page 100)
(3) Diffusion and dissemination: What is the nature of the diffusion process, and in particular how does social influence promote the adoption of innovations? (Chapter 6, page 114)
(4) The inner context: What elements of the inner (organisational) context influence the adoption and assimilation of innovations in organisations? (Chapter 7, page 134)
(5) The outer context: What elements of the outer (environmental) context, including aspects of interorganisational communication, influence the adoption and assimilation of innovations in organisations? (Chapter 8, page 157)
(6) Implementation and institutionalisation: What are the features of effective strategies for implementing innovations in health service delivery and organisation and ensuring that they are sustained until they reach genuine obsolescence? (Chapter 9, page 175)

Chapter 10 (page 199) draws together the results of the empirical studies into a single model (which is not intended to be prescriptive) and describes four illustrative case studies of how the model can be used to explain (and to a limited extent predict) spread and sustainability of a particular innovation in a particular context. Chapter 11 (page 219) discusses the overall messages of the report and provides recommendations for practice, policy and future research; it considers both the content of this review (spread and sustainability of innovations) and the process of undertaking synthesis of complex evidence.

We have also included four appendices:
(1) Appendix 1 (page 232) – data extraction form for primary studies;
(2) Appendix 2 (page 234) – critical appraisal checklists for different research designs;
(3) Appendix 3 (page 245) – descriptive statistics on the included sources, and
(4) Appendix 4 (page 255) – tables of included studies.

Finally, we have included a glossary (page 293), which summarises the definitions of the key terms used in this review.

Chapter 2
Method

Key points

1. The literature relevant to our research question was extremely heterogeneous, methodologically diverse, difficult to classify and seemingly contradictory. It lacked a coherent theoretical framework. Because of this, our initial progress was slow and frustrating. The conventional formula for 'Cochrane' style systematic reviews of simple interventions was clearly inappropriate, and we found that existing approaches to the review of complex evidence were also problematic.

2. Drawing on Thomas Kuhn's notion of scientific paradigms, we developed a new method – meta-narrative review – for sorting and evaluating the 6000 sources identified in our exploratory searches. We took as our initial unit of analysis the unfolding storyline of a research tradition over time. We mapped these storylines by using both electronic and manual tracking to trace the influence of seminal theoretical and empirical work on subsequent research within a tradition. Once the initial mapping phase was complete, we used more conventional synthesis techniques to analyse and combine primary studies.

3. We identified 13 key meta-narratives (listed on page 38) from research traditions as disparate as rural sociology, clinical epidemiology, marketing and organisational studies. Scientists in different traditions had conceptualised, explained and investigated diffusion of innovations differently – and had used different criteria for judging the quality of empirical work. Moreover, they told very different overarching stories of the progress of their research. Within each tradition, research papers and book chapters described human characters emplotted in a story of (in the early stages) pioneering endeavour and (later) systematic puzzle-solving, variously embellished with scientific dramas, surprises and 'twists in the plot'.

4. By first separating out, and then drawing together, these different meta-narratives, we built up a rich picture of our field of study. We were able to make sense of seemingly contradictory data by systematically exposing and exploring tensions between research paradigms as set out in their overarching storylines. In some traditions, 'revolutions' were identifiable in which breakaway scientists had abandoned the prevailing paradigm and introduced a new set of concepts, theories and empirical methods.

5. We believe that meta-narrative review should be added to the methodological toolkit for systematic review. It takes an interpretive rather than a logico-deductive frame of reference, and adds particular value to the synthesis of heterogeneous bodies of literature in which different groups of scientists have conceptualised and investigated the 'same' problem in different ways. Meta-narrative review has many parallels with realist review; we discuss the similarities and differences in Section 2.7 (page 42).

2.1 Outline of method

We began this review in late 2002, at a time when the literature on evidence synthesis had begun to recognise the major challenges associated with producing systematic reviews of complex evidence for broad policymaking questions (see Section 2.7, page 42).[118,140,141] There were already some well-established general principles, such as that
(1) the review process should be multi-disciplinary, exploratory, flexible and reflective;[118]

(2) the preferred approach to evidence should be broad and inclusive rather than narrow and dismissive, and bear in mind the audience for the report;[118] and
(3) researchers who use a formulaic, checklist-driven approach to evaluation and synthesis will produce findings of dubious validity.[142]

Many sources implicitly or explicitly recommended making judicious use of interpretive skills and common sense, and being prepared to defend intuitive judgements. But the literature fell short of offering a formal method for sorting out and pulling together studies undertaken by different groups of scientists who had formulated a particular problem in widely differing ways, asked comparable but not identical questions, and taken contrasting methodological approaches.

It became apparent early in this study that considerable preliminary work would be needed to 'map' the different aspects of the literature so that we could make sense of it. After considering a number of different methodological approaches to the synthesis of complex evidence,[12,115,117–119,142–148] we developed a six-phase process that we have called a meta-narrative review, summarised in Box 2.1. The first five phases are described in detail in Sections 2.2 to 2.6 and the justification of

Box 2.1 Phases in meta-narrative review.[149]

(1) *Planning phase*
(a) Assemble a multi-disciplinary research team whose background encompasses the relevant research traditions (an initial scoping phase may be needed before the definitive research team is appointed).
(b) Outline the initial research question in a broad, open-ended format.
(c) Agree outputs with funder or client.
(d) Set a series of regular face-to-face review meetings, including planned input from external peers drawn from the intended audience for the review.

(2) *Search phase*
(a) Initial search led by intuition, informal networking and 'browsing', with a goal of mapping the diversity of perspectives and approaches.
(b) Search for seminal conceptual papers in each research tradition by tracking references of references. Evaluate these by the generic criteria of scholarship, comprehensiveness, and contribution to subsequent work within the tradition.
(c) Search for empirical papers by electronic searching key databases, hand searching key journals, and 'snowballing' (references of references or electronic citation tracking).

(3) *Mapping phase*
Identify (separately for each research tradition):
(a) The key elements of the research paradigm (conceptual, theoretical, methodological and instrumental).
(b) The key actors and events in the unfolding of the tradition (including main findings and how they came to be discovered).
(c) The prevailing language and imagery used by scientists to 'tell the story' of their work.

(4) *Appraisal phase*
Using appropriate critical appraisal techniques:
(a) Evaluate each primary study for its validity and relevance to the review question.
(b) Extract and collate the key results, grouping comparable studies together.

(5) *Synthesis phase*
(a) Identify all the key dimensions of the problem that have been researched.
(b) Taking each dimension in turn, give a narrative account of the contribution (if any) made to it by each separate research tradition.
(c) Treat conflicting findings as higher-order data and explain in terms of contestation between the different paradigms from which the data were generated.

(6) *Recommendations phase*
Through reflection, multi-disciplinary dialogue and consultation with the intended users of the review:
(a) Summarise the overall messages from the research literature along with other relevant evidence (budget, policymaking priorities, competing or aligning initiatives).
(b) Distil and discuss recommendations for practice, policy and further research.

the method (including an explanation of its philosophical basis) is given in Section 2.7 (page 42). The sixth phase (developing recommendations) is not described in detail here because it pertains not to the systematic review itself but to its implementation. We refer to this phase in Section 11.2, page 220.

2.2 Planning phase

This phase included constructing the grant application (including seeking collaborations between different institutions and departments so as to provide the appropriate skill mix), and negotiating scope, milestones and deliverables with the funder (the UK Department of Health) prior to the award being made. In addition, we interviewed key stakeholders, especially representatives from the NHS Modernisation Agency (the ultimate service-sector client for the review). In the early weeks of the project, 'scoping the project' and 'refining the brief' might more accurately have been described as 'exposing the differences in our expectations and considering how we might resolve them'.

An important first step in this study, as with all reviews of complex evidence, was to assemble a multi-disciplinary research team whose academic training and practical experience spanned all the main bodies of literature relevant to our question. Briefly, our backgrounds are as follows: TG – biomedicine, social and political sciences; systematic review; GR – history and sociology; PB – management and organisational anthropology; FM – natural sciences, management consultancy and health service management; OK – psychology and organisational behaviour. We worked closely with Richard Peacock, a health informaticist and librarian skilled in database searching. In the early exploratory phase of the project, we also employed two external consultants: Anna Donald (medicine and social policy) and Francis Maietta (project management).

In a conventional systematic review of a simple intervention (such as a drug), the research question is set more or less firmly at the outset. But at the time of the initial planning meeting for this project, the research question proved surprisingly elusive. At that time, we were working with much fuzzier and contested definitions of key terms than those set out in Chapter 1 (see page 20), and this ambiguity made it almost impossible to focus the study or set tight inclusion criteria for primary sources. We initially had no clear idea where to look for the 'good research studies' – or even how to define a good study on this complex and seemingly chaotic topic area. In addition, it was evident that if we kept a very narrow focus to our study (e.g. if we restricted our review to research undertaken in public-sector health care), we would miss studies from non–health-care sectors or from the private sector – which might well prove the best source of original ideas for our client, since the best 'new ideas' are very often from initiatives *unlike* one's own.

Given this background, we initially set ourselves two very broad research questions:

(1) What bodies of knowledge and specific research traditions are relevant to the analysis of diffusion, dissemination and sustainability of innovations in health service delivery and organisation?*

(2) To what extent are the notions 'diffusion', 'dissemination' and 'sustainability' adequate for conceptualising and analysing the processes by which new practices are taken up and embedded into everyday practice in the context of health service delivery and organisation, and are there other conceptual or theoretical models in the literature which we should explore further?

At an initial scoping meeting, we planned a number of project review meetings, including a presentation of our emerging methods to a group of external stakeholders (selected academic and service colleagues whom we collectively called 'the fishbowl') one-third of the way through the 9-month project period.

*We explicitly excluded the diffusion of health technologies such as new drugs or procedures from this review since it had been covered elsewhere.[89,150] However, in some areas, notably guideline development and implementation (discussed further in Chapter 3), there is a large area of overlap between the diffusion of the technology and the diffusion of new models of service delivery.

2.3 Search phase

A vast literature was potentially relevant to our research question, and our initial search methods were highly exploratory (involving, for example, what might be called 'systematic browsing' in libraries, bookshops and on the Internet). The early part of this phase was laborious and often disheartening, since we were initially a long way from focused and targeted searching (indeed, there were good methodological reasons *not* to focus too early on particular sources or databases).

We undertook an initial 'territory mapping' exercise and explored a different area of possibly relevant research using informal and unstructured methods. We asked colleagues, sent emails to academic lists, browsed libraries and the Internet, and built on our own prior knowledge. One of us began, for example, with the literature on EBM and guideline implementation,[11] which led serendipitously to another literature on health promotion campaigns[102] (the spread of 'innovative messages' about healthy lifestyles). One of us was directed by a colleague towards work on technology transfer to developing countries,[9] and discovered a huge 'grey literature' in the databases of international development agencies. Another had previously completed a PhD that involved exploring social network theory in relation to the spread of medical technologies.[151] By exploring all these (and more) avenues, we gained a feel of the overall literature.

Our searching gradually became more systematic as the emerging storylines (see Section 2.4) of the different research traditions served as a powerful focusing device for refining some areas of enquiry and rejecting others. Once we had begun to find fruitful sources, we were able to use conventional 'snowball' tracking methods (e.g. pursuing references of references, identifying key index terms and using citation-tracking databases) to locate other quality sources, after which this first stage became progressively easier.

As we had anticipated, the tacit knowledge and informal contacts we brought from our professional and disciplinary backgrounds formed an important starting point for further exploration. We made a strategic decision to search some sources (especially the health services research and organisation and management literature) thoroughly, while drawing more selectively on sources that were likely to have a lower yield. Once we had identified key areas for further study, we used the following methods to refine our searches:

(1) Formal search methods
   (a) Hand searching of 30 key journals (Table A.3, page 249, in Appendix 3)
   (b) Electronic searching of 15 databases, including index terms, free text and named author (Table A.4, page 252, in Appendix 3)
   (c) Reference scanning: we scanned the reference lists of all the papers that we ranked as 'essential to include'
   (d) Citation tracking: we used electronic search methods to forward-track the 20 papers published more than 3 years previously that we had classified as both centrally relevant and methodologically outstanding, thereby identifying papers in mainstream journals that had subsequently cited those seminal papers (Table A.5, page 254, in Appendix 3). Pilot searches demonstrated that citation tracking of papers less than 3 years old produced low yields.
(2) Informal methods
   (a) Our existing knowledge and resources
   (b) Our personal contacts and networks (direct and via email lists) within and beyond our own disciplines
   (c) Serendipitous discovery (e.g. finding a relevant paper for this review when looking for something else).

Electronic searches were undertaken by an experienced librarian (Richard Peacock) in close liaison with the core research team. He refined electronic search strings iteratively in response to emerging data. The search string was modified for different databases to take account of different index terms (e.g. in the educational databases there was an index term 'educational innovation').

The final search string for the Medline database (OVID database) was:

(1) exp. Diffusion of innovation (MeSH)
(2) diffusion of innovation$
(3) 1 or 2
(4) service delivery

(5) service organi#ation (# = wildcard to cover z or s)
(6) SDO
(7) exp. *Delivery of health care (MeSH)
(8) 4 or 5 or 6 or 7
(9) sustainab$
(10) spread
(11) 9 or 10
(12) 3 and 8
(13) 3 and 11
(14) 12 or 13

An earlier, less specific search had yielded several thousand articles, many of which could not be confidently rejected on title and abstract alone (see 'first sift' criteria on data extraction form in Appendix 1, page 232). The string shown above is, however, a somewhat idealised version of the searches we actually made, which included additional exploratory searches in an attempt to capture additional sources. For example, when we identified a good paper by a particular author, we returned to the appropriate database and searched for that author by name. We have a bank of saved search strings for the different stages of the search and for different databases covered; these can be supplied on request.

Our initial searches were limited by theoretical and organisational models (i.e. we restricted the search to studies that had developed and tested models for disseminating, implementing and routinising innovations). However, this limiting concept was removed from later searches – both because we found very few models and because the models we found did not address our research question.

The contribution from different sources to our final report is summarised in Fig. 2.1. Having browsed a total of 6000 abstracts, we pulled just over 1000 full-text papers (including book chapters, monographs, dissertations and so on), of which around 25% were empirical studies and 70% were editorials, opinion articles and non-systematic reviews. We rejected papers that were clearly irrelevant or superficial on abstract alone, and for pragmatic reasons we also rejected all titles whose full-text paper was not available in languages spoken fluently by the authors (English, French, German or Greek). Furthermore, because of the resource constraints of this review, we did not pull primary studies if a high-quality systematic review or meta-analysis had included them, unless they were centrally relevant to our own research question.

As explained in Section 2.3, the wide range of research traditions, professional perspectives and environmental contexts represented in these

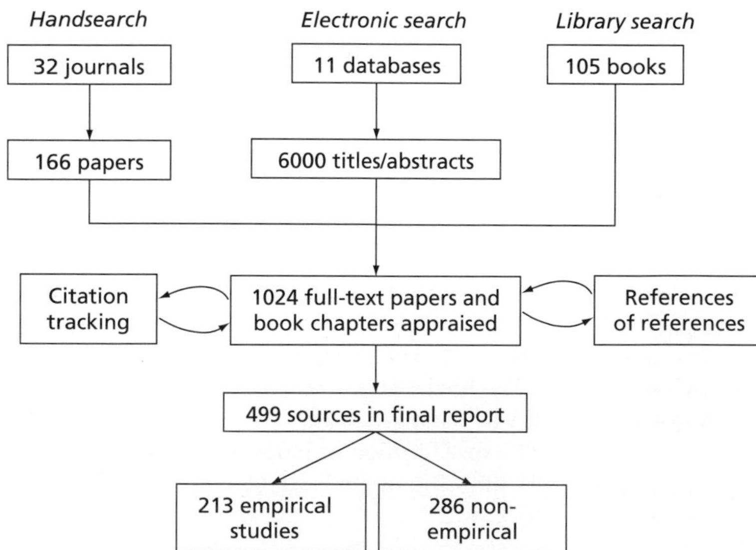

Fig. 2.1 Contribution of different sources to final report.

sources precluded the use of a highly prescriptive list of inclusion criteria. We used a simple, semi-structured checklist (Box 2.2) to guide our academic judgement and exclude sources that were unlikely to add value to our own review.

The checklist in Box 2.2 was specifically designed to capture multiple perspectives on the problem. Rather than applying a strict criterion-based framework to all theoretical sources, we judged them according to how they were received *by their academic peers* within a particular research tradition. This approach is discussed further in Section 2.7 (page 42). It allowed approximately 70% of our full-text theoretical papers to be rejected, mainly on the grounds of lack of originality. A quarter of the papers in this category were checked by two different raters, giving an inter-rater reliability of 91%, with differences resolved by discussion. However, this level of consistency does not necessarily reflect a high degree of accuracy in sorting the papers. It could also be explained by two raters coming at an unfamiliar literature with similar observer biases. In a small pilot study on 25 papers, addition of a third rater did not alter the final judgements reached by the first two.

We used a similarly open-ended checklist to exclude empirical papers we had pulled from our 'first sift' search but which were unlikely to add value to this review (Box 2.3). These questions allowed us to exclude around 50% of the full-text empirical papers, with an inter-rater reliability of 92%.

The taxonomy of studies that contributed to our final report is shown in Table A.2 (page 248) in Appendix 3.

2.4 Mapping phase

It proved a major challenge to classify the vast number of books and papers accumulated for this review and extract the key information from them under topic headings. One problem was that different groups of scientists used different terminology (and, confusingly, sometimes used the same terminology to refer to different concepts). A major methodological breakthrough occurred when we decided to undertake a preliminary mapping exercise to group together studies whose authors were likely to be looking at the problem in the same way, attending the same conferences, reading the same journals and otherwise influencing each other's work and perspective.

The goal of this mapping phase, therefore, was to gain an overall picture of the historical and theoretical context of the various research traditions that had explored the diffusion, dissemination and implementation of innovations. In this phase, drawing on Thomas Kuhn's seminal work on research paradigms (see Section 2.7, page 42),

Box 2.2 Initial inclusion criteria for theoretical papers and reviews.

(1) Is the paper part of a recognised research tradition – i.e. does it draw critically and comprehensively upon an existing body of knowledge and attempt to further that body of knowledge?
(2) Does the paper make an original and scholarly contribution to research into the diffusion, dissemination or implementation of innovations?
(3) If more than 3 years old, has the paper subsequently been cited as a seminal contribution by respected researchers in that tradition?

Box 2.3 Preliminary inclusion criteria for primary research papers.

(1) *Relevance.* Is the paper about (or otherwise relevant to) the diffusion, spread or sustainability of innovations in service delivery or organisation?
(2) *Depth.* Does the paper go beyond superficial description or commentary – i.e. is it a broadly competent attempt at research, enquiry, investigation or study?
(3) *Utility.* Will the paper offer added value for our client, given the policy context and priorities of our own research?

we took our unit of analysis as the research tradition, which we defined as 'a coherent theoretical discourse and a linked body of empirical research in which successive studies are influenced by preceding inquiries'.*

We approached each research tradition with five questions in mind:

(1) What are the parameters of this tradition – i.e. its scope, its historical roots, its key concepts and assumptions, and its theoretical basis?

(2) What research questions (in what priority†) have scientists in this tradition asked about the topic area? What methods and instruments have they used to answer these questions, and by what criteria has 'methodological quality' of primary studies generally been judged?

(3) What are the main empirical findings of relevance from the 'quality' literature in this research tradition?

(4) How has the tradition unfolded over time (i.e. in what way have the findings of earlier studies led to refinements in theory or influenced the design and direction of later empirical work)?

(5) What are the strengths and limitations of this tradition, and in the light of these, what is its likely overall contribution to the body of knowledge on this topic area?

We used this method for the sources we had classified as 'theoretical papers', and also for the discussion sections of primary research papers. All theoretical sources were considered by at least two of the research team and discrepancies resolved by discussion. Whilst there were many instances when we disagreed on the detailed interpretation of a theoretical paper, there were no instances when we remained in disagreement over the fundamental theoretical perspective of a particular author. Similarly, we sometimes had high levels of disagreement on the exact classification of a paper (e.g. whether it counted as 'knowledge utilisation' or 'health services research'), but we attributed this to the fuzzy nature of the taxonomy and not to fundamental differences in how we interpreted the meaning of the paper. A striking finding, discussed in several places in the Chapters 4–9, was the atheoretical basis of so many papers – in other words, the authors did not hypothesise any explicit mechanism by which an intervention had an impact.

We identified 13 traditions (some overlapping) that were of central relevance to the focus of this report: rural sociology, medical sociology, communication studies, marketing and economics, development studies, health promotion (including social marketing), EBM and guideline implementation, studies of organisational structure, studies of organisational culture and process, interorganisational studies, knowledge-based organisational studies, narrative organisational studies, and complexity theory as applied to organisational change. As descriptions of these traditions in Chapter 3 illustrate, the unfolding of the conceptual, theoretical and empirical basis of research on diffusion, dissemination and sustainability of innovations in any particular tradition can be presented as a historical story (meta-narrative) in terms of where a particular group of scientists was (or is) 'coming from'. The results of the mapping phase formed an important background to our review, most significantly because they crucially informed our own *understanding* of the primary literature and the structuring of our empirical results.

2.5 Appraisal phase

It was reassuring that scientists in widely differing traditions used very similar quality criteria to evaluate studies of comparable designs. For example, a survey of organisational attributes in the management literature[62] would be judged by similar methodological criteria by those within that tradition as a survey of consumer views in psychology would be judged by other psycholo-

*We adapted this definition from Rogers, who, drawing on Kuhn, defined a research tradition (page 38) as 'a series of investigations on a similar topic in which successive studies are influenced by preceding inquiries.'[3]

†Since the number of questions in a review of complex evidence may be almost infinite, a pragmatic decision may well have to be made about which ones to omit within the constraints of the project.

gists[152] – namely, appropriateness of sampling frame, validity of questionnaire items, completeness of response and so on.* But different groups of scientists were widely divided on whether a particular research design was appropriate at all. For example, whilst all traditions whose methodological toolkit included the survey classified this as a potentially high-quality research tool, those traditions whose toolkit did *not* include surveys were often dismissive of any work based on this method, regardless of the research question being considered.

These discrepancies are discussed further from a philosophical perspective in Section 2.7 (page 42). From the more prosaic perspective of appraising the primary studies, we accepted as a valid research design any study that was seen as such by the experts within a particular tradition, and dismissed as non-valid any study that those scientists would be unable to defend in front of their own peers.

We evaluated experimental research designs (randomised controlled trials (RCTs), non-RCTs) and quasi-experimental designs (interrupted time series) using modified versions of the quality criteria developed by the Cochrane Effective Practice and Organisation of Care Group for interventions in service delivery and organisation (Boxes A.1 and A.2, respectively, in Appendix 2, pages 234 and 235). As set out in Appendix 2, the main modifications made were:

(1) We did not make firm quantitative cut-offs for such variables as completeness of follow-up. This was because we had so few relevant controlled trials that we felt we should include mention of as many as possible; hence we opted to present their details descriptively to allow readers to interpret the evidence in the light of any limitations.

(2) We included several additional questions, indicated with an asterisk in Boxes A.1–A.7.

Most primary studies of diffusion were attribution studies – i.e. studies that asked: 'What perceived attributes [in terms of relative advantage, compatibility, etc.] of innovation X influence its adoption by adopter group Y?' Also included in this category were studies of organisational innovativeness – i.e. studies that looked at the characteristics of organisations with high (and low) levels of adoption of new ideas and practices. For such studies, we used the criteria developed by Tornatzky and Klein[62] (the only researchers to have undertaken a formal meta-analysis in this area; Box A.3, page 236, in Appendix 3). Many questionnaire surveys were in fact retrospective attribution studies (i.e. respondents were asked to rate aspects of an innovation that had led to adoption or non-adoption); these were assessed (and, where appropriate, rejected) using the Tornatzky and Klein criteria. For other questionnaire surveys, we used new criteria developed independently[153] (Box A.4, page 237). We evaluated qualitative research studies (e.g. interviews) using Mays and Pope's checklist[154] (Box A.5, page 238).

For in-depth case studies and other complex, process-focused qualitative designs, we drew on three checklists,[142,154,155] which have previously been discussed and compared by Mays *et al.*[118] We extracted the most relevant questions from this list for our own review; added some additional specific questions (e.g. about the nature of the innovation), and (following a pilot phase) inserted one or two additional questions (e.g. funding source). Our final list of questions for case studies is shown in Box A.6 (page 239).

For comparative studies that had compared two or more process evaluations asking the question of the general format 'Was programme A (tested in setting X) more successful than programme B (tested in setting Y)?', we adapted the questions developed by Pawson and Tilley[120] for realistic evaluation and modified by Gomm[116] in the 'Would it work here?' framework. Our questions are listed in Box A.7 (page 240).

Finally, for action research initiatives, we modified slightly the list of quality criteria developed by Waterman *et al.* in their systematic review of the action research literature. Our questions are listed in Box A.8 (page 242).

Having applied these criteria, we often discovered that no studies remained for inclusion in

*We do not know if this will be an invariable finding in other comparable reviews, but if that were shown to be the case it would be evidence for the robustness of this method.

a particular topic review. In such instances we broadened our inclusion criteria (most usually, by including high-quality studies from outside the health service field, and occasionally from beyond the service sector; and sometimes by including – with caveats – studies that we had classified as methodologically doubtful).

Having completed the appropriate checklist, we asked a summary question: 'Does the paper meet the established criteria for methodological quality that would be used by a competent peer reviewer in the appropriate research tradition?' Using this question, we classified papers as either 'outstanding', 'some limitations' or 'many important limitations'; we also rated their relevance as 'essential to include', 'relevant but not essential' or 'marginal relevance'. Our inter-rater reliability for this task was 94% for quality and 95% for relevance. We flagged studies ranked as 'outstanding and essential to include', plus meta-analyses ranked as 'some limitations and essential to include' for citation tracking (see Section 2.3, page 35). We rejected almost all studies ranked as 'many important limitations',* but otherwise considered all papers marked 'relevant' for inclusion in the report.

Three members of the research team (TG, GR and OK) completed detailed data extraction sheets (based on Boxes A.1–A.7 in Appendix 3) for the primary research papers on our final list, each concentrating mainly on a particular research tradition. We presented and discussed 'critical examples' from different research fields in face-to-face meetings and by email. In all, three-quarters of all empirical studies were independently assessed by a second researcher (we initially selected a random one in three sample but we also frequently used our judgement to seek a 'second opinion' when necessary).

*Three studies from this group were included for reasons set out in the relevant section of the results. Briefly, we judged the parts of the paper that we drew upon as methodologically adequate even though the paper as a whole was ranked as poor. This flexible approach to methodological quality is an established technique in realist review, as discussed in Section 2.7 (page 42).

2.6 Synthesis phase

The goal of this phase was to draw together, contextualise and interpret the findings from the separate research traditions with a view to building a rich picture of the field of enquiry. We sought to describe and compare, rather than attempt to unite within a single conceptual framework, the different streams in the relevant literature. The synthesis phase was characterised by four key questions:

(1) What is the range of research questions that different groups of scientists have asked about diffusion, dissemination and sustainability of innovations? Can these questions be meaningfully grouped and classified across traditions?
(2) What are the commonalities of research findings across traditions, and where the empirical findings from different traditions are conflicting, to what extent can discrepancies be explained?
(3) Given the 'rich picture' of the topic area achieved from these multiple perspectives, what are the overall key findings and implications for practice and policy?
(4) What are the main gaps in the evidence on this topic and where should further primary research be directed?

As anticipated, we found that different groups of researchers had asked similar but not identical questions and used similar but not identical designs and methods, so a high level of abstraction of results was generally not possible. In most cases, we used simple description and tables of disaggregated data (a technique that Dixon-Woods *et al.*[2] have called 'narrative summary') to build up a rich picture of the topic area from multiple perspectives and to capture and describe rather than 'average out' the heterogeneity between studies. Specifically, we did not undertake additional meta-analyses of either experimental or non-experimental data, nor did we attempt to make any other statistical generalisations. This descriptive approach is strongly favoured by Egger *et al.*,[156] who warn of the dangers of spurious precision if statistical generalisations are made inappropriately on heterogeneous observational studies.

We took the overall question of diffusion, dissemination, implementation and sustainability of innovations, and broke it down into six themes that were more or less common across the different traditions. These were innovations, adoption and adopters, communication and influence (including both passive diffusion and active dissemination), the inner (organisational) context, the outer (environmental) context, and the implementation process (covered in Chapters 4–9, respectively). We grouped within each topic heading all the different questions addressed by different groups of researchers; and commented on the different methods and approaches used by researchers in different traditions. For example, under the broad theme of 'diffusion and dissemination' we considered specific topics such as 'opinion leaders', 'champions', 'boundary spanners' and so on from a range of perspectives.

As a crucial part of the synthesis phase, we compared and contrasted the different research traditions in terms of the questions they asked about a particular topic, the research designs they selected, the criteria they used to distinguish 'quality' studies, and their interpretation of their findings. The goal of this stage was to find epistemological (and indeed pragmatic and realistic) explanations that could illuminate and challenge the differences in the findings and recommendations made by researchers from widely differing traditions on a supposedly common topic area. In this way, the many contradictions we were finding in our sources could be turned into data and analysed systematically (using principles similar to those applied to the analysis of contradictions and 'disconfirming cases' in qualitative research[157]), thus allowing us to go beyond concluding statements such as 'the findings of primary studies were contradictory' or that 'more research is needed'.

A good example of how we used 'conflicting' evidence from different traditions to enhance understanding of a phenomenon is that of opinion leadership. Whilst some traditions – especially EBM – saw opinion leaders as an 'intervention' that could be manipulated by the research team (e.g. through training or through briefing those in positions of influence), other traditions – especially medical sociology – saw opinion leadership as a subtle phenomenon in a delicate social system, which the research team might observe *without* attempting to influence. The former researchers undertook RCTs ('opinion leader on' vs 'opinion leader off', with predefined outcome measures)[54] whereas the latter conducted ethnographic studies of real-world social influence.[53]

As explained in Section 6.2 (page 118) these different approaches to the study of opinion leaders produced apparently contradictory findings. RCTs undertaken within the EBM tradition have consistently shown that opinion leaders have a relatively small impact on the adoption of innovations,[54] but research from medical sociology has produced the opposite conclusion – that opinion leaders often have profound and far-reaching impact on precisely this process.[53] By nesting each primary study within its paradigm, we could systematically explore these differences in terms of how 'opinion leadership' had been differently conceptualised and explored. In this example, a key explanatory variable was the degree of agency of the opinion leader. We concluded that (on the one hand) individuals identified by experimenters as opinion leaders cannot be injected into a complex social situation and reliably manipulated to influence a predefined outcome, but that (on the other hand) certain people have considerable social influence on their peers, and this influence can sometimes be the making or breaking of a complex intervention programme.

Before using the individual primary studies to build up a rich picture of different aspects of the diffusion of innovations, we applied an appropriate critical appraisal checklist. For example, in relation to the studies on opinion leadership, we evaluated randomised trails according to the criteria in Box A.1 (page 234) and qualitative studies according to those in Box A.5 (page 238).

Because of the highly complex (and in some cases, contested) nature of the evidence, we did not use a strictly hierarchical system for grading it (i.e. we did not grade the evidence 'A', 'B', 'C', etc.). Rather, we provided a brief descriptive commentary for each statement, which is based on a modified* version of the World Health Organisation Health Evidence Network criteria for evaluating public health research (Box 2.4).[158] In this taxonomy, 'limited evidence' generally indicates that insufficient research has been undertaken to draw firm conclusions, and that 'moderate direct evidence' may sometimes be more persuasive than 'strong indirect evidence' and vice versa.

The recommendations in Chapter 11 were developed through discussion within the team, as well as formal consultation with stakeholders from the service sector.

Box 2.4 Descriptive grading system for strength of evidence (developed by modifying the WHO HEN criteria for public health research cited in Øvretveit[158]).

Strong direct evidence – consistent findings in two or more empirical studies of appropriate design and high scientific quality undertaken in health service organisations
Strong indirect evidence – consistent findings in two or more empirical studies of appropriate design and high scientific quality but not from health service organisation
Moderate direct evidence – consistent findings in two or more empirical studies of less appropriate design and/or of acceptable scientific quality undertaken in health service organisation
Moderate indirect evidence – consistent findings in two or more empirical studies of less appropriate design and/or of acceptable scientific quality but not from health service organisation
Limited evidence – only one study of appropriate design and acceptable available, or inconsistent findings in several studies
No evidence – no relevant study of acceptable scientific quality available

2.7 Meta-narrative review: philosophical origins and links with other approaches to the synthesis of complex evidence

We drew on a theoretical approach developed by Kuhn[159] in the *Structure of Scientific Revolutions*. Kuhn introduced the notion of 'normal science' – that most science, most of the time, is conducted according to a set of rules and standards that are considered self-evident by those working in a particular field, but which are not universally accepted. Any group of researchers views the world through a particular 'lens' or paradigm. Paradigms, which Kuhn defined as 'models from which spring particular coherent traditions of scientific research', have four dimensions:
(1) conceptual (what are considered the important objects of study – and, hence, what counts as a legitimate problem to be solved by science);
(2) theoretical (how the objects of study are considered to relate to one another and to the world);
(3) methodological (the accepted ways in which problems might be investigated); and
(4) instrumental (the accepted tools and techniques to be used by scientists).

Kuhn's most radical and enduring proposition is the notion that a scientific paradigm is a necessary (though arbitrary) meaning-system without which scientific endeavours *cannot* be focused. He showed, using historical examples from the physical sciences, that the progress of any scientific paradigm in any field follows a very predictable pattern – from pre-paradigmatic (a creative, exploratory phase in which scientists play with ideas and develop methods) through paradigmatic (rule-following, puzzle-solving and incremental theory-building – the phase in which most conventional scientific careers are built and in which apprentices to the discipline are introduced to the rules using an accepted body of jargon) to post-paradigmatic (a decline phase in which anomalies begin to appear in the collected data that demand new concepts and theories to explain them fully – thus setting the stage for scientific revolution).

Kuhn believed that paradigms are to a large extent incommensurable – i.e. an empirical discovery made using one set of concepts, theories, methods and instruments cannot be satisfactorily

*The division of evidence into 'strong', 'moderate', 'limited' and 'none', and the notion of 'high' and 'low' quality is from the WHO classification; the qualifiers 'highly appropriate' and 'less appropriate' for study design and 'direct' and 'indirect' for the study source are our own.

explained through a different paradigmatic lens. This claim for the incommensurability of paradigms is no longer accepted by many philosophers, but this small-print controversy has no direct implications for meta-narrative review. Incidentally, the term 'meta-narrative' was originally introduced by the French philosopher Jean-Francois Lyotard in his seminal work on *The Postmodern Condition*[160] to indicate the grand cosmological and ideological 'lens' through which a group of people views the world. Lyotard's meta-narratives included Judao-Christianity, Marxism, feminism, modernist–rationalist science and psychoanalysis. We use the term in a slightly more prosaic sense to depict the overarching 'storyline' of a research tradition: where did it come from and why; what is its core business; and where is it headed? Thus, 'meta-narrative' in our sense is a research tradition with a time dimension – the *historical unfolding* of ideas, empirical findings and theory refinement.

The two curves in Fig. 2.2, showing the number of papers on diffusion of innovations published per year in two separate traditions within rural sociology, demonstrate this cycle[161]:

(1) publication of an initial 'breakthrough' paper that provided model problems and solutions;

(2) a sharp increase in intellectual effort as promising young scientists were attracted to the new field;

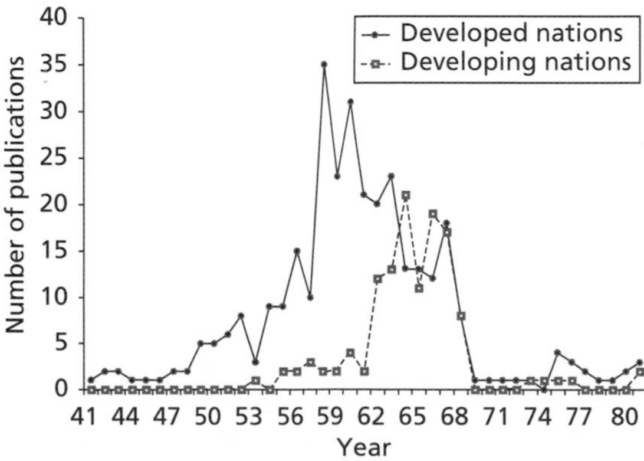

Fig. 2.2 Emergence and decline of two research traditions on diffusion of innovations in rural sociology (data taken from Valente and Rogers[161]).

(3) a steady accumulation and exchange of ideas within the field; and

(4) decline, in which exciting new findings became less and less common and new scientific blood was attracted to different problems.

Figure 2.3, drawn from our own data, maps the publications on diffusion of innovations in four different traditions within health care research, and shows a similar rise and fall pattern. Because of the complexities of modern publication patterns and indexing schemes, Fig. 2.2 is only an approximation of the accumulation of studies within particular traditions. Nevertheless, the trajectories closely mirror those found by Valente and Rogers from a very different tradition in a previous generation. By 2004, research publication on diffusion of innovation in both nursing and medical education had fallen considerably from a peak in 1996–7, whereas comparable research in relation to EBM appeared to have recently reached a peak, and in relation to the EHR it had entered an accelerated phase in 2004.

Having demonstrated that research on diffusion of innovations waxed and waned within different scientific communities at different times, we decided to take the research tradition as the initial unit of analysis for our review. In other words, rather than identifying, evaluating and comparing data from primary research studies (as is standard practice for Cochrane reviews[162]), we set out to collect and compare the different overarching storylines of the rise and fall of diffusion research that we judged relevant to our overall research question.

The systematic review described here drew centrally on the Kuhnian notion of the research tradition and its historical progression from pre-paradigmatic through to post-paradigmatic phases, and on his axiom that any body of science can only be understood (or at least, is best made sense of) through its own paradigmatic lens. In the laborious fieldwork phase of this study, we had to prepare data extraction sheets for hundreds of primary studies as well as sift through overviews and commentaries. The more papers we read, the more confusing the field appeared. Developing an initial taxonomy by research

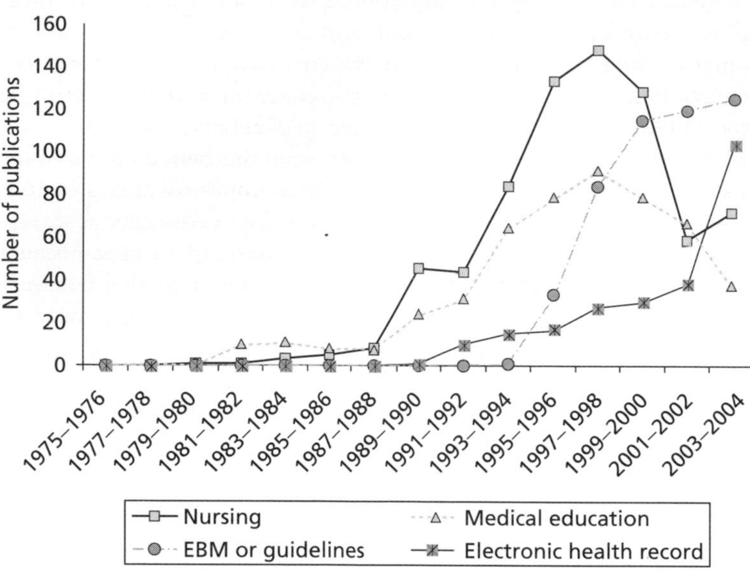

Fig. 2.3 Publications indexed on Medline with 'diffusion of innovations' as a central focus in different branches of health sciences 1975–2004.*

tradition (rather than, as we had previously attempted, by topic area, research question, or study design) enabled us to *make sense* of the vast and apparently incoherent pile of papers.

As set out in the earlier sections of this chapter, we developed a systematic method for identifying and following the development of the different research traditions. This method made explicit use of both informal and intuitive exploration and formal search and appraisal techniques based on hand searching, electronic tracking, and structured checklists. We then used an established synthesis method (narrative summary – see below) to demonstrate how the different traditions contributed to the overall 'rich picture' of a defined topic area and to compare and contrast their findings in the light of their different conceptual, theoretical and methodological bases. In this way, we were able to extract meaning from what appeared to be 'conflicting' theoretical perspectives and primary studies.

Dixon-Woods *et al.*[163] have recently published an overview of synthesis methods for complex evidence. Implicit in their work is a distinction between 'review' (a generic term that can refer to just about any summary of the literature) and 'synthesis' (a technique for producing knowledge that is in some sense more than the sum of its parts[146]). In any taxonomy of review methods, critical emphasis must be placed on the technique used to achieve synthesis over and above summary. In reviews of quantitative evidence, for example, the main synthesis method is statistical meta-analysis, in which the point estimate and confidence intervals of effect size in individual studies all contribute to a new point estimate and (more precise) confidence interval.

Synthesis techniques that can be used across primary qualitative studies include meta-ethnography,[146] cross-case analysis using the expanded matrix technique[164] and grounded theory applied across studies.[147] Techniques for synthesising data from both qualitative and quantitative primary studies include 'quantifying' qualitative data using either content analysis[165] or Bayesian

*These graphs were produced by searching the Medline database for diffusion of innovation (MeSH term or text word), and combining this data-set, respectively, with the exploded MeSH terms 'Nursing', 'Education', 'Evidence-based medicine' or 'Practice guidelines' or 'Guideline implementation'; and 'Electronic health record'. Searches were repeated in 2-year time bands from 1975 to 2004.

meta-analysis,[166] 'qualitising' quantitative data,[167] or using a matrix approach to combine themes derived from quantitative data with a separate thematic analysis of qualitative data (a technique that is becoming known as 'the EPPIcentre method'[168]). In addition, Mays *et al.*[169] have argued that narrative synthesis (a formalised version of the expert overview, in which 'qualitative and quantitative evidence are juxtaposed as text and numbers, but with increasing use of techniques and presentational devices such as conceptual mapping and tabular summaries') constitutes a synthesis method in its own right.

The choice of narrative summary as a synthesis method, in preference to the various more focused (and in some ways more sophisticated) methods listed in Table 2.1, was predicated on the diversity and complexity of the field. Arguably, all the synthesis methods in Table 2.1 are 'within-paradigm' methods (i.e. they require a set of studies that share a conceptual and theoretical basis, make more or less the same assumptions, and use similar methods of investigation and data analysis); narrative synthesis is an 'across-paradigm' method that allows differences in these various parameters to be highlighted, described and explored, thereby producing higher-order data.

In some ways, our approach was comparable with that of Paterson *et al.*[119] on meta-theory, but their approach, as the name implies, is designed to

Table 2.1 Synthesis methods for different types of research question.

Research question type	*Preferred research design*	*Preferred synthesis method*
Does intervention X produce predefined outcome Y (and how large is the effect)?	RCT	'Cochrane' style systematic review of RCTs with meta-analysis if appropriate[162]
Do attributes A, B, C, etc. account for event D?	Prospective or concurrent attribution study	Correlational meta-analysis (e.g. Tornatzky and Klein[62])[a]
What are the beliefs, perceptions, experiences, etc. of group G?	Qualitative methods (semi-structured interview, focus group, observation, etc.)	Several potential methods including grounded theory,[147] meta-ethnography,[146] meta-synthesis[145] and meta-study[170] – see Dixon-Woods *et al.*[2] for discussion of relative merits of each in particular situations
What is the nature of process P and is it transferable to context Q?	In-depth case study, usually with mixed methods[171,172]	Realist review[140,173]
What research has been done into complex field F?	Wide range of different designs	Structured approaches to combining qualitative and quantitative findings in a single synthesis (including 'qualitising' quantitative data and 'quantitising' qualitative data – see text for examples)[163] *or* Narrative summary, in which qualitative and quantitative findings are presented in disaggregated form with interpretive commentary[163]

[a]Tornatzky and Klein, who published their landmark meta-analysis on diffusion of organisational innovations in 1982, acknowledged that at the time, the science of meta-analysis of non-experimental data was in its infancy.[62] For a more up-to-date review of such approaches see the *Cochrane Reviewers' Handbook*.[162]

compare different theoretical approaches with the same question (e.g. they give an example of a particular question through a 'Marxist' interpretive lens and the same question through a 'feminist' lens), whereas our own approach does not privilege the theory over other aspects of the research tradition, and it places critical importance on the description of the historial unfolding of the tradition (including the theory) over time.

The meta-narrative approach also overlaps considerably with realist review, a method proposed by Pawson[140] in 2002. Pawson was one of the original referees for the systematic review reported here, and has subsequently worked with one of us to produce an updated monograph on realist review as applied to health services.[173] Realist review, a development from the well-established technique of realist evaluation,[120] was designed to *critically examine the mechanisms of success or failure* of complex social interventions (such as a community development or health promotion programmes) by exploring the interactions between context, mechanism and outcome. Realist evaluation begins by teasing out the programme theory – i.e. the mechanism by which the instigators of a particular programme intended it to work – and then sets out to test this theory. Realist review takes the same approach across more than one study of a comparable programme.

The central question of both realist evaluation and realist review is: 'what works, for whom, under what circumstances, and why?' Realism strongly rejects experimental approaches in which contextual elements are 'controlled for' and thus stripped away from subsequent analysis. Rather, the realist reviewer engages with the messiness of real-world context, including the idiosyncrasies and discontinuities of the actors implementing the programme, the mismatch between the programme-as-conceived and the programme-as-implemented, any attrition and adaptation of elements of the programme as time unfolds, resource constraints and any resulting compromises, and the detailed nature of the social systems in which the programme is embedded. Not only can these quirks never be fully 'controlled for', they embody the explanation for why – and to what extent – the programme succeeds or fails.

Realist review is discussed further in Section 11.3 (page 225). Whilst it has many parallels with meta-narrative review, and indeed a meta-narrative review might be produced by applying the general principles of realist synthesis, there are three key differences in emphasis:

(1) Whereas realist review focuses centrally on the programme theory (i.e. the mechanism by which the programme produces its effect), meta-narrative review is concerned with the package of concepts, theories, methods,and instruments – i.e. with the four defining elements of a scientific paradigm as set out by Kuhn. Thus, for example, the empirical work on opinion leadership undertaken by the EBM tradition (page 41) implicitly embraces a particular programme theory (that an opinion leader can be identified by researchers, trained to follow a particular guideline, reinserted into a social setting of clinicians, and their behaviour in following the same guideline influenced), which the realist approach is well poised to test. The meta-narrative approach also addresses how opinion leadership was conceptualised and framed by the EBM community, including the words and phrases used to define the concept of opinion leader, the methods considered by scientists as most appropriate to test the theory (the RCT), and the measures of success (in general, a particular behaviour change, often judged 'present' or 'absent'). That is not to say that realist review is entirely unconcerned with this wider package, but its emphasis differs slightly.

(2) Realist review does not explicitly take account of the historical unfolding of research ideas and methods over time. Again, realist review does not reject the importance of a historical dimension, but it does not place central importance on this dimension. Meta-narrative review, in contrast, sees the time dimension as critical to achieving an understanding of the work of a particular group of scientists, since only by placing empirical studies in historical order can the reviewer trace the *development* of science (including the framing of the 'puzzles' to be solved, the formulation and rejection of successive hypotheses, the refinement of theories, and, eventually, the appearance of

inconsistent results that lead to the demise of the paradigm). Using the opinion leadership example again, the meta-narrative approach allowed us to place the various RCTs in historical order, showing how successive groups of clinical epidemiologists attempted to refine the concept of an opinion leader, but failed to 'solve the puzzle' of making this intervention more effective.

(3) Realist review is explicitly designed to test programmes (hence, is limited to – or at least, best suited to – the study of complex social interventions). Although we developed the meta-narrative technique to aid a particular review of programmes (i.e. empirical studies of the introduction of service-level innovations in health care organisations), the same technique could equally be applied to any area of scientific enquiry.

However, it should be recognised that both realist review and meta-narrative review are new synthesis techniques, and firm statements about their respective strengths and limitations (and their areas of overlap) are not possible at this stage.

These differences notwithstanding, it might be asked whether meta-narrative review is merely a specific application of realist review. Certainly, if the research question – as ours did – arises out of a pressing policy question and focuses on the implementation of complex interventions in different contexts, realist criteria (what works, for whom, under what circumstances, and how?[173]) will run through every phase of the review. But there is no a priori reason why the research storyline should not be used as the initial unit of analysis in the scoping phase, and as a key theme in the synthesis phase, across the wider range of review methods illustrated in.

We are still developing and refining the technique of meta-narrative review and placing it appropriately alongside other approaches to the synthesis of complex evidence. We provisionally conclude that in situations where the scope of a project is broad and the literature diverse, where different groups of scientists have asked different questions and used different research designs to address a common problem, where different groups of practitioners and policymakers have drawn on the research literature in different ways, where 'quality' papers have different defining features in different literatures, and where there is no self-evident or universally agreed process for pulling the different bodies of literature together, meta-narrative review has particular strengths as a synthesis method.

However, it should be noted that the method arose in a pragmatic way within the course of a single project; it has not yet been tested prospectively. We invite other research teams working on the systematic review of complex evidence to explore this new method with a view to testing both its theoretical robustness and its practical applications.

Chapter 3
The research traditions

Key points

1. This chapter gives a brief historical overview of the 13 research traditions we drew upon for this review. These traditions overlap with one another but are based at least partly on incommensurable conceptual models and theoretical frameworks from a wealth of primary disciplines, as summarised in Table 1.1 (page 23).

2. Classical diffusion research has roots in sociology, anthropology, physical geography and education. Early sociological studies among US farmers (Section 3.2, page 51) and doctors (Section 3.3, page 53) led independently to the finding that the adoption curve is S-shaped, that interpersonal influence is critical on the adoption decision, and that some individuals (opinion leaders) are more influential than others. Similar findings were demonstrated using different empirical methods in communication studies (Section 3.4, page 55), in relation to the spread of media stories, and in marketing (Section 3.5, page 56), in relation to consumer behaviour.

3. As discussed in Section 3.6 (page 58), these early research traditions were all characterised by a pro-individual, pro-innovation bias and took little account of the wider context (historical, political, ideological, organisational) in which adoption decisions were made or of the unintended consequences of innovation.

4. One early tradition to challenge these biases was development studies (Section 3.7, page 60), which exposed the imperialist assumption that underdevelopment is due to an 'innovation gap' that can be made good by the transfer of the right technologies and ways of working from the West. An alternative model sees development as a participatory process of social change by an informed, active and empowered community.

5. The history of disseminating health promotion messages (Section 3.8, page 62) mirrors this shift in ideology. Early campaigns were couched in terms of a knowledge gap (people engage in unhealthy lifestyles because they do not know any better), and targeted with techniques borrowed from marketing. These early programmes largely ignored the social and political causes of particular behaviours and lifestyle choices. More contemporary approaches to health promotion are aimed at community development and long-term social change.

6. An important research tradition in health care innovation is EBM and the related study of guideline dissemination and implementation (Section 3.9, page 64). These traditions have firm roots in epidemiology and – at least until recently – adopted a highly rationalist, experimentalist and behaviourist approach. Efforts to disseminate innovations (such as guidelines) were evaluated by means of RCTs with little systematic attention to either process or context. More recently, some EBM researchers have broken from this rationalist approach and begun to use ethnographic methods to explore the construction and use of evidence in particular clinical and policymaking contexts.

7. The study of how organisations adopt (or assimilate) innovations has been addressed in several research traditions including studies of the structural determinants of organisational innovativeness (Section 3.10, page 66), which considered the association of different structural features (such as size or centralisation) with organisational innovativeness. More recent traditions within organisational studies have focused more on the process of innovation, the culture, climate and leadership of the organisation (Section 3.11, page 68), and the role of interorganisational networks in establishing norms and spreading 'organisational fads and fashions' (Section 3.12, page 70).

8. The knowledge utilisation tradition (Section 3.13, page 70) takes the view that organisational innovation is centrally to do with the construction and transmission of knowledge within and between organisations. Key concepts include the distinction between explicit (codifiable, easily transmitted) and tacit (embedded, situational, 'sticky') knowledge; the importance of social interaction in the construction and transmission of knowledge; and the notions of sense-making (linking new knowledge meaningfully with existing mental schemas) and absorptive capacity (the knowledge-creating capability that is needed for new knowledge to make sense).

9. Narrative research traditions (Section 3.14, page 77), which seek to understand specific phenomena in terms of unique human purpose and meaning (rather than in terms of scientific causality), use the story both as a research tool and as the vehicle for driving innovation and change. Stories are humanising, sense-making, creative and adaptive. They embrace complexity, celebrate initiative and provide a moral mandate for the organisational rule-breaker. Hence, they are potentially both subversive and innovative.

10. Complexity theory (Section 3.15, page 79) is beginning to influence a new tradition of organisational research in health care. Complex systems are characterised by multiple independent parts, dynamic relationships, patterns (but not predictability) of behaviour, adaptiveness and emergence. In complex emergent situations, the approach to innovation (like any change) must focus on relationships; be exploratory, intuitive and responsive; and make judicious use of rapid-cycle feedback to inform emergent decisions.

3.1 The origins of diffusion of innovations research

Our inability to find a single, all-encompassing theoretical framework to underpin the diffusion of innovations as applied to health service organisations is consistent with previous attempts to review similar bodies of literature.[41,59,174,175,*] As explained in Chapter 2, we have based this overview broadly on the defining characteristics of the research tradition suggested by Kuhn[159] – i.e. for each tradition we describe briefly the historical context, conceptual basis, theoretical framework and preferred methods and instruments used by researchers. We also give a brief outline of the empirical findings for each tradition, but detailed results are described in more detail in Chapters 4–9.

The history of conventional diffusion of innovations theory has been clearly set out by Rogers in the four editions of his book, *Diffusion of Innovations*, published in 1962,[176] 1972,[177] 1983,[178] and 1995,[3] respectively. Rogers was a US postdoctoral student of rural sociology in the 1950s. As a young academic, he found it ironic that researchers in his discipline failed to learn lessons from work in other disciplines and vice versa. As he says in his 1995 edition[3] (page 38):

> My main motivation for writing the first book on this topic ... was to point out the lack of diffusion in diffusion research, and to argue for greater awareness among the various diffusion research traditions.

This chapter draws extensively on Rogers'[3] grand narrative as well as on summary papers by others.[102,179–181] The earliest scholarly tradition influencing diffusion research was probably European sociology in the late nineteenth century. Tarde,[182] a French lawyer and social psychologist, was interested in why a minority of ideas, products and practices spread widely while most did not. He believed that few individuals or societies invent products or practices *de novo*, but that imitation is ubiquitous and the root of social change:

> Renewing initiatives stand as a starting point. They bring new needs and new satisfactions to the world, then spread or tend to do so through forced or spontaneous, chosen or unconscious, quick or slow imitation, always responding to a regular pace, as a light wave or a family of termites.

*We believe that published meta-analyses in the organisation and management field show a greater degree of consistency in the findings of organisational research than most other commentators have suggested exists.[14–16] These papers are discussed in detail in Chapter 8 (page 157).

Tarde formulated what he called the laws of imitation, which include the concept of both invention and imitation (adoption) as fundamentally social acts; the concept of adoption or rejection as a key outcome variable in the diffusion process; the fact that most diffusion curves are S-shaped (as in Fig. 3.1, page 52); the importance of socially esteemed opinion leaders in achieving the crucial 'take-off' phase in the S-curve; the role of geographical proximity in the imitation process; and the increased probability of adoption if the innovation is similar to ideas that have already been accepted.[182]

Tarde was an intellectual liberal and social reformist, arguing that new ideas spread through a trickle-down process in which 'inferiors' imitated 'superiors'; hence (he argued) imitation would eventually lead to assimilation and elimination of the lower social classes. His book *The Laws of Imitation* was ahead of its time, and it was not until 40 years after it was published that sociologists developed the empirical methods (see below) to test its key theoretical concepts.

In a separate tradition (and without knowledge of Tarde's work), anthropologists in Britain, Germany and Austria in the early 1900s began to develop concepts of social change that were based on the notion of adoption of innovations from other societies. Like Tarde, these European diffusionists held the view – now largely discredited – that invention (i.e. discovering or creating new ideas or products) was very rare and that most social change occurs by diffusion from a single central source. It is now generally accepted that at an anthropological level (i.e. the level of human society) parallel invention is very common and true diffusion of innovations relatively rare.[3] However, within a particular society (in which there exist social networks linking individuals and organisations), diffusion by imitation is a critical source of change.

The roots of modern anthropology were established in the 1920s, when the technique of participant observation – in which an anthropologist would spend years living in a particular community *as a member* of that community – became popular. Participant observation generally restricted the researcher to the study of small social systems (such as a single village), but allowed a rich picture to be built not just of the patterns of adoption and spread (i.e. whether and when people had adopted an innovation) but also of *how and why* adoption did or did not occur. This early tradition of in-depth, highly contextual and interpretive research is re-emerging in modern organisational anthropology, and is discussed further in relation to health care organisations in Section 3.11 and also in Chapters 7–9. As Rogers[3] comments (page 46):

> If the anthropologist is successful in attempting to empathise with the respondents of the study, the ensuing account of diffusion will tell the story from the respondents' viewpoint, conveying their perceptions of the innovation and of the change agency with a high degree of understanding. This perspective helps the anthropologist overcome the pro-innovation bias that is displayed in much other diffusion research.

The meticulous qualitative methods used by the early anthropologists allowed them to document in detail the features of an innovation that increased (or decreased) the chances of its being adopted, and also the process of adaptation (reinvention) that successfully embedded an innovation in a new context. Indeed, many of the qualitative methods that are regaining popularity in health services research were originally described in relation to the study of the adoption of new customs, technologies or practices by remote tribal communities (see Rogers,[3] pages 46–51 for examples).

It is worth mentioning in passing the research tradition on diffusion of innovations in the discipline of geography. Like the early anthropologists, early geographers studying the spread of innovations believed that innovation originated at a single point and diffused outward.[183] Using simulation techniques, Hagerstrand[184] developed the urban (or central place) hierarchy model, which states that innovations begin in the largest, most cosmopolitan cities (notably ports and market towns), and spread to smaller, more remote areas. There is also an interesting literature on the impact of the physical environment on adopter curves, which we have not gone into here (see Wejnert[41] for an overview).

Geographical patterns of diffusion (based on physical distance) have more recently been distorted by air travel, through which highly mobile 'vectors' can spread certain innovations (such as illicit drugs) very rapidly;[179] by cultural globalisation, in which it becomes fashionable (particularly amongst the educated classes) to adopt 'chic' innovations from distant countries and regions;[185] and by the telecommunications revolution, in which physical distance is increasingly irrelevant compared with technical access and expertise.[186] Later studies have demonstrated that the more complex and sophisticated the innovation, the more spatial distance between innovators is overshadowed by (and is sometimes a proxy for) *structural equivalence* – i.e. connections based on higher-order conceptual ties that bind together individuals, organisations, or countries, including cultural, political, ideological, philosophical and economic connectedness;[41] these are discussed below in relation to social network analysis.*

A final strand of early diffusion research was education, which has been addressing the spread of innovations in teaching, assessment and school management for almost a century – from local control of school finances (1920s) to modern mathematics (1960s) to Web-based educational technologies (1990s). Teachers and curriculum developers, of course, differed from farmers in that they were not self-employed and hence not independent, autonomous decision-makers. Rather, they worked in large, hierarchical, bureaucratic and change-resistant organisations whose physical space, administrative constraints and organisational culture and climate had a major impact on the adoption decisions of individual staff. Indeed, Rogers'[3] classification of adoption decisions in complex organisations as collective, contingent, or authority-dependent (see Section 4.2) was based on early work in schools.

In Chapters 4–9, we draw extensively on the findings of educational research since several school-based studies from the 1970s and 1980s provide critical empirical or methodological insights for our own research question. Schools were the focus of the earliest research into organisational adoption of innovations.[63] The school (rather than, say, the individual teacher) became the unit of analysis, and the method of investigation moved from the individual interview to the postal questionnaire. Researchers sought descriptive demographic data from head teachers (such as the school's size, catchment mix and financial status) and relatively superficial indicators of a particular adoption decision (i.e. the fact of adoption rather than the reasons for it). Interesting correlations were quickly found, which led to a new raft of hypotheses. For example, in one landmark study in Columbia, the most powerful predictor of innovativeness in schools was found to be financial expenditure per pupil (in other words, rich suburban schools adopted innovations quickly; poor inner city schools lagged behind).[187] This type of study led to the wider research tradition exploring the determinants of organisational innovativeness (see Section 3.10, page 66).

3.2 Rural sociology

Rural sociology is the study of the social structures, networks and customs of rural communities. Just as health services research is funded predominantly by central government and directed at evaluating health technologies and improving health gain, much research in rural sociology is aimed at improving the effectiveness and cost-effectiveness of farming technologies and practices.

The classic study of the spread of an idea in this field – and probably the most widely cited diffusion of innovations study of all time – was Ryan and Gross's[188] painstaking investigation of the adoption of hybrid corn by Iowa farmers in the 1930s. Iowa is a large state in central USA,

*For example, in the historical example of GP fundholding described in Chapter 6, geographical 'pockets' where the innovation was widely adopted (e.g. Hertfordshire) contrasted with areas where almost no practices adopted (e.g. Tower Hamlets). Geographical proximity here was almost certainly a proxy for structural equivalence – the former practices were affluent, semi-rural and sited in strongholds of the political right; the latter were poor, inner city and sited in left-wing areas.

composed almost entirely of isolated corn farms, whose proprietors had few social contacts except with one another and the representatives of seed companies. Traditional corn seed gave reasonable crops and could be re-seeded every year by open pollination. A new, hardier hybrid had been developed that gave reliably higher yields and withstood drought better, but new seed (first marketed in 1928) had to be purchased every year – hence an initial buy-in to the idea was needed.

A core concept of the emerging paradigm was interpersonal communication and influence. The underpinning theoretical model was that people adopt a new idea by copying others who have already adopted it (usually, those who hold privileged social status – a group subsequently given the label 'opinion leaders'). The preferred method was the mapping of social networks (who knows whom, and who views whom as influential), for which the preferred instrument was the sociological survey. Ryan (a recent PhD graduate) and Gross (an impecunious MSc student who had sought a summer job) conducted face-to-face interviews with all Iowa corn farmers in the early 1940s, recording basic demographic information (such as age, income and years of education), social information (notably how frequently they visited the state's main town of Des Moines), and what year the farmer recalled first becoming aware of, and using, the hybrid corn. The innovation adoption curve is shown in Fig. 3.1.

Ryan and Gross's simple technique of the 'one-shot interview' elegantly demonstrated that it had taken 20 years for 99% of farmers to adopt the new seed for 100% of their crops. Some farmers – the 'innovators' and 'early adopters' – had adopted it only a year or two after first encountering it via the seed reps.[3,188] Most (the early and late majority) had taken between 4 and 9 years, usually trying it out on a small field before switching to it for the entire crop. A few had delayed the switch for over a decade, and two (out of 259) never switched at all. This observation, and the discovery that early adopters were richer, better educated, more cosmopolitan (i.e. they visited Des Moines more frequently) and had wider social networks, led to a couching of adoption decisions in terms of personality type – with 'late adopters' and 'laggards' presented in stereotypical and somewhat disparaging terms (uneducated, socially isolated and so on).

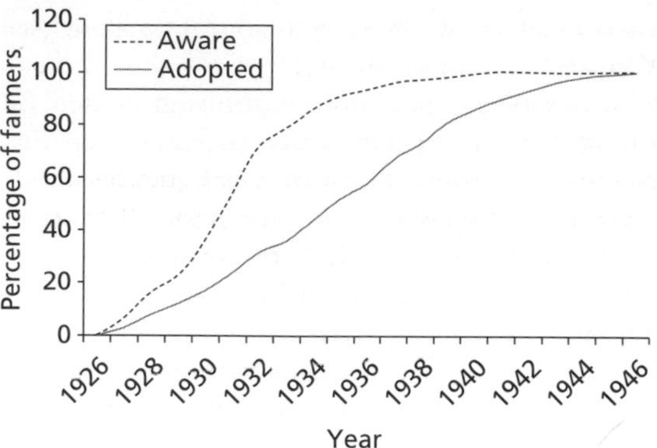

Fig. 3.1 Percentage of Iowa farmers classified as (a) aware of hybrid corn and (b) using it on all fields from 1926 to 1945 (from Ryan and Gross[188,189]).

Ryan and Gross's research, and the spate of similar studies that followed in the rural sociology tradition, occurred in a very particular historical and political context. In the USA in the 1940s and 1950s, fears of a national food shortage had made it a political priority to modernise remote farming communities and improve the nation's crop yields. Colleges of agricultural innovation were established, and were closely linked to academics who were charged with studying how to spread the innovations efficiently from the agricultural colleges to the practitioners in the field – a linkage that was termed 'agricultural extension'. Innovations, emanating from government-funded centres of excellence, were widely viewed as 'progress'.

Ryan and Gross's landmark study had a powerful influence on the methodology of subsequent diffusion research, especially within the wider discipline of sociology. The one-shot research interview, in which respondents were asked to recall decisions made months or years earlier, worked well enough for the Iowa corn study and was adopted somewhat uncritically in later studies (when recall and contextual biases might well have been more influential).

The Iowa hybrid corn had a clear advantage over the previous product and produced, as predicted, both private benefits (to the farmer) and public benefits (to the local economy). But many other agricultural innovations of the day, whose roll-out was planned along similar communication lines, did not produce the same benefits and sometimes had unanticipated consequences elsewhere in the system (e.g. 'miracle' crops that consumers found unpalatable; labour-saving devices that put farm labourers out of a job; and new technologies that farmers could not afford or did not understand[3,190]). The negative findings of the later studies helped to rock the prevailing paradigm, which was gradually revealed as being couched in a powerful meta-narrative of growth, productivity, domination of the rural environment, and 'new is better'.

Rogers, reflecting some 40 years later on the unconscious pro-innovation bias that had prevailed in his discipline, describes how political ideology and scientific priorities were subsequently revisited when agricultural overproduction, rather than food shortages, became America's key farming problem.[3] His description (page 425) of his first piece of fieldwork – a time when the meta-narrative of rural sociology had changed to one of conservation and sensitivity to natural processes – is particularly telling:

> Back in 1954, one of the Iowa farmers that I personally interviewed for my PhD dissertation research rejected all of the chemical innovations that I was then studying: weed sprays, cattle and hog feeds, chemical fertilisers, and a rodenticide. He insisted that his neighbours, who had adopted these chemicals, were killing their songbirds and the earthworms in the soil. I had selected the new farm ideas in my innovativeness scale on the advice of agricultural experts at Iowa State University; I was measuring the best recommended farming practice of that day. The organic farmer in my sample earned the lowest score on my innovativeness scale, and was categorised as a laggard.[3]

3.3 Medical sociology

At around the same time as US rural sociologists were exploring diffusion of innovations in farming, a parallel tradition was developing amongst medical sociologists, which focused on doctors' uptake of powerful new drugs (especially antibiotics) in the mid twentieth century. This early research must be interpreted in the light of changes in the innovativeness of drugs over the past half century. Keenness to prescribe the latest antibiotic in the 1950s (when common infections often killed, antibiotic resistance was unknown, few effective drugs existed and pharmaceutical marketing was relatively unsophisticated) was a very different phenomenon than it is today (when common infections are much less virulent; resistance is a major public health threat; 'new' antibiotics rarely have proven advantages over established products; and the marketing tactics of the pharmaceutical industry are, in many eyes, an international disgrace).

With this historical context in mind, the diffusion study on prescribing of tetracycline, conducted by sociologists at Columbia University in the early 1950s, was designed to identify how quickly a pioneering medical innovation spread amongst doctors. It was assumed, with some justification, that the quicker a doctor started to prescribe the drug, the better. The study, though rigorously conducted and described by Rogers[191] as 'one of the most important diffusion studies of all time', should be interpreted with caution. It was funded by a grant of $40 000 (equivalent to $1.6 million in 2005) from Pfizer, the manufacturer of tetracycline, whose goal was to determine the extent to which advertisements they had placed in medical journals had influenced doctors' decisions. Columbia's researchers, who quickly discovered the importance of personal contacts in influencing doctors' decision-making, extended the study into an exploration of the detailed social networks of potential prescribers of the drug.[5]

An initial sample of 125 doctors were interviewed in four Illinois cities, and (through what we might today call a snowball sampling method), these individuals identified a further 103 doctors whom they indicated had influenced their decision to adopt the drug. The researchers drew up a sociogram (i.e. a diagram of the doctors' social networks). They obtained independent evidence of the time of first prescribing tetracycline using local pharmacists' dispensing records. An additional key finding was a 'profile' of those doctors identified by their colleagues as influencing their decision to prescribe – the individuals whom we would now designate 'opinion leaders' but who were then classified in terms of 'high interpersonal influence'. This aspect of the study is discussed in Section 6.2 (page 118) in relation to empirical studies on opinion leadership.

The study by Coleman *et al.* had many parallel findings to the Iowa corn study published 15 years previously: the adoption curve was S-shaped; time-to-adoption depended heavily on the size and quality of the doctors' social networks; and early adopters had higher incomes and went to more out-of-town medical meetings. A fascinating claim by Coleman and his team is that they were *not* aware of the theoretical and methodological work of Ryan and Gross – in other words, they had come up with an almost identical theoretical framework, research design and instrument (and, incidentally, shown an almost identical S-shaped adoption curve) in a different field of enquiry. The common social, historical and ideological context to these landmark post-war US studies – each of which was paradigm-shifting in its separate tradition – is surely evident. The medical sociologists of the 1950s took a similarly uncritical view of 'innovation as progress' as was taken by the US rural sociologists. Just as the meta-narrative of scientific progress in rural sociology has moved in the last half century from one of domination of the land to the achievement of harmony with it, so a major meta-narrative in medicine has moved from domination of the body by artificially developed pharmaceuticals to the promotion of healthy lifestyles, the development of 'natural' remedies and the boosting of innate immunity.

The Coleman study, groundbreaking in its day, was taken up by mainstream sociology as a paradigm for studying the social networks of potential adopters, as described in Chapter 6. It also had a critical influence on the pharmaceutical industry's marketing strategies. Advertisements had been shown to create awareness but adoption itself required interpersonal contact – a scientific discovery that supported the use of pharmaceutical representatives or 'detailmen'. The pivotal influence of opinion leaders justified efforts by pharmaceutical companies to identify and influence such individuals. And the social nature of prescribing knowledge probably spawned a tradition of pharmaceutical sponsorship of social gatherings of doctors – the now-ubiquitous 'drug lunch'.

A subsequent tradition has, incidentally, emerged (led largely by the EBM movement) of anti-innovation strategies (i.e. those directed at stopping doctors adopting new, expensive products with marginal additional benefit over older, cheaper drugs) and is based on the same sociometric principles. Approaches such as academic detailing, use of 'evidence-based' opinion leaders, and social marketing of best practice have all been evaluated extensively in RCTs; some of which are discussed further in Chapter 6 (for a recent systematic review of these strategies, see Grimshaw *et al.*[11]).

The work of the early medical sociologists, as well as related work by Rogers and Kincaid[7] on spread of family planning methods in developing countries, and Becker's[52,192] landmark study of adoption of public health innovations led to more detailed work on the nature and workings of social networks (defined by Valente[4] as 'the pattern of friendship, advice, communication or support which exists among members of a social system'). Burt,[6] for example, reanalysed the data used by Coleman *et al.* using sophisticated mathematical methods, and developed many of the principles of what is now known as social network theory shown in Box 3.1.

Central to the social network model is the notion that network interconnectedness or 'embeddedness' of an individual in a social system (i.e. the number and extent of their relationships) is positively related to their innovativeness in adopting innovations.[5,194] The 'weak ties' concept is somewhat counter-intuitive, but makes sense because individuals with strong interpersonal ties (spouses, best friends, people who work in the same office) already share large amounts of information, whereas those with weak ties (past acquaintances, friends of friends) have potentially more information to exchange. Hence, the best source of new ideas is often someone one hardly knows.[19,196]

Valente's[4] 'threshold' model differs from earlier social network approaches in that it explicitly

Box 3.1 Principles of social network theory.[4,4,6,98,193–196]

(1) All behaviour is *embedded in social relationships*, hence the adoption and diffusion of innovations are driven by the social relationships among actors.
(2) *Strength of weak ties*. The links in a social network are classified primarily according to the degree to which they convey new information. Individuals who are linked by weak social ties potentially have more information to share with one another.
(3) *Structural equivalence*. Structural equivalence is the degree to which two individuals have the same relations with the same others. People with structural equivalence tend to adopt an innovation with a similar level of exposure.
(4) *Threshold models*. We each have a threshold for adopting an innovation depending on how many others have already done so. Early adopters are those whose threshold for adopting the innovation is low (they will do so when only a few people in the social system have already done so); late adopters will only adopt once most others in their social system have done so.
(5) *Opinion leadership*. An opinion leader is an individual who has unusually high influence over the behaviour of others in his or her social network, by virtue of charisma, competence, embeddedness and perceived homophily.

includes the influence of non-adopters on adopter decisions. His key contribution was to distinguish between the adopter status of any particular individual and that of an entire social system. He showed that individuals do not accurately monitor the adoption behaviour of everyone else in the system, hence when assigning adopter status there is a need to relate it to the adoption patterns shown by those in a particular individual's personal networks, rather than the overall pattern of adoption shown in the social system.*

The conceptual framework of social networks has been extensively applied to the adoption of particular health technologies,[197] but as explained in Chapters 4–9, we found only a sparse literature relating it specifically to diffusion of innovations in service delivery and organisation. A number of comparable concepts at the organisational level (such as interorganisational fads and fashions, and the notion of 'opinion leader' organisations) are discussed in Section 3.12 (page 70) and summarised in Box 3.5 (page 70). For a more detailed exposition of social network theory as it relates to the spread of innovations, see the series of papers by Valente.[4,98] For a contemporary critique of social network theory, see Van den Bulte's overview.[198]

3.4 Communication studies

The development of communication as a distinct academic discipline was closely linked to journalism and media studies. Early diffusion research in this field related to the spread of news stories such as the death of a US president or explosion of a spaceship. Because such spectacular stories spread very rapidly (95% of Americans knew of the shooting of President Kennedy within 90 min of the happening), conventional retrospective surveys were impossible. Communication scholars developed the 'firehouse research' technique, in which cadres of graduate students were trained to conduct standardised telephone interviews with large numbers of respondents within 24 h of a spectacular news event. Such research was popular in the 1960s and 1970s,[199] but waned in the 1980s when it was found that little could be added to the knowledge that the diffusion curve for news was, like other diffusion curves, S-shaped, and that early 'adopters' were better educated and had wider social networks.[200] After all, news can be said to have diffused once people have heard it (unlike other fields when the innovation requires a change in behaviour), so there was little more to research.

The subsequent development of communication science and its relation to diffusion research has been well summarised by Macdonald.[201] At its

*This, incidentally, explains another tactic of pharmaceutical sales representatives – the attempt by various means to persuade a doctor that homophilous individuals are already prescribing a particular product.

simplest, communication (which is the basic building block for all social relationships) involves a sender, a message and a recipient. The message contains information, which is to some extent encoded (in metaphors, nuances of language, pictures, symbols and so on). The recipient must decode the message and, if motivated, act on the information received. Thus, communication is about persuading as well as informing. Drawing on McGuire's seminal work,[202] Macdonald has set out the key input and output variables of communication, each of which has a number of dimensions (Box 3.2).

For example, in relation to a health education message (such as a healthy eating campaign), the input variables comprise who (from what organisation) is saying what, how and in what way, and what they intend people to do as a result. The output variables comprise whether people received the message, how they perceived it (e.g. did they find it offensive or threatening), whether the intended information got across, whether people accepted the information, whether they changed their behaviour, and whether the change was sustained.

Communication theory has early roots separate from diffusion of innovation theory, but the two became closely linked in the early 1970s when Rogers, along with co-author Shoemaker, recouched his textbook on diffusion of innovations in terms of communication theory (indeed, the title of the opus was temporarily changed to *Communication of Innovations: a cross-cultural approach*).[177] Diffusion became defined as the process by which an innovation (that is something that is perceived as new) is *communicated* by various channels over time within members of a social system. Rogers and Shoemaker recognised the crucial elements of receiving and decoding the message, being (or not being) motivated to change, and taking action. They described four key stages of adoption (awareness, persuasion, adoption and maintenance, as described in Chapter 5, page 100). As several field studies had already shown by the 1970s, mass media channels are more influential for creating awareness, whereas interpersonal channels are more influential at the persuasion stage.[177]

Box 3.2 Key variables in communication.

Input variables:
- Source of the message (credibility, likeability, power, quantity and demography)
- The message itself (appeal, style, organisation, quantity)
- Communication channel (mass media or one-to-one, spoken or written, etc.)
- Receiver (demographic characteristics; personality traits; attitudes/beliefs)
- Destination (the intended cognitive/behavioural targets; the intended outcome as either product or practice)

Output variables:
- Exposure to the message
- Perception of the information
- Encoding (the essentials of the message must be coded and stored)
- Acceptability of the message
- Behaviour change (i.e. in line with the intentions of the sender)
- Post-behavioural consolidation

3.5 Marketing and economics

Marketing is much more than the attempt to persuade a potential consumer to purchase a product or service (which for the purposes of diffusion research might be termed the innovation). It is the development and utilisation of a sophisticated infrastructure for matching the basic economic functions of production and consumption, including the identification of consumer requirement, translation of this into produces and services, announcement of availability, transport to convenient locations, display at retail outlets and after-sales care, and the overall coordination and seamless alignment of these activities with one another.

Early marketing research (before 1930) focused on the production and distribution of particular goods (i.e. the product was deemed to have been 'marketed' when it was seen to be widely distributed in a range of retail outlets). In the 1930s, marketing research increasingly emphasised efforts (such as advertising) aimed at increasing sales; consumer orientation (finding out what consumers wanted and tailoring the product of service to fit that – hence 'market research'); and, most recently, social orientation (the evaluation of the social and environmental impact of commercial activities and unrestrained consumer demand – hence increasing emphasis on reducing pollution during production, recycling packaging and so on).[203]

Marketing, particularly sales-oriented marketing, is closely linked with economic modelling. Only a tiny fraction of product innovations are a commercial success. In the 1960s, there was considerable interest amongst business analysts for a presentation of diffusion theory in terms of a mathematical equation that would predict whether and to what extent a particular innovation would 'catch on'. Such a model – now known as the Bass Forecasting Model – was provided by Professor Frank Bass of Purdue University. The model is described in detail elsewhere;[3,8] its main principles are given in Box 3.3.

The Bass Forecasting Model predicts the rate and extent of subsequent adoption of a product from its measured market potential, m, its coefficient of mass media influence, p, and its coefficient of interpersonal influence, q. This model depends on a number of key assumptions, for example, that the market potential of the innovation remains constant over time; that the nature of the innovation does not change with time; and that there are no restrictions on supply.

Provided these assumptions hold, the model appears robust for predicting the success of commercial product launches, and has also been used to predict the spread of educational ideas and agricultural innovations.[3] Forecasting models have not been widely used in health care diffusion research. There may be unpublished literature in the pharmaceutical sector, but an informal approach to senior colleagues in this industry drew no specific examples and a comment from one analyst that such models are likely to have little utility in highly regulated markets.

The concept of adopter categories (innovator, early adopter and so on) is used in marketing to target different strategies to different types of individual. Section 5.1, page 100, presents the characteristics and the standard recommended approaches in marketing literature (although it must be emphasised that we have found little empirical evidence in the primary studies for this review to support these recommendations).

Marketing theory has some important implications for the diffusion of innovations in health services. See, for example, the advice provided by the EUR-ASSESS subgroup on health technology

Box 3.3 Principles of the Bass Forecasting Model.

(1) Adoption of a new product depends crucially on its *market potential*, which can be estimated by measuring sales in the first few time periods of diffusion.
(2) Potential adopters of the product are influenced by two key communication channels: mass media and interpersonal (word of mouth).
(3) *Mass media* are relatively more influential in the early stages of the adoption curve, but have a small, continuing influence throughout.*
(4) *Interpersonal channels* expand exponentially initially (one person tells two people, who each tell two people and so on), then begin to decline as the channels become saturated.†
(5) The *rate of adoption* during the first half of the diffusion process is symmetrical with the rate during the second half (which means, of course, that much can be predicted from the careful study of the early stages).

*Bass calculated the average coefficient of mass media influence in 15 different diffusion studies to be 0.03. Note, however, that this coefficient relates to innovations with mainly private consequences. According to Wejnert's[41] systematic review of the wider literature, mass media influence becomes vastly more important when the 'innovation' is a well-defined and broadly popular societal issue – e.g. the environmental movement. It was beyond the scope of our own review to address such literature, but we should note that the numerical coefficients reproduced here are highly contextual and should not be cited indiscriminately.

†The average coefficient of interpersonal influence in Bass's studies was 0.39, confirming the qualitative impressions of sociologists that interpersonal channels were far more influential overall for the innovations studied.

assessment (HTA) programmes on how to disseminate HTA reports.[89] However, it should be noted that most research in marketing has been undertaken or commissioned by the manufacturers of particular products who seek to influence the behaviour of others – in other words, marketing research is sponsored by marketeers. Market researchers might conduct rigorous focus groups to determine the preferred colour and flavour of fish fingers, but the intended consumer might be more interested, for example, in finding how to resist the impact of convenience food advertising, or how to evaluate the nutritional quality of such products. As Rogers[3] has observed (page 86):

> The source bias in marketing diffusion studies may lead to highly applied research that, although methodologically sophisticated, deals with trivial diffusion problems in a theoretical sense.

The marketing research tradition developed separately from, but had a powerful influence on, the tradition of social marketing in health promotion, which is discussed in Section 3.7.

3.6 Limitations of early diffusion research

Conventional diffusion research (as set out, for example, in Sections 3.3 and 3.4) has a number of limitations as an explanatory framework for the diffusion, spread and sustainability of innovations in organisations – especially those concerned with the delivery of health services. In particular, the following problems should be borne in mind:

Confusion between descriptive, explanatory and intervention models

The S-shaped diffusion curve and the adopter categories based on it were originally developed as a descriptive model; this model has no direct explanatory power and it cannot predict outcomes (such as who will adopt a particular innovation). Analysis of the adoption curve for any given innovation in a given population of adopters in a particular context can suggest hypotheses about the reasons for adoption (or non-adoption or rejection), which might then be tested empirically. But the curve does not itself provide an explanation of either *how* or *why* people adopt particular innovations at particular rates, nor, of course, does it predict whether efforts to influence adoption will meet with success. In our review, we encountered a number of superficial overview articles that extrapolated unjustifiably from adoption curves.

The historical and sociocultural context of early diffusion research

As described above, diffusion of innovations theory was developed and used in several overlapping and converging research traditions in the second half of the twentieth century. It is probably no accident that the seminal work in several different traditions was done in the USA at a time of exceptionally high economic growth and (arguably) an ideological climate that celebrated innovation and change for its own sake. Publications like *The Limits to Growth*[204] began to appear in the 1970s, and there are strong counter-traditions that call for a careful assessment of the value of innovation or that promote stability rather than innovation as a social ideal. Furthermore, as discussed in Section 3.7, developing countries had important differences in social structure that called into question some of the assumptions implicit in the classical diffusion paradigm – e.g. about the value of innovations and the nature of social influence.

Pro-innovation ('measuring the measurable') bias

The early research traditions described above had a pro-innovation bias, since it is easier to study some phenomena than others. For example, we know more about

- innovations that have spread successfully than those that have not;
- innovations that have spread rapidly than those that have spread more slowly;
- innovations that spread from the centre compared with those that arise and spread peripherally;

- adoption than non-adoption or rejection;
- continued use than discontinuation; and
- the fact of adoption than the reasons for it.

Pro-innovation bias is a particular problem with retrospective research designs, which take as their starting point an established innovation and look backwards to determine its pattern of uptake. In the remaining sections of this chapter, we describe some traditions that have attempted to move beyond this pro-innovation perspective, and in Section 11.3 (page 225) we suggest some additional ways of remedying the bias in future research.

Individual blame bias

The conceptual framework implicit in many diffusion research studies places all individuals in particular descriptor categories ('early adopters', 'laggards' and so on). In Chapter 1, we emphasised that the categories were *mathematically* not psychologically defined by the original exponents of the theory. Nevertheless, the terms cannot be separated from their common linguistic meaning – and hence are implicitly value-laden. Because the S-shaped diffusion curve focuses on individual adoption and labels people according to where they are placed on the curve, there is an implication not only that individuals are to 'blame' for slow adoption, but that only individuals are amenable to change. Individuals are arguably easier (and cheaper) to study, so a 'measuring the measurable' bias enhances individual blame bias. As we discuss in detail in the later sections of this chapter and elsewhere in this book, there are many alternative approaches that focus less on the individual and more on system variables.

Notion of the innovation as fixed

With the wisdom of hindsight, the types of innovation studied in the early research were somewhat fixed and static. You cannot do much with a packet of hybrid corn seeds except plant them. Research in such fields as technology transfer,[205] which although undertaken at a similar time took longer to influence other traditions, showed that innovations are very often modified as they are disseminated, and that the process of modification merits study in its own right. On page 84, we discuss the critical importance of reinvention, an attribute of innovations that Rogers admits to being blind to in the early years of his research.

Linear relationship bias

In most of the early diffusion studies, different variables were treated as independent, and there was little consideration of how these interacted with one another. Indeed, it could be argued that the most famous diffusion study was conducted in the sociological equivalent of laboratory conditions, since the intended adopters (Iowa corn farmers in the 1940s) were perhaps uniquely autonomous, socially homogeneous and geographically isolated, and the innovation (hybrid corn) was uniquely advantageous, compatible, simple, trialable and observable. As Chapters 4 to 10 argue, few if any innovations in health service delivery and organisation fulfil all these criteria. In Section 11.1 (page 219) we discuss in more detail our finding that most of the empirical literature we uncovered in this review made unjustified causal inferences between hypothecated determinants of innovativeness and measured outcomes.

Context-transferability bias

It might be shown in a rigorous and systematic research study that a particular innovation is readily adopted (and that it is effective, efficient, acceptable, cost-effective and so on). But this in itself does not mean that an innovation that is adopted and works well at site A will be adopted equally readily and work equally well at site B, nor that an innovation delivered by team X will work well when delivered by team Y. The early diffusion traditions reviewed above, and to some extent those that have developed more recently, made very little concession to the influence of context. A useful framework for considering the transferability of innovations is the realistic evaluation matrix developed by Pawson and Tilley[120] (and modified by Gomm[116]) and adapted for this review in Box A.7 (page 240). In Section 11.3 (page 225) we consider further potential for a realist approach in future research into the context-transferability of innovations.

Lack of attention to consequences

Innovations, especially complex ones, have both intended and unintended consequences. As described above, the US rural sociologists found a negative knock-on impact of wonder crops developed in centres of agricultural excellence.[190] To this day, remarkably few studies have systematically documented the downstream human, financial and organisational consequences of so-called 'good ideas' – an omission that we highlight in Chapters 4–9.

The convergence of different research traditions in diffusion research has thus been, according to Rogers,[3] a mixed blessing. He observes (page 39) that

> ... diffusion studies now display a kind of bland sameness, as they pursue a small number of research issues with rather stereotyped approaches. ... Perhaps the old days of separate and varied research approaches were a richer intellectual activity than the present well-informed sameness.

To summarise the overview of research traditions covered so far in this chapter, the historical roots of diffusion of innovations theory provide important insights into how the S-shaped adoption curve has been discovered and explored in different research traditions. It is important, however, to be aware that the ubiquitously cited 'landmark' studies of diffusion of innovations,[5,182,188] although outstanding in their own context, were the product of particular social and intellectual trends. Because they focused exclusively on individuals and relatively fixed and simple innovations, their findings have limited transferability to the spread of organisational innovations in twenty-first century health service. Hence, while they set the stage for this review, they only inform our own conclusions to a limited extent.

Whereas the research traditions described above are either 'variations on the theme' of classical diffusion theory or the explanatory framework it offers for individual adoption, those that follow have drawn on additional conceptual frameworks either as well as or instead of diffusion theory as set out in Section 1.1. To a greater or lesser extent, the traditions described in the rest of this chapter have addressed dissemination, implementation and reinvention as well as passive diffusion.

3.7 Development studies

There is a vast literature on diffusion of innovation in development studies, which is beyond the scope of our study. The most relevant aspects of this literature relate to development initiatives around health-related activities, such as the Rogers and Kincaid[7] study and Rogers' overview[206] on dissemination of family planning practices in third world countries. Initial research into diffusion of innovations in developing countries occurred a decade or two later than parallel traditions in the West, but followed similar research methods and took on similar assumptions (e.g. the pattern of rural sociology research as shown in Fig. 2.2, page 43). The S-shaped adoption curve was shown to describe, for example, the diffusion of contraceptive methods in peasant villages in Latin America[7,206] even though the communities themselves were very different in terms of financial resources, access to mass media, educational background and so on.*

From the 1970s, however, it was increasingly recognised that the methods and theoretical models exported to developing countries had, in the words of Rogers[3] (page 125) 'a strong stamp of made in America' about them. In the 1976 version of his book, he had reflected on four key issues relevant to developing nations when the theory was being introduced there: a rapid degree of economic growth, equivalent to the Industrial Revolution that had occurred in the West; the introduction of multiple, labour-saving technologies, mostly from the West; centralised planning by governments and their appointed agencies, intended to speed up the process of economic and technological growth; and

*On one level, this is hardly surprising, since the S-shaped diffusion curve is essentially a mathematical phenomenon and makes no claims to explanatory power.

the root causes of underdevelopment, which were attributed to factors (such as adverse physical environment, political corruption and so on) intrinsic to the developing country.

These issues (and this frame of reference) allowed classical diffusion theory to be 'grafted on' to the problems of third world countries: underdevelopment was effectively couched in terms of an 'innovation gap', and the well-intentioned West was offering to fill that gap by going through the now-familiar steps of marketing the benefits of each innovation, identifying channels of communication, harnessing the influence of opinion leaders and so on.[9]

A more radical discourse on development,* which was to make diffusion of innovations a very different field of enquiry in the developing world, began in the early 1970s. It became recognised that the social structure of underdeveloped countries was often fundamentally different – with power, money, education and information concentrated in the hands of a small elite. 'Early wins' for the diffusion of innovations could often be achieved by dealing exclusively with these privileged few (indeed, because windfall profits tend to accrue to early adopters, diffusion of innovations has a tendency to benefit these elite few at the expense of others and thereby *increase* socioeconomic inequalities). But more widespread diffusion was inextricably linked with the need to recognise and address these pervasive social inequalities.

Thus, in the second half of the twentieth century, development gradually ceased to be defined as a deficiency that could be made good by the transfer of the right technologies and ways of working, and came to be defined as – necessarily – a participatory process of social change intended to bring about both social and material advancement (including greater equality, freedom and other valued qualities) for most or all of the population.[9] The crucial *mechanism* of development (see Rogers,[3] page 127) was reframed as fundamentally to do with empowerment – 'the people gaining control of their environment'.

It became increasingly unacceptable to view the introduction of new technologies in a development context as simply 'adoption of innovations' in an ideologically neutral context, and new insights into the consequences of innovation diffusion were quickly sought and gained as a more radical conceptual lens drove research into new domains. In a review of the impact of technological innovations in the third world, for example, Brown[205] describes how the assumed benefits of new technologies often failed to accrue in practice, and instead led to an increase in regional inequalities and elitist entrenchment. Rogers[3] gives a wealth of examples, such as:

- The introduction of snowmobiles not only wrecked the economy in a rural Lapland community but also (through their polluting impact) drove reindeer stocks to near extinction (page 408).
- So-called labour-saving technologies offered to technologically primitive communities often increased rather than decreased the subordination of women to men (page 421).
- The introduction of wet rice cultivation in Madagascar (described in a detailed historical anthropological study) had not only a direct and immediate effect on people's daily lives (e.g. it triggered the change from nomadic to settled existence), but also a knock-on effect on first-generation (e.g. breakdown in kinship clans), second-generation (e.g. new social bonds formed on the basis of economic interests) and third-generation (e.g. changes in patterns of warfare; slaves became important economically) communities (page 416).

Bourdenave (cited in Rogers, page 127[3]) has set out a contemporary agenda for diffusion research in developing countries that takes account of the wider needs of the adopting system (Box 3.4).

Interestingly, field studies in developing countries that succeeded in terms of the Bourdenave criteria (i.e. successful introduction of an innovation that benefited local people and narrowed socio-economic gaps) attributed their success to four factors:

*This radical perspective, whilst in some ways of marginal relevance to our own research question, may have important parallels when considering how to spread 'innovations' to parts of the health service that some might classify as 'underdeveloped' – e.g. primary care in under-resourced inner city areas.

Box 3.4 Criteria for a diffusion research agenda in the developing world.

(1) *Selection of the innovation.* What criteria guide the choice of innovations that are to be diffused? (e.g. is the desire to spread the innovation driven by public welfare, producing goods for export, keeping prices low for locals or increasing profit for industrialists?)
(2) *Social structure.* What influence does society's social structure have on an individual's desire (and capacity) to innovate?
(3) *Stage of development.* Are the technological innovations appropriate and adequate for the stage of socio-economic development of the nation or region?
(4) *Consequences.* What are the likely consequences of the innovation (e.g. in terms of unemployment, migration to already-overcrowded urban areas, subjugation of vulnerable groups, and redistribution of income)? Will the innovation widen or narrow socio-economic gaps?

(1) meticulous preliminary research into the needs of the user system, including the use to which the proposed innovation would actually be put, and the meaning that it is likely to have for them;
(2) nesting the specific innovation within a wider programme of community development and capacity building;
(3) strategies designed specifically with an equalities agenda in mind (notably the use of mass media to create awareness amongst the less well connected in terms of social networks); and
(4) involvement of members of the user system in the planning and implementation of dissemination strategies.[207,208]

There are direct parallels here with the linkage activities discussed in Chapter 9 (page 175) in relation to health services development.

3.8 Health promotion

'Diffusion' research has been popular in health promotion since the 1970s, and has covered a diverse range of public health, health education and 'healthy lifestyles' initiatives.* Until relatively recently, this research tradition rested centrally (although not exclusively) on the concept of social marketing – i.e. the application of basic communication and marketing principles (see above) to persuade individuals to change their behaviour towards healthier lifestyles and choices.[210] Lefebvre[211] has defined social marketing as

> ... an orientation to health promotion in which programmes are developed to satisfy consumers' needs, strategized to reach the audience(s) in need of the programme, and managed to meet organisational objectives.

The social marketing approach (described in detail elsewhere[3,210,211]) has been widely used in campaigns relating to contraception, smoking, breast-feeding, cot death, sexual health, drug abuse, safer driving and so on.† The most crucial element of a successful social marketing is probably client orientation – i.e. understanding the needs, preferences, perspective and concerns of the intended user.

Social marketing is based on exchange theory – i.e. the notion of *exchanging* one behaviour or attitude for another. Whilst there may be clear short- and long-term benefits in this exchange (e.g. in giving up smoking, money saved on cigarettes, fresher breath, longer life expectancy), there is also an immediate cost to the participant (expense of cognitive and physical effort, disapproval of peers, withdrawal symptoms), which must be recognised. Exchange theory as applied to health promotion is about creating awareness among the audience that they have a problem and then offering a solution.‡

Another key concept is *market segmentation.* Even if the goal is to change the attitudes and

*In an overview, Oldenberg *et al.*[209] lamented that only 1% of health promotion research concerns diffusion and 5% concerns implementation of programmes, but these proportions are probably higher than in many comparable fields.

†For a good worked example of social marketing in health promotion, see Farquhar *et al.*[212]

‡See Lefebvre[211] (page 222) for an insightful discussion of the limitations of uncritical, 'politically correct', bottom-up approaches to social marketing, and also a discussion on how professional and organisational politics can weaken a well-intentioned social marketing campaign.

behaviour of society at large, the marketing task must be tailored differently to different segments of society. Segmentation is often done in relation to individual characteristics, especially demographic (age, gender, ethnicity, socio-economic status, etc.), behavioural (current smoking status, exercise level), psychological (readiness to change) and so on. But if the goal is organisational change (e.g. introduction of anti-smoking policies), segmentation might be by sector (educational, industrial, governmental, etc.), location (urban, rural), type (manufacturing, service, agricultural), size, current policy or practice, organisational variables (innovativeness, leadership style, etc.) and so on.

The goal of segmentation, of course, is to offer a different marketing package to each segment in order to maximise success. There should be homogeneity within segments and heterogeneity between segments, and each segment should be large enough to justify a separate allocation of resources and energy. Segmentation analysis will include initial assessment of market characteristics and needs of different segments; market analyses to determine positioning strategies; pilot tests of message/product/service acceptability and effectiveness and so on. In general, qualitative methods such as in-depth interviews and focus groups are particularly important at this stage to gain detailed understanding of the segment and its responses.

Marketing mix is the combination of message content (particularly, how it is couched as a benefit and the specific reasons why this matters), action (precisely what is the audience being asked to do); persuasion strategies (empathy, concern arousal, believability, etc.), message design (idea, language, style, symbolism, distinctiveness, cultural appropriateness, situation and character identification, etc.), and memorability (idea reinforcement, minimising distractions, repetition).

Cost is often a major barrier to lifestyle changes. Health promotion campaigns often centre round efforts to distort the financial market for products (condoms, exercise programmes, nicotine patches) and services (counselling, vaccination, training) through subsidies – at least until a critical proportion of the target audience has adopted them. In marketing terms, 'cost' also includes geographical distance ('How far do I have to travel to get free condoms?'); social costs ('What will my partner think if I use a condom?'); behavioural costs ('Does this mean I will have less casual sex?'); psychological costs ('What if it kills my sex drive?') and so on.[57]

The development of appropriate channels for disseminating a social marketing message requires an analysis of different media and their ability to transmit complex messages, the reach of particular target groups, the requirement for intermediaries, and overall cost. As will be shown in Chapter 6, the selection of appropriate agents for interpersonal communication – i.e. those with a high degree of common ground (homophily) with the individuals whose behaviour is being targeted – is a key success factor. The possibility of saturation (when people have heard a message so much that they 'turn off') is also important, as is the selection of a communication channel that the social marketer can control – even if it means eschewing sponsored channels in favour of paid advertising or agents.

The central importance of process tracking has parallels with the well-established finding that audit and feedback are fundamental to good management practice more generally (see, for example, Sections 3.13 and 3.14). Monitoring systems for social marketing campaigns must be tailored to individual programmes, but generic templates are available (see, for example, Lefebvre, page 237[211]). Particular attention must be given to quality control – for example, that the message does not become distorted or diluted as different teams attempt to deliver it in different contexts.

The theoretical development of health promotion as a field of study in many ways closely parallels that of marketing (Section 3.5, page 56) and EBM (Section 3.9, page 64): there was an early focus on establishing the knowledge base and developing robust interventions based on high-quality evidence (in this case, about what behaviours and lifestyles led to health gain). This was followed, as described above, by a focus on how to influence individuals with a view to behaviour change – initially somewhat naively through the provision of information about what was good for people, and later using increasingly sophisticated social marketing methods to target different influence strategies.

More recently, as with development studies (see Section 3.7), there has been a much greater focus on community development (defined as 'a process that seeks to facilitate community self determination and build community capacity to confront problems'[213]) and efforts to address the social causes of health inequalities and 'ecological' factors such as the obesogenic environment in developed countries. Increasingly, health promotion programmes now overlap with more broad-based community development and regeneration programmes.[214]

Two good examples of this 'paradigm shift' are the change in name and mission of the UK Health Education Authority to the Health Development Agency in 1999 and the Health Action Zones initiatives in inner cities, funded and implemented jointly by local public-sector health and social care organisations. Table 3.1 shows some of the key shifts in emphasis reflected in these initiatives.

3.9 Evidence-based medicine and guideline implementation

EBM – the attempt to get health professionals consistently to base their decisions on the results of scientific research studies – has its roots in rationalist science, and particularly epidemiology (the study of diseases in populations). The mathematical basis for the S-shaped diffusion of innovations curve was set out in Section 1.1 (page 20) and illustrated in Fig. 1.1 (page 21). When a bacterium divides, or when one person with influenza coughs on two others, a doubling phenomenon begins and continues until the curve levels off at maximum saturation.

Interestingly, epidemiologists sometimes use the language of contagion to talk about the spread of ideas as well as the spread of disease. They talk, for example, of 'susceptibility' of individuals to a new idea, the corresponding 'contagiousness' of that idea. It was hardly surprising, then, that epidemiologists have continued to use the language of contagion when analysing the diffusion of non-infectious health problems such as smoking and illicit drug use. We have not covered this literature in detail here but recommend a thorough review by Ferrence.[179] The term 'viral marketing' has even been coined to describe the powerful influence of social movements on individual adoption decisions. Such metaphors implicitly play down the notion of individual agency (after all, you cannot *decide* whether you catch a cold!) and prompt a mental model of adoption 'just happening' once contact has been made.

Table 3.1 Shifts in emphasis in health promotion (adapted from Riley[215]).

Characteristic	*Traditional health education model*	*Health development model*
Unit of analysis	Individuals	Populations or defined target groups
Main focus of change	Risk factors and individual lifestyle or behaviour choices	Patterns of health-related behaviours in particular vulnerable groups
Dominant public health strategies	Health education, screening, mass protection (e.g. vaccination)	Range of 'joined up' educational, environmental and policy initiatives linked to a developmental and community empowerment agenda
Responsibility for public health	Public health agencies	Multiple sectors and agencies including involvement of user and voluntary groups
Role of the professional	Educator and teacher	Facilitator and partner
Preferred infrastructure	Hierarchies and disciplinary divisions	Semi-autonomous, inter-agency task groups

It is hardly surprising, then, that research on the spread of EBM was predicated on a highly rationalist conceptual model that saw adoption of the idea (in this case, new scientific knowledge about drug treatments or surgical procedures) as the final stage in a simple linear algorithm (research → published evidence → change in doctors' behaviour). The problem of 'getting evidence into practice' was initially couched in terms of an innovation gap (lack of high-quality research evidence). Research activity focused on producing the evidence (e.g. the UK's extensive HTA Programme, which began in the early 1990s – see http://www.hta.nhsweb.nhs.uk/) and on developing methods and systems for packaging and distributing the results of such programmes to fill the evidence gap and make it available in the clinic and at the bedside.

A theoretical paper by Haines and Jones (cited by 149 subsequent papers in the EBM tradition) illustrates how the link between *provision* of best evidence and the *making* of an evidence-based decision was at one stage considered unproblematic by leading medical scientists,[216] although both authors subsequently moved on from this position. Objective and context-neutral evidence was seen to 'drive' the evidence-into-practice cycle by a mechanism described by Williams and Gibson (cited in Dawson[217]) as 'like water flowing through a pipe'.

As the EBM tradition developed, the conceptual model shifted slightly and the problem of getting evidence into practice changed from being framed as an 'innovation gap' (lack of evidence on what works) and became a 'behaviour gap' (doctors' failure to seek out or use this evidence). Research activity focused on finding ways to fill the assumed knowledge gap (via mass media[218] or formal education[219–221]) and the motivation gap (e.g. using the social influence of opinion leaders[54]), and on providing a variety of behavioural incentives,[11] with the ultimate goal of changing clinician behaviour in line with the evidence.[150] As the systematic reviews referenced above show, although the empirical research drew variously on a host of theories of communication, influence and behaviour change, almost all were designed as RCTs, for which the model study to set the paradigm was Sibley *et al.*'s[222] RCT of educational interventions for doctors published in 1982 and cited by 150 subsequent papers. Many of these RCTs (including the early work done by this pioneering team) had surprisingly low success at prompting doctors to implement the innovations supported by the evidence.

An overview by Grol[223] summarises the reasons why intervention studies to promote implementation of 'evidence-based' innovations were so ineffectual. Many 'evidence-based' guidelines were ambiguous or confusing; the guideline usually only covered part of the sequence of decisions and actions in a clinical consultation; they were often difficult to apply to individual patients' unique problems; they generally required changes in the wider health care system; and their implementation was rarely cost-neutral. In other words, the mental model on which the paradigm was built (research → evidence → implementation) was critically flawed and needed more than just reframing: there simply is *no causal link* between the supply of research evidence and the implementation of evidence in clinical decision-making.

Another important programme of work which might be deemed paradigm-shifting in EBM, described in more detail in Chapters 5–9, was undertaken by Fitzgerald, Ferlie and colleagues, who challenged the concept of interventions as dichotomous variables (i.e. the putative mechanism for promoting the spread of an innovation was classed as 'present' or 'absent'). Rather, these researchers rightly claimed, these are complex, multifaceted issues to be explored, understood, contextualised and richly described.[12,32] However, Ferlie *et al.* were not themselves epidemiologists (and few of them were clinicians). Arguably, because of this lack of homophily with the mainstream EBM community, their work has far less impact in the EBM tradition than it deserves.

Methodologically and instrumentally, the standard approach of the EBM movement to diffusion of innovations research is something of a curiosity. Epidemiologists, trained to undertake controlled experiments of disease treatments on populations of patients, had transferred this conceptual model and research methodology wholesale to the new problem of spreading innovations: their new 'population' was the doctors whose behaviour needed to change; their 'experimental intervention' was some sort of incentive or educational package to prompt the following of a guideline; and their anticipated 'outcome' was adoption of the guideline or other behavioural protocol deemed by the researchers as desirable.

It is one of the hallmarks of traditional epidemiology that RCTs are considered 'best evidence' for evaluating interventions. But few scientists from other traditions would support the notion that RCTs are the most appropriate design for exploring the practicalities of implementing innovations (including those concerned with clinical decision-making).[115,118,224,225] The argument might be framed thus: whilst the RCT simulates 'laboratory' conditions and minimises the effect of bias, making the outcomes of a particular experimental study highly *reliable*, such conditions often exclude the very things that influence implementation in the real world, producing little or no data on complex processes or contextual variables and thereby reducing the *validity* of findings.

This deep methodological tension is summed up by two opposing 'mission statements'. The first, from a wide-ranging systematic review on the dissemination and implementation of health technology reports undertaken by members of the Cochrane Collaboration, which was based on a strict hierarchy of evidence (with RCTs explicitly privileged as 'best evidence'), states: 'Experimental studies are the most reliable designs for evaluating the effectiveness of dissemination and implementation strategies'.[89] This reflects mainstream EBM thinking of the mid-1990s. The second statement, from a senior policy researcher in the complex field of community-based mental health, and a clear dissenter from the EBM tradition, states: 'The RCT model is unable to control for the effect of social complexity and the interaction between social complexity and dynamic system change'.[224]

If we look for the underlying metaphor for change in the meta-narrative of diffusion of innovations in EBM in the 1990s, it is surely the experimental scientist interjecting a clever intervention, and then standing back to measure the impact of his or her work. As Fig. 2.3 (page 44) shows, the rationalist model linking evidence to implementation in EBM and guidelines research has probably had its day.[226] As described in the sections that follow, the research agenda on implementing best practice has begun to move into other traditions with quite different key concepts, mental models and overarching storylines, and led by scholars who are not generally from an epidemiological background.

3.10 Structural determinants of organisational innovativeness

As described in Section 3.6 (page 58), early diffusion studies focused almost exclusively on the individual adoption decision in relation to a well-defined and easily measurable innovation. This focus was partly because individual adoption is an important and elementary aspect of all diffusion research, and partly because the early studies focused on primitive communities (anthropology), independent farmers or medical practitioners (sociology), or the public as individuals (communication and marketing). It was some time before organisational theorists began to draw attention to the possible effect of organisational variables and factors on diffusion processes.

In a historical overview of diffusion research, Pettigrew *et al.*[78] suggest that a major problem with the rational, linear diffusion models that were popular with sociologists in the 1960s[5,176] is the difficulty of distinguishing adopters of innovations from non-adopters in terms of key characteristics, and of explaining different rates of diffusion in different groups or markets. Previous reviewers have noted that not one of the 52 major propositions that formed Rogers' research conclusions in his original 1962 review[176] and only 17% of studies reported in his 1983 revision[178] referred to a complex organisation as the innovation adopter or to organisational features as independent variables affecting the process.[63,125] As one organisational theorist[63] expressed:

> Research on the diffusion of innovation and organisational change had too often focussed on the wrong cluster of variables. In particular, the orientation toward the early phases of

> the innovation cycle, the concentration on small-scale technical innovations, and the individualistic biases has hindered our understanding of major organisational innovation.

In later editions of his book, Rogers[3] acknowledged these criticisms by including a chapter on innovation in organisations and highlighting that 'teachers are school employees and that most doctors work in hospitals or in a group practice' (page 376) as opposed to acting simply as individuals. However, the organisation and management literature includes a number of important subtraditions that add to (and in some cases challenge) the perspective offered by Rogers. Their approximate historical evolution is summarised in Fig. 3.2, but they should not be thought of as leading directly and sequentially into one another.

The search for the characteristics of organisations that make them innovative - i.e. for the determinants of an organisation's propensity to generate and adopt new ideas – was an early, popular theme in mainstream organisation and management research. As Section 3.2 described briefly, this tradition began in schools[63] (and, somewhat later in hospitals[59]) in the USA, and involved the distribution of postal questionnaires to large numbers of organisations to determine the characteristics of the more- and less-innovative ones. By the early 1990s, as summarised by Rogers[3] (see page 380), it had been established that organisational innovativeness was associated with characteristics of its leader (positive attitude towards change) as well as with structural features of the organisation (large size, presence of complex knowledge and expertise, decentralised power and control, informal rules and procedures, well-developed interpersonal networks, slack resources and cosmopolitanism) and the exchange of information across interorganisational boundaries (a characteristic known as 'system openness'). The empirical basis of these findings is discussed in detail in Chapter 7 (page 134).

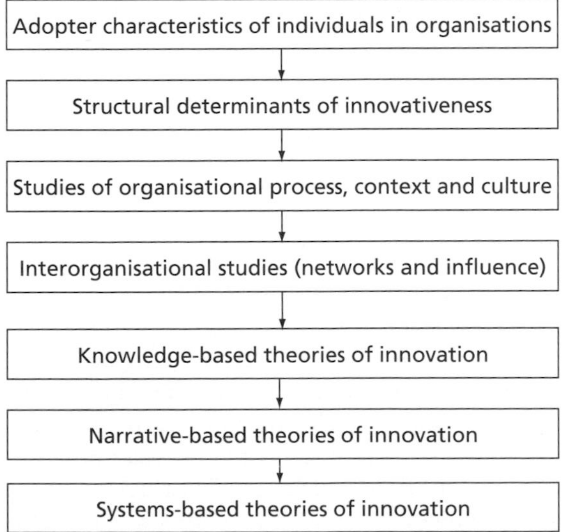

Fig. 3.2 Evolution of research subtraditions on innovation in the organisation and management literature.

Until the 1970s, researchers simply transferred to the study of organisations the models and methods that had been developed earlier for individuals. The early research that attempted to characterise organisational innovativeness had conceptual limitations comparable to earlier sociological research that had tried to classify individuals according to their 'adopter characteristics': it was predicated on the notion that a certain 'type' of organisation behaves in a certain way. As such, it was inherently both simplistic and deterministic, especially given the main empirical instrument – the self-completed questionnaire comprising entirely of closed questions. Researchers typically considered innovativeness as a general organisational 'trait' rather than in relation to specific innovations or types of innovation, and they concentrated attention on the 'event' of adoption by a key individual within the organisation. This approach left many questions unanswered about what exactly 'adoption' meant at the organisational level, and on the complex post-adoption processes and consequences within the firm.

The key studies in this tradition have been well summarised by Damanpour in three meta-analyses described in detail in Section 7.2 (page 135). Additional studies published since Damanpour's work, and focusing specifically on service-sector innovations, are summarised in Section 7.3 (page 140). All these studies considered the organisation as a whole as the unit of analysis, and consequently revealed little about the *process* of innovation within the organisation or about the complexity of the interaction between different structural factors. For example, a particular variable may have been positively or negatively related to innovation during the initiation phases of the innovation period but have the opposite effect during the implementation phases. So, for example, whilst low centralisation, high complexity and an informal rule structure may facilitate initiation in the innovation process, these same characteristics may make it difficult for an organisation to *implement* an innovation.[227,228] But early researchers in this tradition were constrained by their chosen methods of enquiry and analysis and were unable to analyse these complexities.

3.11 Studies of organisational process, context and culture

Organisational process

By the mid-1970s, the key focus of research in organisational studies had largely moved from determining the variables related to more-innovative and less-innovative organisations and to tracing the *process* of innovation – and particularly the process of developing, adopting and implementing ideas – in single organisations over time.[3] In a landmark study of the innovation process in US and French hospitals (described in more detail in Chapter 7), Kervasdoue and Kimberly[229] examined the extent to which variability in rates of adoption of innovations in medical technology could be accounted for by variations in their structure. They concluded that it is necessary to go beyond the structuralist paradigm and ask questions about socio-political, historical and cultural influences in and around organisations.

By the mid-1970s, it was established (to the surprise of many researchers) that the characteristics of individuals within a given organisation did not fully explain the innovative behaviour of people in an organisational context. A methodologically seminal research was Walton's[230] detailed work in the private sector, which used qualitative methods to highlight the social and organisational dimensions to diffusion. Walton tracked the diffusion of particular innovations over time in a dozen companies and found an extraordinarily high failure rate. Whilst pilot projects were successful in their own area, they generally failed to spread because of wider organisational resistance. His work emphasised the important role played by choice and social process within the firm, especially around the rate of diffusion of an innovation. Walton's later work emphasised the role of institutions in the innovation process, especially in their ability to shape learning mechanisms (see Section 7.8, page 154) and to create cohesion or fragmentation among a variety of stakeholders.

The principles of process-based research (and what distinguished this tradition from the studies of structural determinants that preceded it) are:

(1) it focuses on organisational events in their natural settings;

(2) it explores these phenomena at both vertical and horizontal levels;

(3) it examines their interconnections over time; and

(4) it develops a systematic description of the properties and patterned relationships of the process, which is critical to theory development.

The organisational process is conceptualised as an interlocking cycle of social actions by individuals, situated within an organisational context, and unfolding dynamically over time. Both the organisational process and its context are seen as socially constructed, with specific meanings attached to the involved organisational actors. The goal of process-based research is to enable the researcher to 'get inside the research situation' " and to systematically develop theories (which might subsequently be tested in formal experiments). Unsurprisingly, then, process-based research uses predominantly qualitative methods.

Thus, from the 1970s onwards, and using what were then considered radical new methods, important insights were gained into the nature of the whole innovation process. One very important development was the notion of sustainability of implementation, which organisational theorists began to consider in terms of organisational routines and 'institutionalisation'. The emerging focus on the process of innovation within single organisations also led researchers to explore aspects of organisational structure in more depth and to consider the impact of the wider environmental context on the adoption/implementation process. Early structural contingency theorists had proposed that the innovation potential of an organisation depends not merely on its own structure but on its relationship to its wider environment.[231–233]

From the 1980s, process studies increasingly stressed the various stages involved in putting an innovation into sustained, committed and routine use in an organisation. A landmark study in this tradition was Meyer and Goes' extensive in-depth case study of 12 medical innovations as they were adopted in 25 hospitals in a US city (Chapters 4–9).[38] Another major contribution to innovation process research was made by a team of 30 scholars at the University of Minnesota in a programme led by Van de Ven. They conducted in-depth case studies on 14 innovation projects across a range of different fields in industry, education and health care,[123] and probably spawned or inspired a much wider stream of research. Indeed, the late 1980s saw the publication of some 1299 journal articles and 351 dissertations addressing 'organisational innovation' during the period 1984–9, many of which were oriented towards the innovation process.[174]

More recently, research into the process of adoption of innovations has also focused less on the organisation as a whole and more on the teams actually implementing new technologies and ideas. A good example of this more restricted focus is the study of 16 US hospitals implementing an innovative technology for cardiac surgery by Edmondson *et al.* (see Section 8.4), which focused on those directly responsible for implementation – the team that initially used, communicated beliefs about and transferred practices related to the new technology – rather than on broad organisational characteristics and processes.[95] Fitzgerald *et al.*[234] similarly addressed the team rather than the wider organisation in their studies of adoption of primary care innovations.

Organisational context

Understanding the process of adoption in a single individual requires in-depth understanding of that individual in his or her social context, including the meaning of the innovation to that individual (see Section 5.2, page 103). Similarly, an understanding of how and why innovations are adopted and sustained within an organisation or organisational sector requires in-depth study of organisational culture, climate and processes, and the construction and negotiation of meaning by different individuals and groups within – and between – organisations.[227,235–237] The work by Pettigrew *et al.*[78] on receptive and non-receptive contexts for change is important in this respect, with concepts of 'implementation failure', 'drivers and barriers,' 'embeddedness', 'interconnectedness' and 'rate and pace of change' as the primary concerns. Pettigrew's work stresses the cultural, political and strategic contexts, although it tends to address change in general rather than innovation specifically. In contrast, Kanter's[238–240] work is much more closely focused on innovation and innovation contexts, being especially strong on the cultural barriers and supports to innovation. These important issues are considered in detail in Chapter 7 in relation to our empirical findings.

Organisational culture and leadership

Leadership has long been a central interest of organisational researchers, and we have only covered this topic briefly in this review. Leaders within organisations are critical, firstly, in creating a cultural context that fosters innovation (e.g. Kanter's[17] work on fostering creativity for innovation) and, secondly, in establishing organisational strategy, structure and systems that facilitate innovation:

> [Innovation] is a network-building effort that centres on the creation, adoption and sustained implementation of a set of ideas among people who through transactions, become sufficiently committed to these ideas to transform them into 'good currency' ... this network-building activity must occur both within the organisation and in the larger community of which it is a part. Creating these intra- and extra-organisational infrastructures in which innovation can flourish takes us directly to the strategic problem of

innovation, which is institutional leadership.[123] (page 601)

Beyond a leader's role in facilitating a climate for innovation, the extent to which the innovation process can actually be controlled and directed by senior management within an organisation has been questioned.[27] In this regard Kling and Anderson[241] coined the term the 'illusion of manageability' (see Fig. 3.5, page 82). The empirical research into the 'manageability' of innovation in relation to health service organisation (which, incidentally, we found surprisingly sparse) is covered in Chapters 7 (page 134) and 9 (page 175).

3.12 Interorganisational studies: networks and influence

In the 1980s and 1990s, as well as developing greater interest in developing process theory within single organisations, institutional theorists suggested that innovations spread through organisational fields via mimetic (copying) processes. According to the 'fads and fashions' theory proposed by Abrahamson,[21] decision-makers feel impelled to move closer to received institutional norms and fashions as some practices come to be seen as more modern, professional or 'leading edge'. Prevailing organisational theory generally emphasised the role of social factors rather than economic or efficiency factors in driving organisational action, including external uniformity pressures from regulatory bodies or parent organisations, social pressures from other organisations with ties to the focal organisation, as well as collective, interorganisational processes in which norms were socially constructed.[81] As Box 3.5 shows, there are obvious parallels here to the models of individual social networks described in Section 3.3 (page 53).

Box 3.5 Some organisational parallels from social network theory.[21,81,193,242–244]

(1) *Organisational fads and fashions* – innovations spread between organisations by copying.
(2) *Organisational opinion leadership* – certain organisations come to be seen as 'leading edge'.
(3) *Organisational ties* – the extent and direction of flows between, and closeness among, organisations. Ties can be indirect (mediated through a third party) or direct (expected to be stronger). The stronger the ties, the more innovative the organisation.
(4) *Organisational centrality* – i.e. its position within a network, measured by resource and information flows and social ties (the greater the centrality of the organisation, the more innovative it might be expected to be).
(5) *Redundancy* – where two organisations provide a third with the same information.
(6) *Structural holes* – where two organisations are tied to a third but not to one another.

3.13 Knowledge-based approaches to diffusion in organisations

As the previous sections in this chapter have shown, 'communication and influence' was for many years the dominant metaphor for researching the spread of innovations in sociology-based traditions, communication studies, and classical organisational studies (in this last tradition, 'influence' was seen as a property of the organisation), and the parallel 'contagion' metaphor was until recently dominant in more medically based traditions. In knowledge utilisation research, scholars use a very different metaphor for depicting the spread of innovations: the creation and transmission of knowledge. Organisations are conceptualised not in traditional terms (as places of work or collections of formal roles and relationships) but as knowledge-producing systems and as nodes in knowledge-exchanging systems.[245,246] Innovations are seen as spreading by two mechanisms: *organisational learning* (defined as a change in the state of an organisation's knowledge resources[247] – see page 74), and the *embedding* of knowledge in an organisation's product and service outputs.[248]

It is, incidentally, something of an oversimplification to suggest that knowledge utilisation (once described as 'a conceptual cartographer's nightmare'[249]) is a distinct body of theoretical knowledge that informs a clearly demarcated tradition of empirical research. Indeed, knowledge utilisation might be better thought of as a contemporary cross-cutting theme in many professions and academic disciplines,[250] or, alternatively, as a complex application that draws variously on a range of primary disciplines including philosophy, psychology, linguistics, political science, and education.[102] Nevertheless, we did identify a more or less distinct group of researchers who influenced one another's work and who contributed to a definable body of empirical literature on knowledge-based diffusion of innovation in organisations; the key findings in this tradition are presented in Section 7.5 (page 146).

A key concept in the knowledge utilisation tradition is the notion that knowledge exists in two modes: tacit and explicit.[22,251] Explicit knowledge can be expressed in symbols (codified) and is (therefore) easy to communicate and transfer. Tacit knowledge, in contrast, is difficult and costly to codify and transfer between individuals (and especially between organisations) because of the following properties:

(1) It is inextricably woven with the experiences and situational contexts within which it was generated, and is often attached to the practical wisdom of a particular individual (a phenomenon known as 'stickiness'[252]).

(2) It deals with the specific and the particular, consists of various small increments, and is dependent for its meaning on interpretation and negotiation by individuals in a particular context.[253]

(3) The person (and indeed, the organisation) receiving the knowledge needs to have some prior knowledge and experience for the new knowledge to make sense.

Nonaka and Takeuchi[22] contend that the tacit–explicit distinction is at the root of organisational knowledge creation. They propose that 'organisational knowledge is expanded and diffused through social interaction between tacit and explicit knowledge' (page 61). In this sense, the diffusion of innovations may revolve around an interaction between two dimensions: conversions and codifications from tacit to explicit knowledge and vice versa; and transfers between individual, group, organisational and interorganisational levels.

Codifying knowledge into explicit forms renders it more fluid (i.e. less 'sticky'), thereby facilitating its dissemination, communication, transformation, storage and retrieval. Thus, codification is likely to enhance innovation flows between organisations. Formally codified knowledge (such as a protocol) is not quite the same as explicit knowledge, since tacit knowledge can be made explicit using informal linguistic devices, e.g. metaphor or stories.

It should be mentioned in passing that as knowledge has come to be viewed as a critical organisational resource, there has been a corresponding tendency towards what might be termed a 'quantitative approach' to the relationship between knowledge diffusion and innovation in much of the literature. According to this, knowledge is assumed to have a direct, linear and positive relation to the diffusion of innovation and organisational performance. The role of knowledge management then is to enhance the production, circulation and exploitation of knowledge. By capturing, stockpiling and transferring greater quantities of knowledge the ability of the organisation to diffuse innovation will be automatically improved. This quantitative approach has led to numerous general and prescriptive models aimed at increasing the quantity and circulation of knowledge within the organisation.[254]

The problem with such quantitative approaches is that, whilst they assume a positive relationship between the accumulation of knowledge and improvement in diffusion capability and organisational performance, this relationship is rarely examined analytically. In the simplistic 'quantitative' approach, knowledge is treated as valuable in its own right, divorced from the social action and tasks that actually generate changes in performance, the assumption being that the more knowledge an organisation has, the more innovative and therefore more successful it will become. But a more sophisticated view holds that knowledge can only generate and contribute to the diffusion of innovations if we acknowledge the essentially social nature of knowledge and explore knowledge within its social context and action.[255]

Knowledge then, even individual knowledge, is seen as socially constructed, produced and negotiated through social action, action that is anchored in a social context and connected to specific purposes.[256] According to this view, knowledge lacks meaning if divorced from the context of action in which it has been produced and accepted and its diffusion becomes impossible.

Knowledge manipulation activities

To be of any use in an organisation, knowledge must be manipulated (i.e. found, sorted, processed, applied, negotiated, transmitted, reframed and so on). Since the sharing and transformation of knowledge facilitate the diffusion of innovations, enhancing this process depends on finding effective ways to support these activities. This process relies heavily on appropriate leadership, because knowledge creation activities are facilitated in an environment that discourages knowledge hoarding and rewards knowledge sharing.

Osterloh and Frey[257] have argued that whereas the manipulation of explicit knowledge is largely externally motivated (i.e. done for rewards such as pay or the approval of one's boss), the manipulation and transfer of tacit knowledge is generally internally motivated (i.e. done for personal fulfilment and valued for its own sake). In plain English, we might distribute a new protocol to all our junior staff because that is on our job description, but when we 'show someone the ropes' we do it because we gain personal and professional satisfaction from this activity. This underlines the critical need for positive social relationships and culture of reciprocity in the organisation as well as the presence of formal knowledge transfer systems.

Table 3.2 provides a summary of knowledge manipulation models identified in the literature; we briefly expand on two of these in the text.

In 1990, Cohen and Levinthal[265] introduced the concept of *absorptive capacity* to denote the capacity of an individual or organisation to 'value, assimilate and apply new knowledge'. In a more recent (and very comprehensive) overview of the knowledge utilisation literature, Zahra and George[23] redefined absorptive capacity as 'a dynamic capability pertaining to knowledge creation and utilization than enhances a firm's ability to gain and sustain a competitive advantage'. They propose four dimensions: acquisition (the ability to find and prioritise new knowledge quickly and efficiently); assimilation (the ability to understand it and link it to existing knowledge); transformation (the ability to combine convert and recodify it); and exploitation (the ability to put it to productive use). Acquisition, of course, requires social contacts outside the organisation, whereas assimilation and transformation are critically dependent on the quality of social interaction *within* the organisation.

A comparable model has been proposed by Nonaka and Takeuchi,[22] whose theoretical work on knowledge utilisation is extensively cited in the organisational literature. They outline four stages in the knowledge creation cycle:

- *Socialisation*, in which members of a community share their experiences and perspectives and the tacit knowledge of one person is converted into tacit knowledge for another person. An example might be when a student nurse shadows a more experienced colleague and 'learns by osmosis'.
- *Externalisation*, in which the use of metaphors, stories and dialogue lead to the articulation of tacit knowledge, converting it to explicit knowledge. An example of this would be when the more experienced nurse jots notes on the back of an envelope for the novice to keep as an aide memoire.
- *Combination*, in which explicit knowledge is converted into another form of explicit knowledge, such as occurs when community members interact with other groups across the organisation. An example of combination is when a nurse collects various ward protocols into a folder to be used as a reference resource.
- *Internalisation*, in which individuals throughout the organisation learn by doing (and perhaps through listening to stories of how others have learnt by doing), and hence are able to create knowledge, usually in tacit form. Internalisation is demonstrated when a person reads a protocol or other piece of formalised knowledge and can perform the procedure described in it, as when a

Table 3.2 Different taxonomies of 'knowledge manipulation' for organisational learning.

Author/year	*Knowledge manipulation described in terms of*
Choo 1998[258]	1. Sense-making (includes 'information interpretation')
	2. Knowledge creation (includes 'information transformation' '')
	3. Decision-making (includes 'information processing' '')
Holsapple and Winston 1987[259]	1. Procure; 2. Organise; 3. Store; 4. Maintain; 5. Analyse; 6. Create; 7. Present; 8. Distribute; 9. Apply
Leonard-Barton 1995[260]	1. Shared and creative problem-solving
	2. Importing and absorbing technological knowledge from the outside of the firm
	3. Experimenting prototyping
	4. Implementing and integrating new methodologies and tools
Nonaka 1991[261]	1. Socialise (convert tacit knowledge to tacit knowledge)
	2. Internalise (convert explicit knowledge to tacit knowledge)
	3. Combine (convert explicit knowledge to explicit knowledge)
	4. Externalise (convert tacit knowledge to explicit knowledge)
Szulanski 1996[262]	1. Initiation (recognise knowledge need and satisfy that need)
	2. Implementation (knowledge transfer takes place)
	3. Ramp-up (use the transferred knowledge)
	4. Integration (internalise the knowledge)
van der Spek and Spijkervet 1997[263]	In the Act Process
	1. Develop; 2. Distribute; 3. Combine; 4. Hold
Wiig 1993[264]	1. Creation; 2. Manifestation; 3. Use; 4. Transfer
Zahra and George 2002[23]	Absorptive capacity
	1. Acquisition; 2. Assimilation; 3. Transformation; 4. Exploitation

nurse who is new to a ward correctly follows an algorithm in a reference folder.

When all four of these processes coexist, they will, according to Nonaka and Takeuchi,[22] produce knowledge spirals that result in accelerated organisational learning and diffusion of innovation. Figure 3.3 shows diagrammatically how interorganisational links via boundary-spanning individuals can enable knowledge to be captured and added into the cycle. This serves as an explanatory model, in knowledge utilisation terms, for such initiatives as interorganisational collaboratives, Beacons and networks discussed in Section 8.2 (page 163). Related models include Weick's[137] focus on knowledge as sense-making (i.e. fitting the new idea within an existing conceptual schema, with or without concomitant modification of the schema), Leonard-Barton's[260] notion of the problem-solving cycle, and Hansen *et al.*'s[266] emphasis on the need for 'personalisation' of tacit knowledge.

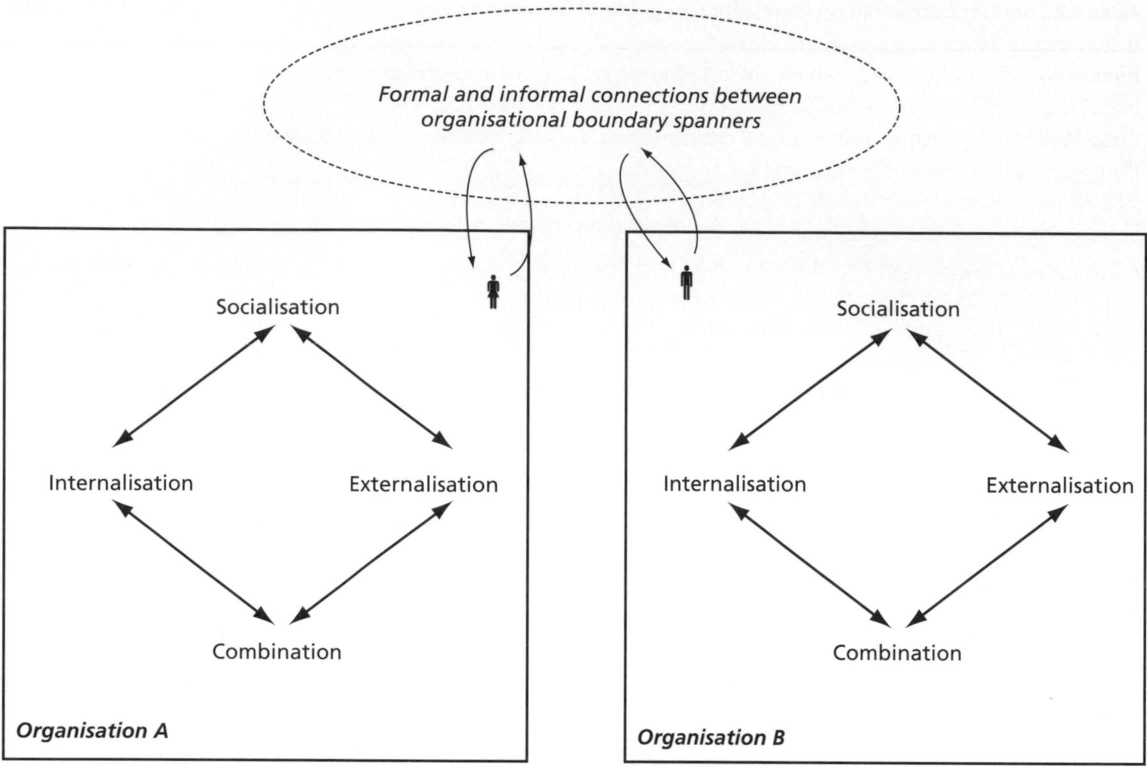

Fig. 3.3 The knowledge creation cycle in organisations and the role of organisational boundary spanners in capturing knowledge (based on Nonaka[261]).

An inherent tension in knowledge utilisation research (perceived in this tradition as the core task of spreading innovations) is the complex and fuzzy nature of much of the knowledge associated with 'ideas' or 'innovations', which makes them difficult constructs to research empirically – especially in the field of technology-based systems. Knowledge utilisation research has many branches, ranging from the design and analysis of the 'hard systems' (computers and their connections) for the transmission of formal knowledge to the exploration and illumination of the 'soft networks' of individuals through which informal knowledge and organisational wisdom is transmitted, transformed and enhanced.

The latter field of enquiry is located mainly in the wider discipline of organisational anthropology, and uses predominantly in-depth ethnographic methods to build up rich case studies of particular organisations and their various subcultures. One of several seminal works in this area was Brown and Duguid's[186] *The social life of information*, which describes a year-long field study of the men who mend photocopiers for Xerox. The researchers 'hung out' with these technical experts and documented *how* they converted codified knowledge (such as the technical manual) into practical action, and also how they exchanged the richer and more elusive tacit knowledge needed for fixing photocopiers (in informal spaces such as canteens via anecdotes and metaphors, by the provision of 'personalised' solutions to real-life problems presented by one member to the group, and by semi-official apprenticeship and shadowing schemes).

The learning organisation

In a learning organisation, knowledge is systematically captured and shared.[247,267] Learning organisations are skilled at creating, acquiring and transferring knowledge, which is then used to modify the organisation's behaviour.[247] The new behaviour reflects new knowledge and insights. Organisational learning relies on an environment that encourages learning, and which has information processes and systems that promote knowledge acquisition, transfer and use – activities driven by a shared and articulated vision and integrated through an open network of individuals. Designated roles often exist for knowledge workers (collecting and transmitting knowledge) and knowledge managers (facilitating and planning such activities). Learning organisations generally differ in both structure and culture from traditional organisations (Table 3.3).

To be effective, organisational learning must be local and distributed, and it must – at different times – be both continuous and episodic.[247] These requirements pose challenges to those charged with managing knowledge in the organisation, because they require living with change and uncertainty relative to both what needs to be learned, how quickly it must be learned, and how individuals and teams need to apply such new knowledge. While there are established generic knowledge processes such as knowledge creation, sharing and storing (see above) that have generalisable features, successful learning processes are mostly local and depend on the history, nature, local culture and leadership of the organisation and the learning styles and recent experience of individuals. In other words, it is impossible to be prescriptive about how to build a learning organisation. Knowledge managers must be sensitive to the locality of effective learning and to the unpredictable nature of many learning situations.

Fundamental to the learning that contributes to innovation diffusion is the attitude and motivation of the individual knowledge worker. While knowledge managers may influence individual attitudes and motivation, the extent of such influence is limited. Given this limitation, what knowledge managers can do is to support individual learning and organisational learning through the effective nurturing of culture, infrastructure, technology, policies and personal behaviour.

In summary, this tradition is built on the premise that innovative organisations must be learning organisations, and a key role in such organisations is the knowledge manager who has responsibility for building and maintaining an organisation that facilitates individual learning and knowledge distribution. Empirical studies focus on the requirements for effective knowledge sharing, including the needs and capabilities of knowledge workers as they relate to learning, change and risk-taking. However, even in learning-centred organisations, knowledge is developed, transmitted and maintained in particular social situations.[260] This raises the issue of sense-making, which is covered below.

Organisational sense-making

The seminal theoretical work in the area of organisational sense-making is that of social psychologist

Table 3.3 Key differences between a learning organisation and a traditional organisation (compiled from various sources[72, 247, 260, 267])

Feature	*Traditional organisation*	*Learning organisation*
Organisational boundaries	Clearly demarcated	Permeable
Structure of the organisation	Predesigned and fixed	Evolving
Approach to human resources	Minimum skill set to do the job	Maximise skills to enhance creativity and learning
Approach to complex activities	Divide into segmented tasks	Ensure integrated processes
Divisions and departments	Functional, hierarchical groupings	Open, multifunctional networks

Weick.[137] When people are called upon to enact some innovation, they do so by trying to ascribe meaning to it. Organisational members are active 'framers', cognitively making sense of the events, processes, objects and issues that comprise a complex innovation. A schema of a person's construction of reality provides the frame though which he or she recalls prior knowledge and interprets new information. Eveland,[50] writing in the 1980s, uses the example of the personal computer – described variously as a 'typewriter', 'calculator' and 'terminal' by members of one organisation – to show how different linguistic metaphors construct a different reality around the innovation and both create and block opportunities for its use:

> Seeing PCs as typewriters implies one-to-one access, usually by secretaries, on desks or in typing pools with relatively little consultation by system engineers with those who use them except about aesthetics or ergonomics. The 'calculator' metaphor implies that the tools will be used one-on-one in professional offices, with choices about both equipment and usage left largely to the individuals. Others see PCs as 'terminals' – an approach that implies they should be scattered around, spaced roughly equally apart, for open use by anyone who wanders by. None of these metaphors is precisely wrong – but each tends to limit the choices of users in critical ways. ... Sharing information among people (and organisations) requires that all be operating on somewhat the same general level of abstraction, and be using something like the same variety of metaphors. It does not require perfect information, or precise specificity, to be effective – sometimes ambiguity and generality can be very effective, particularly one does not know just what sorts of metaphors an information recipient is applying.

When the potential adopter receives inconsistent information, as is invariably the case in innovation, his or her overall view of the organisation may still reflect the well-ingrained schema that denies the validity of the experiential evidence; the individual retains the schema instead of discarding or modifying it.[268] The result is cognitive inertia (i.e. the tendency to remain with the status quo and the resistance to innovation outside the frame): it is difficult to change a schema once it becomes entrenched.[269] Cognitive inertia leads to resistance to the diffusion of innovation because the innovation-in-use deviates from existing schemas and frames – i.e. an innovation by its newness is necessarily surprising, unexpected or equivocal. To be successfully assimilated, an innovation must somehow make sense in a way that relates to previous understanding and experience.

From the sense-making perspective, the success of efforts to disseminate and assimilate innovations depends not only on the organisation's ability to have in place the appropriate knowledge manipulation structures and activities, but also the ability of stakeholders to understand and assimilate a new conceptualisation of the organisation that accompanies the diffusion of each innovation.* The impetus for the diffusion of innovation often lies with top management who typically are key actors in articulating the nature and the need for the dissemination and spread of specific innovations. However, when innovation programmes are presented as radical departures from the organisation's past, they may fail because the cognitive schemata of members, whose cooperation is necessary for successful implementation, constrain their understanding and support of the proposed innovations. Kanter[239] (drawing on others) has highlighted the highly political and sometimes frankly confrontational nature of innovation in organisations: 'Innovation at its core ... is replete with disputes caused by differences in perspectives among those touched by an innovation and the change it engenders' (page 231).

Weick[137] has emphasised the evolutionary nature of organisational sense-making. It is evolutionary in the sense that people first engage in a continuous stream of action, which generates the

*See Fig. 5.4 (page 112), which shows that an innovation in service delivery and organisation comprises a 'hard core' of its irreducible elements plus a 'soft periphery' of things that have to change – *and be made sense of* – if the innovation is to function effectively in its new context.

equivocal situations they experience in an organisation, and then *retrospectively* impose a structure or schema on the situations they face in order to make them sensible. In other words, new knowledge can be thought of as a *retrospectively imposed interpretation* of our organisational stream of experience. This type of retrospective structuring represents the vast majority of our stock of organisational knowledge. It is a *post hoc* imposition of order that makes plausible sense of the ecological–adaptive field of organisational action. Such an ordering structure might be construed as a personal or organisational narrative (see Section 3.12), as elements are imaginatively selected out of the enacted environment and causal relations impugned between past events in order to deal with perceptions of dissonance and surprise.[186,270]

In summary, the research literature on knowledge management and knowledge utilisation does not represent a single research paradigm. In particular, as Fig. 3.5 (page 82) shows, the various activities that go under the broad banner 'knowledge management' range from planned, controlled managerial initiatives in infrastructure provision and knowledge distribution to much more facilitative and emergent activities in organisational sense-making. Common to most (though not all) of these subtraditions is the view of innovation as knowledge and knowledge as characterised by uncertainty, unmeasurability and context dependence (with adjectives such as 'plastic', 'sticky', 'embodied', 'fuzzy' and 'interpretive'), which contrasts sharply with the rationalist paradigm of traditional EBM (Section 3.9, page 64), in which innovation is seen as knowledge celebrated for precisely the opposite qualities (focus, clarity, transferability, accountability, generalisability and provenance) and with the traditional sociological paradigm in which innovation is viewed as driven by individual behavioural choices driven by a combination of factual awareness and interpersonal mimicry.

3.14 Narrative organisational studies

Narrative approaches analyse organisations (and, sometimes, attempt to drive change) via the stories told about them and the stories told within them. Storytelling is a universal human trait, which has been well studied both psychologically and philosophically. Bruner,[271] for example, distinguished two forms of human cognition: logico-scientific ('the science of the concrete') and narrative ('the science of the imagination'). Each has its own distinctive way of constructing reality; neither is reducible to the other. Logico-scientific reasoning seeks to understand specific phenomena as examples of general laws; narrative reasoning seeks to understand specific phenomena in terms of unique human purpose.[272] A narrative approach has particular appeal in the organisational setting for a number of reasons:

- The story is inherently non-linear – i.e. events are seen as emerging from the complex interplay of actions and contexts. Hence storytelling may be an efficient means of capturing the complexity and non-linear relationships (see Section 3.15, page 79) in organisations.
- The story is a humanising and sense-making device. Storytelling may be essential to adaptation and survival in large, impersonal, bureaucratic and technology-dominated environments.
- Stories – especially funny stories (blunders, comeuppance) – are inherently subversive; they serve as counterpoint to official 'rose-tinted' stories used by senior management in marketing and image-branding. Funny stories assign alternative identities to key characters, and may have particular value for the oppressed and disempowered in an organisation.*
- Stories are memorable (indeed, the story is often the unit of individual memory, and 'organisational folklore' is a key element of institutional memory[25]). Hence, stories have an important potential for education and contribute crucially to organisational culture.

*Gabriel's[25] own fieldwork, for example, highlighted the contrast between organisations' official version of their own story ('well-oiled machine, cutting-edge technology') and the subversive metaphors used by the members ('the [pompous, incompetent] management, nothing works round here'.

• Stories stimulate the imagination, allowing us to envision a different future. Hence stories have powerful change potential.
• Leadership is related to storytelling. 'Leaders are people who tell good stories, and about whom good stories are told'.[273]

The fundamental philosophical difference between scientific truth and narrative 'truth' underpins narrative organisational research. Poetic licence is the essence of storytelling: the telling is an artistic performance and the use of literary devices is part of the art. Stories do not convince by their objective truth but by such literary features as aesthetic appeal, apt metaphor, moral order, and authenticity.[271] A single problem or experience will generate multiple stories (interpretations), and oral stories may change with each telling. Not only is the 'true' version of events an unhelpful concept, but the very plasticity of stories in organisations is the key to what Gabriel[25] has called (page 112) the 'organisational dreamworld'. These principles suggest why (as researchers in other traditions have discovered) organisations cannot be understood via the 'facts' alone. Stories told by members of an organisation interpret events, infusing them with meaning by linking them in temporal (implicitly, causal) sequence, and through distortions, omissions, embellishments, metaphors and other literary devices.[25]

The unique epistemological nature of stories raises unique issues of research methodology. There is little if any *empirical* evidence for the use of narrative approaches in organisational analysis. Czarniawska[24] points out that

> By the criteria of scientific (paradigmatic) knowledge, the knowledge carried by narratives is not very impressive. Formal logic rarely guides the reasoning, the level of abstraction is low, and the causal links may be established in a wholly arbitrary way.

Given that stories are relatively easy to collect and transmit, that the essence of narrative is personal anecdote, and that the narrative turn is currently fashionable in many quasi-intellectual circles, we must be wary of the emergence of 'narrative research studies' that lack a sound theoretical basis.* Both Gabriel[25] and Czarniawska[24] advocate an ethnographic (participant-observer) approach, in which the researcher joins the workforce and undergoes the same kind of prolonged 'immersion in the field' that an anthropologist might undergo when studying a native culture.

In contrast to the prevailing view that the main function of stories in organisations is to entertain (and, implicitly, to give light relief to the daily grind of organisational life),[25] or for senior management to impose a particular institutional identity on staff,[275] Higgins and McAllister[276] identify stories as the key vehicle for the creative imagination amongst organisational innovators. Buckler and Zein also emphasise the key role of stories in organisational innovativeness.[26] Stories, they claim, are inherently subversive. They create the backdrop for new visions and embody 'permission to break the rules'. In an old-fashioned machine bureaucracy, behaviours and events that go beyond the existing structures and systems are implicitly (and often explicitly) 'wrong'. Telling a story about someone with a new idea allows their actions to be imbued with meaning and the change agent to be accorded positive qualities like courage, creativity and so on ('Mrs Smith from the records department went in and told them straight'). The potential of storytelling to capture innovation within and between organisations is discussed below.

Because of their direct relationship to assimilation, narrative and sense-making are crucial (related) theoretical perspectives to take forward when considering the results of empirical work on innovation in organisations. Yet as Chapters 7 and 9 show, we found remarkably few studies relevant to this review that have adopted this perspective – a potentially remediable weakness of the existing literature.

---

*Denning, for example, provides a highly anecdotal account of storytelling in 'igniting action' in developing knowledge management policies in a large international organisation. His stories of storytelling have superficial appeal but he offers little objective evidence to show that it was the stories (rather than, for example, external social, economic or technological forces) that drove the change – or even whether the change occurred (and was sustained) in the way described.[274]

A very different use of the narrative-as-sense-making approach, popular in the USA, is appreciative enquiry (AE) – the search for the 'best stories' in organisations and the systematic use of these stories in shaping organisational destiny.[277] AE thus replaces analytical, problem-solving/fixing approaches with narrative/emotive techniques of *appreciating* (valuing the best of what is); *imagining* (envisioning what might be); and *dialoguing* (describing, negotiating and creating what will be). AE uses an action research framework,[278] in which members of the organisation raise questions and conduct the enquiry, facilitated by external consultants, rather than the traditional consultancy method where the consultant acts as a diagnostician and then 'prescribes' a 'treatment' for the organisation. We did not find any relevant empirical studies that used this approach (indeed, AE seems currently to be the province of management consultants rather than empirical researchers), but there may well be additional material in the grey literature.

3.15 Complexity and general systems theory

A recurring theme in many of the research traditions described in previous sections of this chapter has been their inability to explain the complexity that characterises health service organisations, for which complexity theory offers one model.[27,28,279] A complex adaptive system is defined as a collection of individual agents who have the freedom to act in ways that are not always totally predictable, and whose actions are interconnected such that one agent's actions changes the context for other agents. Complex systems typically have fuzzy boundaries and are embedded in other systems, leading to unexpected outcomes in response to actions. A key concept is individual creativity (which leads to the ideas that become innovations) and the importance of human interaction ('generative relationships') in developing new – usually unanticipated and unplanned – capabilities of the system. Finally, complex systems are adaptive and self-organising, making multiple and dynamic internal adjustments in response to changes in the external (and internal) environment. This last feature highlights the critical importance of feedback loops in informing the organisation's development.

Fonseca has set out the key principles of complexity theory as applied to innovation in organisations.[27] He defines innovation (page 3) as 'the emergent continuity and transformation of patterns of interaction, understood as ongoing, ordinary complex responsive processes of human relating in local situations'.[27] Furthermore, he identifies *conversations between individuals* as the key mechanism for diffusing innovations. The critical characteristic of the innovation process is, for Fonseca, that it is a social process, socially created, socially transmitted and socially sustained. Innovation is primarily to do with social interaction and the exchange of ideas, and only secondarily to do with institutionalisation or process control. The spread (and the sustainability) of innovations results from local, self-organising interaction of actors and units. This contrasts markedly with the conceptual model used by the classical, 'rational' school of management, in which (as Fonseca[27] puts it, page 9) 'Innovation originates as intention in the mind of an autonomous individual and that it is either directly manageable and controllable or indirectly manageable through the assumed ability to design the social conditions in which innovation will emerge'.

Plsek,[28] who makes similar points, argues that there are many situations in which a rational, planned and regulated approach serves an organisation well. Such situations can be summed up as those in which there is high certainty about what the problem is, and high agreement about what to do in those circumstances – the bottom left corner (simple zone) of Fig. 3.4. But a regulatory approach is less helpful where people are uncertain about the nature of the problem or when they disagree about the rules to be followed for that kind of problem (the complex and chaotic zones in Fig. 3.4).

Innovation and the spread of new ideas, of course, tend to occur in the complex zone, where the appropriate approach is therefore exploratory, intuitive and responsive, showing

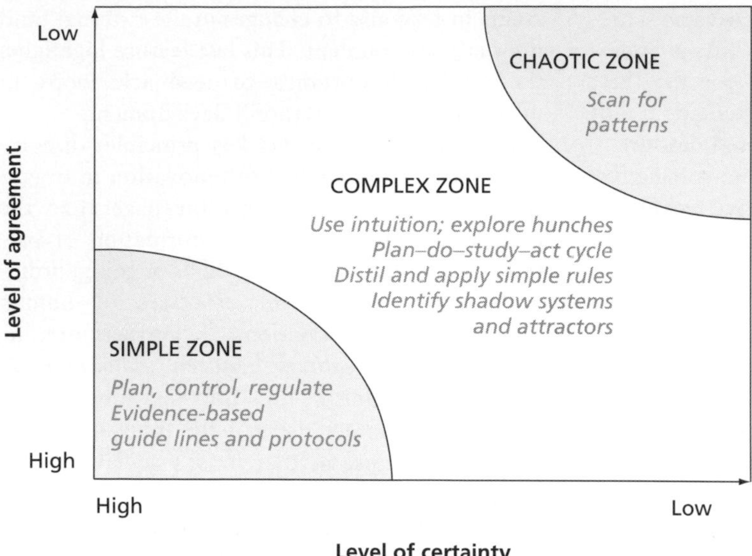

Fig. 3.4 Certainty–agreement matrix (based originally on Stacey[280] and published in this form in Plsek and Greenhalgh[279]).

sensitivity to existing patterns and relationships, and using tools such as the plan–do–study–act cycle or the rapid-cycle test-of-change technique.[84,281] As Fonseca has pointed out, such an approach is very different from the rational, planned and controlled ('managerial') approach advocated in much conventional 'implementation' advice, and which, suggests Plsek, lies at the root of many misguided attempts at introducing innovations into the health service (Table 3.4).

Some of the best empirical evidence on how innovation arises in complex systems has been collected by Kanter,[239] who analysed hundreds of case studies and failed to find any evidence for success of rational planning models in most of them. She argues, however, that whilst it is not possible to manage innovation (since it depends critically on the creativity and initiative of others), it *is* possible to design and control the contextual and organisational conditions that enhance the possibility of innovation occurring and spreading.[17] Although she uses different terminology, Kanter's[17] preconditions for creativity (and the converse conditions – her famous 'rules for stifling initiative') are almost identical to what Pettigrew *et al.*[78] called 'creating a receptive context for change'.

Explicit examples of the empirical application of complexity theory to health service innovation are relatively rare, but the various collaborative improvement projects discussed in Section 8.2 (page 163) draw extensively on this theoretical framework.

3.16 Conclusion

This chapter has covered a vast range of research traditions whose work has a bearing on the spread and sustainability of innovation in health service organisations. Different traditions have been built on very different concepts and theories of what innovation is and how it spreads. Early research on diffusion of innovations in the organisation and management field focused first on structural determinants and later on issues of process, context and culture – including the overlap of implementation with good management practice (including such issues as leadership, resource allocation, teamwork, goals and milestones, training and so on). More recently, several contemporary, and to some extent overlapping, traditions (organisational knowledge creation, narrative organisational studies and complexity theory) have emphasised the dynamic, contestable, socially

Table 3.4 Contrasting approaches to innovation and spread (adapted with permission from Plsek[28]).

	Rational, 'managerial' approach	*Complex adaptive systems approach*
Underlying metaphor	Organisation is a machine	Organisation is an organism adapting to its environment
Implicit mechanism of change	Plan and control	Learn and adapt
Generation of ideas	To be done by creative specialists and experts	Ideas can emerge from anyone; they are often the result of generative relationships (see page 79)
Implementation of ideas within the organisation	Should be thoroughly planned out and be primarily a replication of structures and processes that have worked elsewhere	Can be informed by what has worked elsewhere, but must take into account local structures, processes and *patterns* (relationships, mental models, attractors, etc.)
Widespread adoption across organisations	Primarily an issue of evidence dissemination and motivation	Primarily an issue of sharing knowledge through social relationships and adapting ideas to fit local conditions and attractor patterns
Receptive context for change	Health care organisations are largely similar; there are a small number of key issues that we must address to ensure success	Health care organisations are similar in some ways, but also have important unique characteristics that must be taken into account at times of change

constructed and emergent nature of organisational knowledge and organisational action. These 'constructivist' traditions all couch the discourse of diffusion of innovations in the language and action of human relationships and the construction of shared meaning.

As Fig. 3.5 shows in diagrammatic form, these various traditions might be thought of as lying on a continuum. Whilst the dimension of 'manageability' is not strictly a linear one, nor is it the only dimension on which the traditions differ, it is a key consideration for those who seek to influence the diffusion and implementation of innovations.

At one end of the manageability continuum are the linear and rationalist conceptual models in which an innovation is a 'thing', adoption is an 'event', and implementation is a rational, controllable process that is amenable to advance planning and monitoring against targets. At the other end of the continuum lie the more complex 'ecological' and interpretive models in which innovation, adoption, implementation and sustainability are complex, context-dependent and creative social processes that cannot be planned in detail and are not amenable to external control or manageability. These traditions are generally characterised by a greater emphasis on understanding the adopter and his or her system (asking, for example, what the innovation *means* to them), tapping into the agency and creativity of actors in the organisation and recognising the need to adapt or reframe the innovation and consider its knock-on effects for the wider system.

As Chapters 4–9 demonstrate, the different traditions described above have used very different empirical methods and have sometimes produced apparently 'conflicting' findings. As we

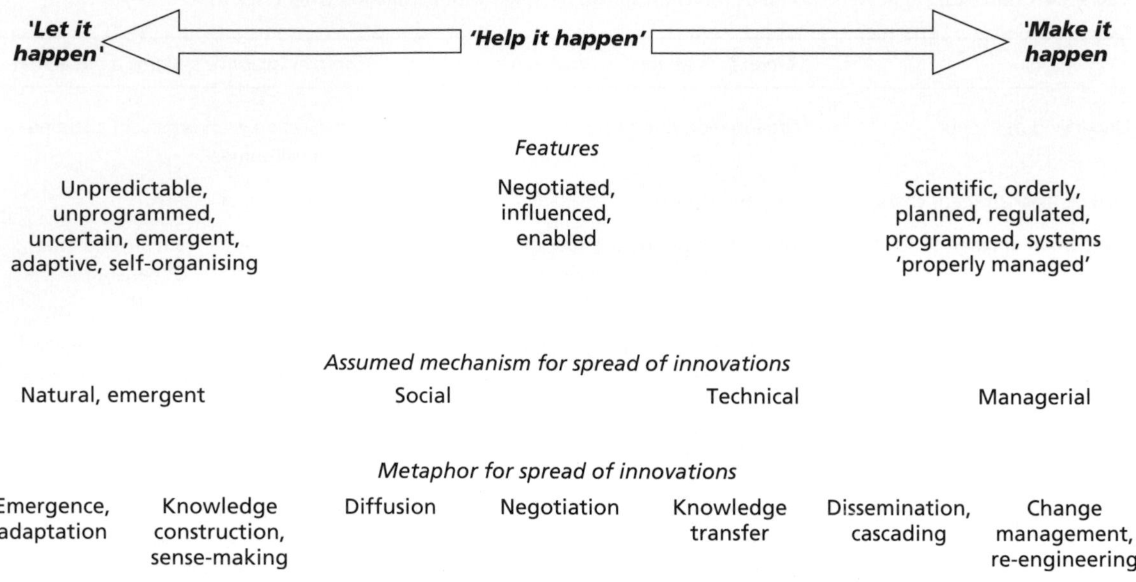

Fig. 3.5 Different conceptual and theoretical bases for the spread of innovation in service organisations.

discussed in Section 2.7 (page 42), these conflicts can be explained in Kuhnian terms, and the apparent discrepancies analysed as higher-order data. Chapters 4–9 attempt to do this by drawing together the empirical findings from different traditions that addressed the same or similar themes.

Chapter 4
Innovations

Key points

1. This chapter is about innovations – studies sometimes referred to under the general heading 'attribution research', concerned with what attributes of innovations, as perceived by potential adopters, are associated with their successful adoption. Hundreds of empirical studies have been conducted on this topic, and although few specifically relate to health service innovations, the conclusions from the wider literature have important messages for this review.

2. Different innovations spread and get adopted at different rates. Some never spread at all. The five key attributes originally described by Rogers (relative advantage, compatibility, low complexity, observability and trialability) are necessary but not sufficient to explain the adoption of complex service innovations. A sixth attribute, potential for reinvention, may be particularly critical in the organisational setting.

3. Additional *operational* attributes, especially relevant for organisational innovations, include the relevance of the innovation to a particular task, the complexity of its implementation, and the degree of risk associated with adoption in a particular organisational and environmental context.

4. Innovations that involve the use of technology are common in health service organisations. They are inherently complex and have an important contextual element. Additional attributes for a technological innovation include visibility (whether others are seen to be using it), voluntariness (whether use of the technology is under individual choice), the nature (tacit or explicit) of the knowledge required to use it, and the quality of support provided. Regular and repeated use is often needed to consolidate the decision to adopt a technology-based innovation.

5. The somewhat reified notion of an innovation with fixed boundaries and measurable attributes that are independent of context has been superseded in the organisational literature by the notion of 'innovation–system fit', which may include adaptation and contingency. These constructs are covered in later chapters in this review.

4.1 Background literature on attributes of innovations

Innovation in service delivery and organisation was defined on page 28. As described in Chapter 3, the attributes of innovations that influence adoption by individuals were a central concern of the early sociologists, a literature that has been ably summarised by Rogers.[3,178] Most of these studies followed the method originally developed in the 1930s by Ryan and Gross[188] (described in Section 3.2, page 51) and independently in the 1950s by Coleman *et al.*[5] (Section 3.3, page 53) – i.e. the researchers interviewed a sample of potential adopters with a view to identifying the perceived attributes of the innovation that had led to their adoption (or non-adoption), and also the interpersonal and other channels through which this influence had occurred.

Sociologists are divided on whether the key construct is the 'absolute' attribute or whether it is the innovation's *perceived* relative advantage, complexity and so on that determines adoption. Rogers[3] (page 209) makes a powerful argument for focusing on perceived attributes. In relation to EBM, for example, there is a well-recognised difference between objective advantage (the research evidence as evaluated by experts) and *perceived* advantage in the eyes of practitioners.

Whilst not every study confirmed every attribute of innovations shown in Box 4.1, there was a remarkable consistency in the overall findings of early sociological research, with these attributes accounting for 49–87% of the variance in rate of adoption of innovations.[3] Rogers has described the six attributes (page 208) as 'empirically linked but conceptually distinct'.

Overall, relative advantage (i.e. whether the potential adopter has seen any advantage over existing practice) was the most significant and consistent attribute determining adoption. Trialability was in many studies closely linked to complexity. The Iowa farmers, for example, whose adoption practices for hybrid corn formed the 'classic' diffusion of innovations study in sociology (see Section 3.2, page 51) could (and did) plant the new corn in just one or two fields at first, thus making this innovation almost uniquely trialable. The importance – and the difficulty – of creating 'trialability space' for complex service innovations is highlighted in our own recommendations.

Box 4.1 Attributes of innovations that have been shown in empirical studies to influence their rate and extent of adoption by individuals (based on an extensive review of the sociological literature by Rogers[3]).

(1) *Relative advantage* (measured, for example, in economic terms, social prestige, convenience or satisfaction).
(2) *Compatibility* (with existing practices and values, past experiences, and needs of potential adopters and their social system).
(3) *Complexity* (the degree to which the innovation is perceived as difficult to understand and use).
(4) *Trialability* (the degree to which an innovation may be experimented with on a limited basis).
(5) *Observability* (the degree to which the results of an innovation are visible to others).
(6) *Reinvention* (the extent to which the innovation is changed or modified by the user in the process of adoption and implementation).

Reinvention was, interestingly, not added to the list of core attributes until several decades after the others, even though there was empirical evidence to support reinvention as an independent attribute. Rogers[3] (page 17) gives an admirably honest description of how he missed descriptions of reinvention by adopters in the early days of the rural sociology tradition because his closed questionnaire had no box for recording the phenomenon even when it was described to him. Section 6.6 (page 131) suggests that reinvention may be particularly crucial for innovations that arise spontaneously through local, unplanned innovation and that diffuse horizontally through peer networks.*

In reviewing the literature on innovation attributes, Rogers warned that they are probably not an exhaustive list, and called for further research to develop a standard classification scheme against which the attributes of innovations in *any* study might be measured. Other writers have echoed this call, and proposed combining Rogers' and alternative classifications to develop an 'accepted typology of attributes' that could lead to greater generalisability of innovation studies.[174] Nevertheless, the attributes listed in Box 4.1 are extensively cited (usually with the omission of reinvention†), and they form the conventional starting point for many studies of innovation characteristics and adoption.

We identified a single study that considered attributes of an innovation in relation to *discontinuance* of use. Riemer-Reiss *et al.* showed that three attributes of assistive technologies (i.e. devices that help those with disabilities lead independent lives) were significantly associated with discon-

*For a fascinating article from the political sciences literature about how political policies are 'reinvented' as they diffuse from one US state to another, and a useful review of the spread of policy as distinct from other innovations, see Hays.[282]

†This is a good example of a 'bibliographic virus' in which successive reviews of the literature have reproduced one another's omissions by failing to verify the primary sources referenced, and underlines the need for systematic reviewers to return to original sources.

tinuance – relative (dis)advantage, (non-)compatibility, and (lack of) involvement of the user in selecting the device.[283] We mention it in passing to highlight this methodological modification – there is no reason why attribution studies might not be undertaken to explain discontinuance as well as adoption.

Innovations in service delivery and organisation often include an information and communications technology (ICT) component. The adoption of innovations in ICT is underpinned by a vast literature on technology transfer and human–computer interaction, which is beyond the scope of this book, but which could be the subject of further secondary research.

A technology, by definition, has two elements – the hardware or physical 'stuff' of the technology, and the information that goes with it (often but not always presented as software). As Rogers has suggested,[3] all technologies potentially solve one problem but create another one – i.e. they offer the potential to reduce uncertainty (by virtue of the information contained within their software), but they also increase uncertainty in other fields (by virtue of their unintended consequences). Thus, for technological innovations, the innovation-decision process is essentially about information seeking, allowing the individual to reduce uncertainty about the advantages and disadvantages of the innovation.

Eveland[50] has pointed out that 'technology is not simply hardware or physical objects; rather, it is knowledge about the physical world and how to manipulate it for human purposes'. Some technologies are composed almost entirely of information (hence, notwithstanding other more complex aspects of adoption of ICT, this will tend to slow their diffusion because of low observability).

Technologies often come in clusters – i.e. one technology has sister products aimed at solving similar kinds of problem. Familiarity with one product in the cluster reduces the uncertainty associated with another. Rogers,[3] drawing somewhat eclectically on empirical studies, noted some particularly prominent features of the adoption of ICT innovations (which are also relevant to many other complex innovations):

- Regular and repeated use is generally necessary to consolidate the decision to adopt.
- A critical mass of adopters is needed to convince the majority of other individuals of the utility of the technology.
- Adoption very often (indeed, usually) requires an element of reinvention.

In 1991, Moore and Benbasat[284] published a landmark study of the adoption of ICT-based innovations. They drew on Rogers' six attributes (as set out in Box 4.1) and also on Davis's[287] (page 985) Technology Adoption Model,* which states that computer acceptability is determined by two perceptions: usefulness – i.e. 'the prospective user's subjective probability that using a specific application system will increase his or her job performance within an organisational context') – and ease of use – i.e. 'the degree to which the prospective user expects the target system to be free of effort'). From these and one or two other sources, they produced a new list of constructs that they then tested empirically.[288] They began with a 44-item survey instrument and found eight separate constructs to be significant in their final model for adoption of ICT innovations. From these, they developed an instrument to measure the Perceived Characteristics of [technological] Innovations (PCI) Scale, shown in Box 4.2.

Most of these empirically developed attributes of ICT innovations have parallels with Rogers' original list of general innovation attributes: compatibility is on both lists and image is closely related to this; ease of use is very similar to complexity, relative advantage is on both lists but in the Moore and Benbasat scale it is split into perceived independent advantage and perceived usefulness for doing a particular job; and there is surely little difference between result demonstrability and observability. Hence, visibility and voluntariness are probably the only attributes unique to ICT innovations. Voluntariness is, strictly speaking, a characteristic of the organisational context rather than the innovation, but it was

*Davis's model drew in turn on the Theory of Planned Behaviour developed by Azjen and Fishbein.[285] For a detailed description of the development of his constructs, see Davis.[286]

Box 4.2 Moore and Benbasat's[284] Perceived Characteristics of Innovations Scale for adoption of information and communications technology.

(1) *Compatibility* (with existing practices and values; see Box 4.1).
(2) *Ease of use* (the degree to which the innovation is expected to be free of effort).
(3) *Image* (the degree to which it is seen as adding to the user's social approval).
(4) *Relative advantage* (split into the degree to which it is perceived as better than its precursor and the degree to which it is perceived as useful – implicitly, for doing one's job*).
(5) *Result demonstrability* (the degree to which it is perceived as amenable to demonstration).
(6) *Trialability* (can be tried out on a limited basis; see Box 4.1).
(7) *Visibility* (the degree to which the innovation is seen to be used by others).
(8) *Voluntariness* (the degree to which use of the innovation is controlled by the potential user's free will).

*Dearing *et al.*[48] also split relative advantage into two separate dimensions: effectiveness and cost-effectiveness – a common distinction in EBM.

included in Moore and Benbasat's[284] scales and found to be a significant predictor of adoption.

Another recently published taxonomy of attributes in relation to ICT innovations is that of Mustonen-Ollila and Lyytinen,[289] who propose four dimensions: factors that are truly inherent to the innovation (ease of use, industry standard), task factor (user need recognition), individual factors (own trials, autonomous work, perceived ease of use, and the opportunity for learning by doing) and organisational factors (the organisation's past technological experience). Whilst they, like most writers on innovation attributes, tend to offer a more complex taxonomy than the previously published literature, Weiss and Dale[290] suggest that the attributes of technological innovations can be collapsed into two core constructs – relative performance advantage (to what extent can the technology perform better than what it replaces?) and operational novelty (to what extent does the user have to learn new skills?). To our knowledge, however, this appealingly simple list has not been empirically tested.

One attribute of innovations that has received surprisingly little attention by researchers is what might be called 'riskiness' – the amount of risk the individual perceives is associated with its adoption. Innovations that are a radical change from what has gone before, and those with a high degree of uncertainty about outcome, tend to be seen as more risky.[291,292] Some authors have seen riskiness as a component of relative advantage, and others have included it in compatibility, but we concur with Fidler and Johnson[292] in viewing it as a separate – and organisationally important – construct. To the extent that it has been studied, perceived riskiness tends to reduce an innovation's chances of successful adoption.[31,292] In Section 7.7 (page 150) we introduce the concept of organisational climate – i.e. the extent to which it is 'okay to take risks' in an organisation. There is some (mostly indirect) evidence, reviewed in Section 7.7, that in organisations with a positive risk-taking climate, perceived riskiness is less likely to inhibit adoption of an innovation.

In summary, the attributes associated with adoption by individuals, discussed above, are well established and broadly consistent between studies. However, an early review of the organisational literature noted that for all of the research that has accumulated on organisational change and innovation, no general theory incorporating the attributes of innovations and their adoptability within organisations has emerged.[293] This is not for want of trying on the part of investigators. The wider literature in organisation and management reveals that innovation attributes that seem positively related to adoption in one organisational study are negatively related in a second, and unrelated in still another. In the words of one research team:

> The literature on innovation has been described as 'fragmentary', 'contradictory', and 'beyond interpretation'. ... From both a theoretical and a practical perspective, our cumulative knowledge of why and how organisations adopt and implement innovations is considerably less than the sum of its parts.[38]

Bearing in mind this general conclusion, the rest of this section considers studies that have looked empirically at attributes of innovations in a specific health service context (whose results, although sparse, closely mirror those of the wider organisation and management literature). We have also included selected studies of organisational innovations in a non-health service context where these add to the analysis.

4.2 The Tornatzky and Klein meta-analysis of innovation attributes

We found only one meta-analysis, from the organisation and management literature, that addressed attributes of innovations and their relationship to adoption and implementation in the organisational setting.[62] Tornatzky and Klein's overview, whose focus was on product innovations in manufacturing industry, was published in 1982 and reviewed 75 primary studies, all of which had asked the question: 'what attributes of innovations increase the rate and extent of adoption?'* This was not in the strictest sense a systematic review since a very limited range of sources was used, but the search strategy was explicit and the analysis of secondary data systematic and reproducible. We were initially surprised not to find a more recent meta-analysis of innovation attributes in the organisational setting, but as this section shows, the primary studies on which such meta-analyses are based are inherently problematic, and more recent research traditions have used different (and, arguably, more robust) approaches, as set out in the subsequent sections and chapters.

Tornatzky and Klein constructed a methodological profile of the studies and assessed the generality and consistency of the empirical findings, as summarised in Table 4.1. Although presented as a meta-analysis of 'organisational' innovations, most primary studies took the individual adopter as the unit of analysis. The scope and methodological quality of the included studies varied considerably. From an initial list of 30 innovation attributes, the meta-analysis considered the ten that had been most frequently addressed in the 75 studies (in order of frequency: compatibility, relative advantage, complexity, cost, communicability, divisibility, profitability, social approval, trialability and observability). It should be noted that this was a somewhat arbitrary selection criterion, since it may have reflected little more than the preconceptions of researchers. As the authors observe, only three of the 75 of the studies presented intercorrelation tables, and the combined data are disappointingly uninformative. They suggest that the interdependence of perceived attributes is a neglected area of research.[62]

Specific points made by Tornatzky and Klein relevant to this review include:

- Only two of the 75 studies were predictive studies – i.e. they looked prospectively rather than concurrently or retrospectively at the different hypothesised attributes.
- Only five of the 75 studies examined the relationship of innovation characteristics to adoption and implementation.
- In most of the studies too few characteristics were studied in too few innovations (35 of the 75 studies had only studied one attribute and 40 had only studied one innovation).
- In 45 of the 75 studies the researchers inferred the importance of the innovation characteristic in the eyes of potential adopters rather than systematically measuring perceived characteristics.
- In more than half of the studies, the adopting unit was an individual; even though the studies claimed to be looking at organisational innovation, only a third of them considered the organisation as the unit of analysis.

Compatibility was the attribute most frequently investigated by the primary studies in the Tornatzky and Klein meta-analysis. Of the 41 studies reviewed, 13 could be included in their statistical analysis, and ten of those found a positive, although not always statistically significant, relationship between the compatibility of an innovation and its adoption. Once these data were

*The principle sources for these references were Rogers and Shoemaker,[177] Rothman,[294] Zaltman *et al.*[227] and Havelock.[295] Additional citations were obtained from researchers working in the field, computer searches and by 'consulting other reviews'.

Table 4.1 Methodological profile of studies of innovation attributes from Tornatzky and Klein's[62] 1982 meta-analysis.

Design attribute	*Actual studies % (number of studies)*				
Predictive vs retrospective approach	Predicted adoption or implementation 2.7% (2)		Explained adoption or implementation in a *post hoc* fashion 90.7% (68)	Data not available 6.7% (5)	
Dependent variables	Adoption 93.3% (70)	Adoption and implementation 6.7% (5)			
Design methodology	Survey 54.7% (41)	Secondary data analysis 20% (15)	Experiment 1.3% (1)	Case study 17.3% (13)	Theory 6.7% (5)
Measure of attributes	Rated by decision-makers 18.7% (14)	Rated by expert judges 5.3% (4)	Cost and profit 10.7% (8)	Inferred 60% (45)	NA 5.3% (4)
Number of attributes considered	One 46.7% (35)	2–5 36% (27)	6–9 10.7% (8)	10 or more 6.7% (5)	
Number of innovations studied	One 53.5% (40)	2–5 12% (9)	6–9 2.7% (2)	10 or more 25.3% (19)	NA 6.7% (5)
Nature of adopting unit	Organisation 33.3% (25)	Individual 57.3% (43)	Other 8% (6)	NA 1.3% (1)	

aggregated, the association just reached statistical significance ($p = 0.046$).

However, there was a problem of inconsistency of definitions. Some studies interpreted compatibility as referring to compatibility with the values or norms of the potential adopters (normative or cognitive compatibility) whilst some took it to represent congruence with the existing practices of the adopters (operational compatibility). This notion of compatibility with *individual* norms and practices should, incidentally, be carefully distinguished from compatibility with the organisation's norms, routines and practices; the latter is discussed in Section 4.3 (page 90). Furthermore, most (26 of 41) of the compatibility studies did not actually measure compatibility objectively, but merely inferred that the innovation was compatible to the potential user group.

After excluding studies that used 'relative advantage' as a proxy for other more specific characteristics, Tornatzky and Klein[62] found that of 29 studies of relative advantage, five reported correlations and all found a positive relationship to adoption ($p = 0.031$). However, as Tornatzky and Klein note, studies of relative advantage typically lacked conceptual strength, reliability and prescriptive power.

Complexity was the third characteristic found in this meta-analysis to be (negatively) related to adoption.[62] The quality of the 'complexity' studies as reviewed was generally higher than that of other studies in that they tended to have more sophisticated designs, used a more robust measure of innovation attributes, and studied more characteristics and more innovations at a single time. Thirteen of the 21 studies of innovation complexity included statistical analyses and seven of these were suitable for inclusion in a meta-analysis. Six of the seven found a negative relationship between the complexity of an innovation and its adoption ($p = 0.062$).

Of the eight studies mentioning trialability, five provided statistical results but only one study reported the first-order correlation. Four of the observability studies reported relevant results, and only one provided any direct correlational measure of the observability–adoption relationship. Thus, little can be concluded from the meta-analysis about this attribute in an organisational setting.

A final attribute addressed by this meta-analysis was communicability (the extent to which the innovation's features can be conveyed to others).* Communicability was discussed in 13 studies reviewed by Tornatzky and Klein but only three reported statistical findings relevant to the communicability–adoption relationship. None of these studies permitted direct statistical examination of their relationship within the meta-analysis.

Overall, Tornatzky and Klein found that only two innovation attributes (compatibility and relative advantage) were positively related to adoption across studies ($p < 0.05$). One other characteristic (complexity) was negatively related to adoption at a 'near-acceptable level of statistical significance' ($p = 0.062$). However, this meta-analysis is arguably an example of spurious precision,[156] since the diversity in scope and quality of primary studies calls into question the validity of summary statistics. As the authors note (page 40):

> [although] the majority of innovation characteristic studies employed defensible designs ... these designs were all too often rendered useless by inappropriate and unsystematic measures of the independent variable, the innovation characteristic(s).

In other words, this early meta-analysis, whose primary studies were mostly based outside the service sector, probably used summative statistics inappropriately and would have had greater validity if the highest quality studies had been weighted appropriately and the lowest quality ones omitted from the summary. Bearing these limitations in mind, a tentative conclusion is that overall, three (relative advantage, compatibility, and complexity) of Rogers' six attributes of innovations were confirmed as influencing their adoption in an organisational setting.

*See Section 3.13 (page 70) for a possible explanation of why this is such a crucial attribute.

4.3 Empirical studies of innovation attributes

Table A.7 (Appendix 4, page 255) summarises the primary studies published since 1982 (i.e. since the Tornatzky and Klein meta-analysis) that addressed attributes of health service innovations in a health care organisational setting. Of these studies, which are discussed in chronological order in the text below, we ranked none as both 'methodologically outstanding' and 'highly relevant'. We have therefore included all studies rated as 'relevant' and as 'some limitations' or as above (i.e. we have excluded only those studies that we rated as having 'many important limitations'). We have commented in the text on the impact of the limitations of these studies on the validity of their findings.

We found very few studies that looked at a service innovation and that addressed individual adoption in a way that was removed from the organisational context. This was undoubtedly because our definition of an innovation in service delivery and organisation effectively precluded an exclusive focus on the individual. As the Grilli and Lomas[37] study illustrates, one area where relevant research did address individual adoption was in evidence-based practice and guideline implementation. However, it is no accident that more recent work in this field (including work by these authors) has focused more centrally on supporting organisational adoption.

One important attribution study to mention here is Meyer and Goes' study of adoption of complex innovations in US hospitals, which is covered in detail in Section 5.3 (page 106). In this large and ambitious study, which was set up mainly to look at adoption decisions rather than innovation attributes, the latter explained 37% of the variance in organisational innovativeness. Innovations that were highly observable, carried low risks and required relatively little skill to use were much more readily adopted. This study is also covered briefly in Section 7.4 (page 141).

In the early days of electronic databases (e.g. Medline) searching, Marshall[30] and colleagues undertook a questionnaire survey of perceptions of 150 users from the health professions. All the participants in the study were early adopters – i.e. they comprised the minority of health professionals who had expressed early interest in using electronic databases. The researchers related actual level of use of the databases to five perceived attributes (relative advantage, compatibility, complexity, trialability and observability), and they also asked about the user's intention to continue using the database. The two attributes of electronic databases that effectively predicted implementation of end-user searching were relative advantage in relation to previous practice and lack of complexity. The attribute that best predicted personal commitment to keep using the databases was relative advantage in relation to access and control. People who were already high information users implemented the innovation most readily. The authors concluded that different strategies need to be deployed when introducing clinicians to databases, depending on the user's perceptions of attributes.*

Arguably, a specific scale for attributes of ICT innovations (e.g. the Moore and Benbasat Perceived Characteristics of Innovations scale, Box 4.2, page 86) might have been more appropriate in the Marshall study. We found very few studies that had used such a scale in a health care setting. Lee[296] and colleagues used this scale to survey a total of 115 health professionals and managers who were being trained in the use of a new electronic medical record (EMR); they describe significant differences between professional groups in different dimensions of the scale (e.g. physicians rated the likely impact of the EMR on their image as considerably lower than did administrators). However, this study had a major methodological weakness in that it did not study the actual adoption of the EMR by the individuals surveyed, but merely asked their intentions. We mention this study here despite its limitations because Lee's[296] survey methodology, if accompanied by a longitudinal follow-up of adoption practices in different groups, could potentially identify specific barriers

*This notion of 'audience segmentation' is discussed further in relation to dissemination of innovations in Section 6.6 (page 131).

to adoption of ICT innovations by health care staff in an organisational setting.

Grilli and Lomas undertook a review of the literature on guideline implementation and found 23 eligible studies. Each author independently graded each guideline according to three of Rogers' six attributes (see Box 4.1) – complexity, trialability and observability (presumably because these were the most inherent to the innovation and could reasonably be estimated by a third party, whereas relative advantage, compatibility and re-invention would require additional research into the perceptions of potential users). They found that recommendations concerning procedures with high complexity had lower compliance rates than those low on complexity (41.9% vs 55.9%; $p = 0.05$), and those judged to be high on trialability had higher compliance rates than those low on trialability (55.6% vs 36.8%; $p = 0.03$). Overall, the three attributes accounted for 47% of the observed variability in compliance rates with clinical guidelines.

A more recent study by Dobbins *et al.*[42] considered a similar question in relation to systematic reviews. They surveyed 147 public health decision-makers and asked a number of questions about factors that might influence self-reported use of systematic reviews. Hence, their study had the advantage that attributes were derived from perceptions of potential adopters rather than from evaluation by researchers, but it had the disadvantage of relying on self-reports of behaviour. Perceived relative advantage was not an independent predictor of use, but perceived ease of use was (perhaps 'relative advantage' was misinterpreted by participants as implying that the review reported positive rather than negative findings, rather than that it had an advantage over other forms of evidence). A smaller (and less methodologically robust) survey of 51 public health nurses identified the *complexity* of guidelines as the only one of Rogers' five core attributes associated with self-reported adoption, but free-text responses suggested two additional perceived constraints: competing agency demands and lack of time – neither of which are, of course, attributes of the innovation but both of which are important adopter characteristics of health service staff.[297]

There is a large and growing 'opinion' literature on clinical guidelines, which we have not covered in detail here since with few exceptions[34,37] the associations made by authors tend to be speculative. 'Non-adoption' of guidelines by clinicians (even when linked to educational initiatives and incentives) is explained in terms of Rogers' key attributes:

(1) The perceived relative advantage of evidence from clinical trials is often hard to discern (indeed, new evidence generally makes work for practitioners who have to seek it out and interpret it).

(2) The evidence is rarely simple (indeed, its interpretation requires skills of critical appraisal that most clinicians do not have and its validity is very often contested by experts in the field).

(3) Recommendations are often perceived as incompatible with prevailing practice and values.

(4) Many recommendations turn out to require unforeseen changes in systems and ways of working (e.g. a patient placed on warfarin will require regular blood tests, which may require a hospital referral), and hence are not perceived as easily trialable.

(5) The perceived observability of much evidence is low (at the level of the individual patient the immediate benefit may be marginal and the long-term benefit not apparent to either patient or clinician).

(6) The potential for reinvention of most clinical guidelines is low – there is little or no scope built into the guideline for local adaptation.

Foy *et al.*[34] undertook a prospective study of the attributes of 42 clinical practice recommendations in gynaecology. They developed and pre-tested (on a sample of experts) 13 attributes of the recommendations (common issue, precisely described, compatible with clinicians' current norms and values, essential to the recommendations as a whole, based on sound evidence, fits patient expectations, observable, requires organisational change, requires changed routines, high profile, complex, trialable, requires new knowledge or skills). Using a panel of seven expert gynaecologists, they rated the 42 recommendations using a modified RAND (structured consensus) method. They then measured two aspects of actual clinical practice: compliance with the recommendation and extent of change following audit and feedback, as measured by independent analysis of 4644 patient records. They found that recommendations that were compatible with clinician values and not requiring changes to fixed routines were associated with greater compliance at baseline and follow-up. Those that were incompatible with clinician values were associated with lower initial compliance but with greater *change* following audit and feedback. The authors concluded that the notion of 'adoption of the innovation' should be unpacked to distinguish between initial compliance and propensity to change, and they note that the widely cited attribute of incompatibility with norms and values appears to be amendable to the intervention of audit and feedback.

In a study in the Netherlands, Dirksen *et al.* looked at six surgical endoscopic procedures: appendicectomy, cholecystectomy, thorax operations, hernia, Nissan fundoplication and large bowel resection. The authors surveyed 138 surgeons and looked at their perceptions of three attributes of the procedure ('extra benefit', 'surgical technique', 'nature of the technology'); six attributes of the system context ('budget', 'patient demand', 'planning/logistics', 'reimbursement', 'support industry', and 'service industry'), three social influence factors ([learnt about the procedure at a] 'training/course', [learnt about the procedure at a] 'conference', [learnt about the procedure through] 'media'), and one attribute of the wider environment ('competition').

The results showed that different endoscopic procedures had widely different adoption patterns, and different attributes had different impact depending on the procedure. Overall, four attributes distinguished between adopters and non-adopters of surgical innovations: 'extra benefit', 'nature of the technology', 'surgical technique' and 'conference'. Perceived 'extra benefit' had an influence earlier in the adoption process and was considered a sine qua non.

The Dirksen study was a retrospective attribution study whose predictive power is therefore weak. All the hypothesised mediators and moderators were measured only in terms of the surgeons' subjective perceptions; no objective measures of costs, patient demand and so on were made. Nevertheless, the finding that few if any attributes consistently apply across different organisational innovations is important and consistent with other studies. The finding that attributes of innovations are evaluated *sequentially rather than concurrently* (specifically, that innovations without any perceived advantage may not be evaluated further) is also important and is supported by empirical studies from the wider literature.*

Meyer *et al.* report a fascinating study of the attempted introduction of three preventive health innovations in the American Cancer Information Service (CIS) – an interorganisational network of researchers and practitioners committed to providing high-quality, free cancer information to the public. Most of the network's activity was providing telephone advice and follow-up information to people who called a helpline number. Three organisation-level innovations were studied:

(1) proactive counselling about mammography (inviting women who called about something else to attend for a routine mammogram);

(2) 'cold-calling' under-represented groups (ethnic minorities and the poor) and offering a free mammogram; and

(3) provision of culturally congruent anti-smoking information to African-American smokers and recent quitters.

Various CIS staff, mostly project directors and senior managers, were sent a questionnaire. Response rate was excellent (96%), and sophisticated factor analysis was undertaken to refine the instrument. Attributes tested were relative advantage, compatibility, complexity, trialability, observability, adaptability (similar to capacity for reinvention), riskiness and acceptance.

---

*For example, Vollink *et al.* (2002) studied the adoption of four different energy conservation measures in the energy industry in relation to four of Rogers' classic attributes (relative advantage, compatibility, complexity and trialability). As in the Dirkson study, these authors found that for each of the different innovations there was a *different relationship* between the perceived attributes and intention to adopt. In two of the four, if perceived relative advantage was low, the respondent did not pursue evaluation of attributes further.[298]

The different projects were differently perceived in terms of the attributes tested. The authors' hypothesis had been that projects (1) and (3) would be perceived as less risky, more acceptable, and more compatible with staff values and ways of working, since the 'front line' of the CIS network is designed as a call centre system, and staff had never previously been asked to cold-call members of the public. Their data broadly confirmed this hypothesis, but their instrument for compatibility proved unreliable. They also showed that different professional groups perceived the attributes of the different projects differently, again confirming that attributes of complex innovations are not fixed and consistent, even within the same organisation or project. Interestingly, they showed no significant association between either trialability or observability and adoption, perhaps because the innovations were presented to staff as large-scale projects that had been strategically selected to go ahead across a wide network of participating organisations.*

Aubert and Hamel[35] studied the use of a 'smart card' patient-held record in a large pilot study in Canadian ambulatory care involving 299 health professionals and 7248 service users. They used three items (compatibility, relative advantage, trialability) from Rogers' attributes (Box 4.1) and a further four (ease of use, image, usefulness, voluntariness) from the Perceived Characteristics of Innovations scale (Box 4.2, page 86) plus several new constructs including information ('perception of the availability, quality and value of the information produced by the innovation'); involvement ('mechanisms through which an individual feels part of the development, design or implementation process of an innovation'); mandatoriness (service users must use the card to gain reimbursement from insurance); membership (sense of belonging to the professional association that uses the smart card); quality of support ('perception of accessibility, rapidity, and how the support is provided'); satisfaction (fulfilment of expectations about the innovation); and visibility (seeing others using the innovation).

They developed a questionnaire based on these constructs and sent it to two groups of professionals – 287 who had been in the pilot study of the smart card, and 2000 who had not. In addition, face-to-face interviews were held with 123 service users who had used the smart card for their own health care during the pilot year. The response rates of the two professional groups were 66% and 26%, respectively (that of the users was not stated). Only the results of the first group (professionals who had used the card) are reported here since these were relevant to our own research question. Five attributes were found to be significantly associated with self-reported use of the smart card – ease of use ($r = 0.38$); compatibility ($r = 0.36$); perceived quality of support ($r = 0.36$); voluntariness ($r = 0.32$);† and information ($r = 0.28$). The smart card innovation was complex in that it required adoption by two different groups (professionals and clients) at once. This is addressed (somewhat speculatively) by the authors in their discussion.[35] Note that there was a possible Hawthorne effect since respondents were part of a high-profile pilot study that had ended by the time they completed the questionnaires for this study.

In a study of the introduction of an IT system for human resource management, Yetton *et al.* tested the hypothesis that perceived attributes of innovation (task relevance and task usefulness) and characteristics of the individual adopter (innovativeness, skill, performance) would be more important influences on adoption than organisational support (management urging, management support, physical access, training and documentation) or informal support (grapevine, network). They justified this prediction on the grounds that the particular innovation had an impact at the level of the individual rather than the group or team. The results strongly supported their hypothesis: the only organisational variable to show significant association with adoption in the multiple regression model was physical access to the innovation; management urging or support had no impact, and neither did informal support through 'grapevine' or networks.

*See Section 5.2 (page 103), in which we introduce the notion of collective, authoritative and contingent adoption decisions in organisations, all of which occur at a level above that of the individual adopter.

†That is, professionals were significantly *more* likely to use the smart card if they perceived its use to be voluntary.

The Yetton *et al.* study showed that even in the organisational setting, attributes of innovations are powerful predictors of adoption, and it raises interesting (and as-yet untested) hypotheses about different implementation approaches for different innovations (i.e. individual approaches for innovations that impact on the individual; team-based implementation for innovations that impact on teams and so on).

Overall, the attribution studies that focused on individual adoption decisions for health service innovations suggest that such innovations have adoption characteristics very similar to those studied in the wider literature – i.e. simple innovations that are perceived to have a clear advantage over what they are intended to replace, which are compatible with the adopter's values, which are easy to use and trialable on a limited basis, which do not require major changes in the organisation or in personal routines, and whose impact is observable, are more likely to be adopted. The empirical studies discussed also suggest that different adopters (and adopter groups – such as different professions) perceive innovations differently. One tentative conclusion from these studies is that we should not think of attributes as fixed qualities of the innovation, but recognise that attributes are primarily *perceptions* of the individual (and hence, potentially amenable to change), as pointed out by Rogers. Another important conclusion is that attributes seem to have a sequential rather than concurrent impact on the adoption decision – in particular, if no relative advantage is perceived, the potential adopter may not explore any of the other attributes.

4.4 Limitations of conventional attribution constructs for studying adoption in organisational settings

The above studies raise a number of important epistemological questions* about the validity and usefulness of the concept of 'attributes of innovations' when considered in an organisational setting. We consider these below in relation to the attributes listed in Boxes 4.1 (page 84) and 4.2 (page 86).

Relative advantage is traditionally defined as 'the extent to which an innovation is perceived as being better than the idea it supersedes'.[3] However, as Tornatzky and Klein point out, relative advantage ('being better') is an ambiguous notion for organisational innovations. Rogers and Shoemaker[177] suggested expressing relative advantage in terms of 'economic profitability', but an alternative conception is that the nature of the innovation will in part determine what counts as relative advantage in that particular case. In other words, the *definition* of the attribute must change with the nature of the innovation and who within the organisation is adopting it.

Whilst an innovation's relative advantage is not always (or indeed, usually) an economic one, it is often helpful to consider the notion of 'costs' versus 'benefits' to the different stakeholder groups (individual adopters within the organisation, the organisation itself, and the clients it serves).† Note also that the same innovation might be advantageous to one stakeholder and disadvantageous to another in the same organisation, leading to a highly complex (and quite possibly unmeasurable) set of opposing forces. Inexpensive health care innovations have sometimes, somewhat surprisingly, diffused less rapidly and less extensively than high-cost, high-technology ones (see, for example Denis *et al.*[33]). The sub-dimensions of relative advantage that might explain this might include: its degree of economic profitability; low *initial* cost; a decrease in discomfort; social prestige; savings in time and effort; and the immediacy of the reward.[43] This last factor explains in part why preventive innovations generally have an especially low rate of adoption. As Adler *et al.*[43] point out (page 22):

> ... innovations that put additional cognitive or economic burdens on professionals will not diffuse effectively unless they afford sufficient

*That is, questions about the nature of knowledge and the extent (therefore) to which we can trust the findings of particular study designs.

†See, for example, the discussion on marketing in Section 3.5 (page 56).

> compensating advantages. Relative advantage helps explain why, for example, so many areas of medicine are under-computerised ... Moreover, diffusion is considerably slowed if it requires learning different kinds of skills. Innovations in hospital practice such as multidisciplinary care teams involve managerial skills for which medical professionals have not been trained. To the extent that the acquisition of these new kinds of skills is more costly in time and resources than the acquisition of new clinical skills, diffusion will be further slowed.*

Wejnert[41] suggests that the diffusion of innovations in professional settings (e.g. health care) will be less sensitive to the innovation's cost advantages for the professional, and more sensitive to (perceived) quality advantages for the patient/client. However, despite looking explicitly for studies exploring these distinctions in perceptions of relative advantage in different members of organisations, we were unable to find any.

There is also the notion that 'relative advantage' as defined by stakeholders outside the organisation can be a driving force for change within the organisation. Adler *et al.*, for example, suggest that, in the health care context,

> under environmental pressure to adopt innovations that offer important advantages to clients and other stakeholders but are less compatible with traditional professional norms, both professional norms and the modus operandi of professional organisations will evolve to facilitate diffusion.

Again, this is an enticing hypothesis that calls for further empirical testing.

The *compatibility* of an innovation has been defined as 'the degree to which an innovation is consistent with the existing values, past experiences and needs of a potential adopter'[3] – and hence has many parallels with the organisational construct of congruence. Rogers suggested that an innovation can be compatible or incompatible with

(1) a person's sociocultural values and beliefs,
(2) previously introduced ideas, or
(3) a client's needs for the innovation.

Psychological theories suggest that employees who perceive the use of an innovation to be congruent with their values are likely to be committed and enthusiastic in their innovation use. In the words of Strang and Soule[124] (page 278):

> Practices that accord with cultural understandings of appropriate and effective action tend to diffuse more quickly than those that do not.

But in an organisational context there is the additional dimension of compatibility with the *organisation's* values, routines, procedures and practices. Klein and Sorra[237] introduce the notion of innovation–values fit:

> The construct of innovation–values fit thus directs researchers to look beyond an organisation's global implementation policies and practices and to consider the extent to which a given innovation is perceived by targeted users to clash or coincide with their organisational and group values.

A contemporary hypothesis on compatibility (and one that has considerable face validity) is that the more an innovation can integrate and coexist with technologies and social patterns already in place in an organisation, the greater its prospects for innovation and diffusion.[299] Klein and Sorra[237] suggest that implementation effectiveness – the consistency and quality of targeted organisational members' use of an innovation – is a function of:

(1) the strength of an organisation's climate for the implementation of that innovation and
(2) the fit of that innovation to targeted users' values.

Thus, in relation to organisational innovations, we should cease to think of compatibility as a fixed (or measurable) attribute of the innovation, and construct instead in terms of the *fit between the*

*For a conceptual model of innovations in service delivery and organisation that takes account of factors such as training needs of staff, see the article by Denis *et al.*,[33] which is described and discussed in Section 4.3 (page 90).

innovation and the organisation (especially the latter's climate and context). The notion of organisational fit is considered in more detail in Section 7.4 (page 141).

Complexity was defined by Rogers as 'the degree to which an innovation is perceived as relatively difficult to understand and use'. He noted – somewhat surprisingly perhaps – that the research evidence supporting an association between complexity and innovation adoption is not conclusive.[3] It is, however, widely believed that the simpler the innovation the more likely it is to be adopted.[300] An alternative definition of complexity, perhaps especially relevant to complex organisational innovations, is the number of dimensions that the potential individual adopter has to evaluate before making the adoption decision.[292]

Van de Ven,[123] who led one of the largest ever research programmes into diffusion of innovations (see Section 3.11, page 69), exhorted researchers to take account of indirect evidence from psychological research (page 594)*:

> Much of the folklore and applied literature on the management of innovation has ignored the research by cognitive psychologists and social-psychologists about the limited capacity of human beings to handle complexity and maintain attention.

An important distinction relevant to the organisational setting is the difference between the complexity of the innovation and the complexity of its implementation.[301] An innovation might be intrinsically simple (e.g. a new system for summoning patients in a GP surgery, in which the name of the patient lights up when the GP presses the buzzer) but complex to implement (since every patient will need to be trained to look for the stimulus and respond appropriately to it). Implementation complexity is discussed further in Chapter 8.

Trialability was defined by Rogers and Shoemaker[177] as 'the degree to which an innovation may be experimented with on a limited basis'. Others, somewhat confusingly, have used an alternative definition: the ability to refine, elaborate, and modify an innovation according to the needs and objectives of the implementor[62,227,302] – a definition that aligns with Rogers' concept of *re-invention*. It is probably no accident that these concepts have been conflated by organisational researchers, since the 'trialing' of innovations at the organisational level tends to go hand in hand with their adaptation to context – i.e. their re-invention. Thus, this is yet another example of a construct that is relatively simple and consistent when applied to individual adoption becoming complex and contested when applied in the organisational setting.

Observability was defined by Rogers[3] as 'the extent to which results of an innovation are visible to others' (assuming, presumably, that the results are seen as positive). The more visible the results of an innovation, the more likely the innovation will be quickly adopted and implemented. But again when transferred to an organisational context this begs the question of observability *to whom*. Meyer and Goes[38] defined observability as 'the degree to which the results of using the innovation are visible to organisational members and external constituents'. But few things in organisations are visible to everyone, and a more useful concept might arguably be the extent to which the impact of innovations can be *made* observable to key stakeholders and decision-makers through demonstration projects and similar initiatives. Incidentally, Damanpour and Gopalakrishnan[130] have shown that product innovations are more adoptable than process innovations because the former are more observable, although as we pointed out in Chapter 1, the product–process distinction is not an especially helpful one in relation to health service innovations.

As Eveland[50] has commented:

*We became aware as we worked through this review that a number of research traditions within mainstream cognitive psychology would have important messages for our own research question, and we recommend that a separate systematic review be commissioned on this.

> By the mid-1970s, we had come to see that this approach [the search for 'key attributes' of innovations that would make them more generically 'adoptable'] terminally complicated by differences in perceptions, or ... by varying metaphors for the new ideas.

Another commentator, Dearing,[48] highlights the conceptual limitations of the notion of attributes:

> Conceptualizing innovations as 'having' attributes is a common heuristic that people employ when they are judging something new. Yet this tendency serves to obscure the importance of human perception in the diffusion of innovations. What is new to one person may be 'old' to another. ... Moreover, the decision to adopt and/or use the innovation is based on individual perceptions of the innovation's worth relative to other ways of accomplishing the same goal. What is easy for one person to use may be exceedingly difficult for another'.

Leonard-Barton and Sinha[303] suggest that the notion of *reinvention* (in which the innovation is modified to fit the organisation) should be replaced by one of mutual adaptation (i.e. the degree to which users refine a system – both the innovation and the context in which it is used – to meet their particular needs). Denis *et al.* address the same notion (the need for mutual adaptation) when they talk about complex service innovations having fuzzy boundaries – i.e. a 'soft periphery' of organisational infrastructure and systems needed to make the 'core' innovation work effectively (see Fig. 5.4, page 112). A closely related concept, innovation–system fit, is explored further in Chapter 9.

In summary, the superficial face validity, conceptual independence, and stability of the innovation attributes set out in Boxes 4.1 and 4.2 have not been borne out by empirical studies of organisational innovations in the health care setting. This may be due to the fact that many studies were small, parochial and preliminary in scope, but it may also be because organisational innovations have additional issues to factor into the picture – most notably that adopters are not homogeneous in their perceptions, that the individual adopter is not the only unit of analysis to consider, and that the organisation may need to adapt as well as (or instead of) the innovation being 'reinvented'. The remainder of this section describes work undertaken since the 1980s that has moved the focus of analysis from the innovation itself to the innovation-in-use in the organisational context.

4.5 Attributes of innovations in the organisational context

In the early days of this review, we loosely – and naively – described our goal as 'to find out what features we might build into innovations to make them spread more effectively'. We can now confidently state that any such search is likely to prove fruitless, since the very notion of static and endurable attributes of innovations in the organisational setting is inherently flawed. Downs and Mohr[293] concluded in a 1975 review that characteristics of the innovation and the adopting agency cannot be studied separately, and that a simple checklist of 'adoptability features' would be meaningless for predicting the adoption (and even more so, the implementation) of organisational innovations. With the benefit of a further generation of empirical studies, we (along with others[41,174]) strongly concur with this early insight. Organisational theorists such as Becker,[52] Kaluzny[304] and Mohr,[305] drawing on contingency theory, have emphasised the need to focus not merely on the attributes of the innovation but also on perceptions of its *compatibility with the institution or environment* into which it was being introduced (see Fennell and Warnecke[36] for a summary), again emphasising that it is not fixed attributes of either the innovation or the organisation that matter, but the fit between them.

Whereas the attributes discussed in earlier sections have related entirely or mostly to the innovation, a set of 'operational' attributes* have

*This is not a term (nor indeed a distinction) that has previously been used explicitly in the literature, but we propose it as an important aspect to consider in relation to innovations in service delivery and organisation.

emerged that relate to the interaction between the innovation and a particular task and context.

Yetton has suggested that the attributes of innovations-in-use can be operationalised by asking two questions: how relevant is the innovation to a particular task or process, and by how much (if at all) does it improve performance on that task? Agarwal *et al.*,[301] taking a similar pragmatic focus, suggests that technological innovations have three key operational attributes – transferability, implementation complexity and divisibility (see Box 4.2, page 86, for definitions).

Finally the knowledge utilisation literature (see Section 3.13, page 70) makes clear that the 'attributes' of a complex innovation crucially include the nature of the knowledge required to use it. In particular, an innovation may include a substantial element of know-how that is not intrinsic to it (and therefore not transferred or diffused with it, or even codifiable and transferable). As explained in Section 3.13, the more tacit and uncodified the innovation, the more slowly it will diffuse and the more it will require hands-on practice and face-to-face interaction. O'Neill *et al.*[44] expresses this well (page 108):

> Where knowledge is tacit, strategies will not travel well ... visible elements of the strategy may travel across organisational borders, but the embedded context of the innovation stays with the originator.

This notion of the 'tacitness' of an innovation's knowledge is related to both the complexity and observability of the innovation, and to what others have termed 'communicability'.[62,301] Tornatzky and Klein considered this attribute in their 1982 meta-analysis (see Section 4.2, page 87), but at the time it was still seen as a construct intrinsic to the innovation rather than contingent on the context, setting, actors and so on. Rothman[294] (page 441) suggested a similar attribute, which he defined as 'the degree to which aspects of an innovation may be conveyed to adopters'.

Adler *et al.* suggest that in the health care context, innovations will diffuse relatively more easily among professionals than among non-professionals because of professionals' relatively codified knowledge base. Diffusion effectiveness will vary between professions as a function of the degree of codification:

> Anaesthesiology is one medical discipline that has codified a relatively high proportion of its core knowledge, and this codification has stimulated the diffusion of quality-related innovations. Similarly, oncology relies to a relatively great extent on treatment protocols, and new cancer treatments therefore diffuse faster than in specialties where knowledge is more exclusively tacit.[43]

Box 4.3 Some operational attributes of organisational innovations (i.e. those relating to the innovation-in-use and the moderating effect of organisational context).[39,301,306,307]

(1) *Task relevance* (the extent to which the innovation is relevant to the performance of the end-user's task).
(2) *Task usefulness* (the extent to which the innovation contributes to improvement in task performance).
(3) *Transferability* – comprising
  (a) *operational feasibility* (the extent to which it has been or can be proved feasible in an operational setting) and
  (b) *communicability* (the degree to which its underlying operating and scientific principles can be communicated to people other than developers).
(4) *Implementation complexity* (the number of response barriers that must be overcome for the technology to be successfully implemented).
(5) *Divisibility* (the extent to which it can be partitioned into modules to allow for its adoption on an incremental basis).
(6) *Nature of the knowledge* required to use it
  (a) *tacit–explicit* (extent to which it can be codified);
  (b) *systemic–autonomous* (extent to which stands independent of other systems in the organisation); and
  (c) *simple–complex* (see definition of complexity, Box 4.1).
(7) *Compatibility* with institutional norms and procedures.

This raises interesting issues around the clinical protocol as an innovation, which are discussed further in relation to one of our case studies (integrated care pathways) in Section 10.2 (page 202). The attributes of innovations-in-use and in relation to a particular organisational context are summarised in Box 4.3. Because these cannot be considered separately from the use of the innovation in a particular context, we consider them in Chapter 5, which covers adopters and adoption.

In conclusion, empirical research that addresses the question 'What makes an innovation more likely to get adopted?' has until fairly recently focused largely on attribution studies that measure the *association* between explicit and predefined variables and the event of adoption or extent of assimilation. Unlike the Perceived Characteristics of Innovations Scale (Box 4.2, page 86), the list in Box 4.3 was compiled from various sources rather than developed empirically. It is therefore unlikely to be either comprehensive or internally coherent (e.g. 'communicability' probably overlaps with the tacit–explicit dimension of knowledge needed to use it). Indeed, almost every contemporary study of organisational innovation introduces at least one new construct to try to capture the innovation–context interaction. We have boxed together these various examples of 'second-generation attributes' to indicate the increasing complexity of the field and the general focus of new research into innovation attributes, and this list should be interpreted in the light of this.

A more recent (and currently very sparse) stream of research, discussed in Chapters 5 and 9, has begun to make use of a range of qualitative methods, notably ethnographic observation and cross-case analysis, to explore the detailed and complex interaction of multiple variables, especially with respect to the operational attributes of the innovation-in-use.

Chapter 5
Adopters and adoption

Key points

1. This chapter addresses the characteristics of individuals who adopt innovations (or fail to adopt them), and also considers research studies of the adoption of innovations in health service organisations. The empirical literature on adopters and adoption is less extensive than that on innovations. The literature on the adoption (or assimilation) process for complex innovations in health care organisations is extremely sparse, but there are some recent high-quality studies.

2. 'Adopter categories' (innovator, early adopter, laggard and so on) are simplistic and value-laden terms that are widely misapplied as explanatory variables. They have never been rigorously tested in relation to service sector innovations and should not be applied in this context. Individual personality traits and other psychological variables (e.g. locus of control) are undoubtedly important in the adoption of organisational innovations and deserve further exploration, but have not been covered in this review.

3. Adoption by an individual in an organisation is a complex process involving several stages. Different concerns dominate at different stages – from an initial focus on information seeking (the nature of the innovation, personal costs and benefits) through task management (how to use it to do a job) to evaluation of consequences, collaboration and adaptation.

4. As Chapter 4 showed, attributes of the innovation (relative advantage, compatibility with individual values and practices, complexity and so on) are critically important in the organisational setting. However, these attributes usually interact in a complex (and sometimes unpredictable) way with adopter and organisational variables.

5. Socially-driven perceptions about 'expected behaviour of someone in my role' may be a more powerful influence on adoption than more rational and logical processes.

6. Different actors attribute different meanings to innovations, and this can inhibit adoption; conversely, initiatives to develop and negotiate shared meanings are associated with greater implementation success.

7. Adoption (assimilation) in organisations is a highly complex and difficult-to-research process involving multiple decisions by multiple actors. Barriers to adoption often occur at several levels and influence both one another and the overall innovation capacity of the system. Except in a minority of circumstances, organisations should not be thought of as rational decision-making machines that move sequentially through an ordered process of awareness–evaluation–adoption–implementation. Rather, the assimilation process should be recognised as complex, iterative, and frequently beset by shocks, setbacks and surprises.

8. The systematic study of non-adoption (and resistance to adoption) may be as crucial as the study of adoption, but is as yet a largely unexplored field.

5.1 Characteristics of adopters: background literature

Adoption was defined on page 28. Innovations are, in general, easier to study than the people who adopt them. As Wejnert[41] has observed (page 320):

> Most accounts of diffusion have focused on the sources and nature of information about an innovation that are available to an actor. What has received much less attention in diffusion research is the actor, per se, as an important contributor to the diffusion process.

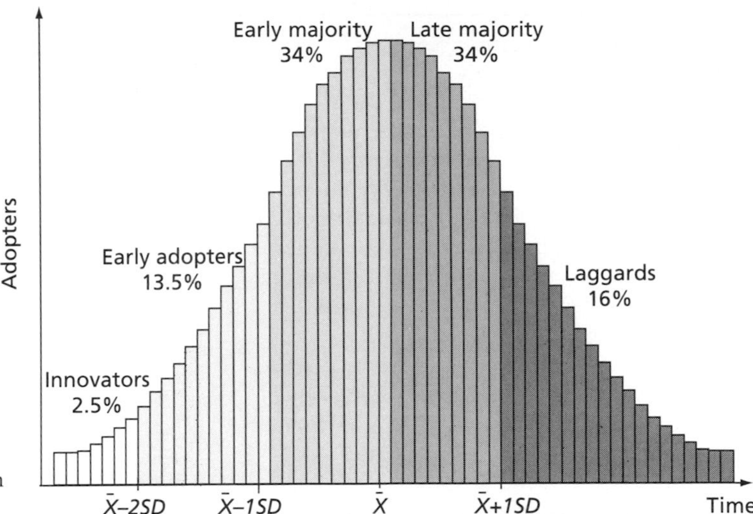

Fig. 5.1 Distribution of new adopters of an innovation against time.*

As shown in Fig. 5.1, and as explained in detail in Rogers,[3] the early sociologists developed standard nomenclature to delineate those individuals who are more than two standard deviations earlier than the mean in adopting an innovation ('innovators' comprising 2.5% of the population), those between two and one standard deviation earlier ('early adopters'; 13.5%), those with one standard deviation on either side of the mean ('early majority' and 'late majority' respectively; 34% each), and those beyond one standard deviation from the mean ('laggards'; 16%).

It is important to note that categories such as 'early adopter' are thus not fixed personality traits of individuals but are mathematically defined cut-offs for the adopters of any particular innovation by a particular population. Early empirical work by rural sociologists (see Section 3.2, page 51, for selected examples and Rogers[3] for an in-depth account) appeared to demonstrate that early adopters consistently shared a number of positive characteristics: they tended to be better off, better educated, more cosmopolitan (as measured, for example, by the frequency of visits to big cities) and had wider social networks. This led to assumptions about the underlying personality traits of the different categories, and this in turn led to different recommendations for marketing innovations (Boxes 5.1 and 5.2).

Because of the constraints of this project, we have not attempted to verify the empirical studies underpinning the recommendations set out in this section (which are derived from market research into the adopters of commercial and technical products). We have included them chiefly to illustrate the 'conventional wisdom' about individual adopter categories, and we caution against their simplistic application in the very different context of a service-sector organisation.

In his book *Crossing the Chasm*, and drawing on a vast literature of empirical market research (perhaps of variable quality), Moore[308] argues that early adopters of high-technology innovations are fundamentally different from later adopters (indeed, that there is a measurable gap, known as 'Moore's chasm', between them), and that persuading the latter to adopt a new technology requires a shift from product-centred values ('fastest/smallest/lightest, most elegant, price, unique functionality', which plays to the individual's desire to be at the cutting edge of technological innovation) to market-centric values ('largest installed base, warranty and service, system integration, training and

*This figure is modelled on the same hypothetical data as Fig. 1.1 (page 21) in Chapter 1. The curve shows the raw data on *new* adopters against time whereas Fig. 1.1 shows the cumulative numbers.

Box 5.1 Marketing strategies suggested for different adopter categories.[3]

- *Innovators* are venturesome information-seekers with a high degree of mass media exposure and wide social networks. They can cope with a higher degree of uncertainty about an innovation than other adopter categories. Mass media channels often work well for them. But because they are ahead of the norm, few others copy them.
- *Early adopters* are open to ideas and active experimenters. They tend to be technology-focused and to seek information. They are self-sufficient and respond well to printed information.
- *Early and late majority* generally require a good deal of personalised information and support (especially supervised trial and error) before adopting, but they are often influential on peers (i.e. they may be opinion leaders). They are risk averse and seek tested applications of proven value.
- *Laggards* have lower social status, sparse social networks and the lowest exposure to mass media; they tend to learn about innovations from interpersonal channels, especially trusted peers.

Box 5.2 Marketing strategies suggested for different adopter categories in the adoption of high-technology innovations.[308]

- *Technology's innovators*: Technology is a central interest in their lives, regardless of its function; they are less interested in the application than in the technology; they are intrigued by any fundamental technology advance; they often buy just for the pleasure of exploring the new advance.
- *Technology's early adopters*: They are more interested in applications than in technologies per se; they easily appreciate the benefits of new technology. They are visionaries (intuitive, contrary, breaking away from the pack; they take risks, are motivated by future opportunities, and see what is possible).
- *Technology's early majority*: They are driven by a sense of practicality (e.g. they know that many new inventions end up as passing fads); they take a 'wait and see' approach and want to see well-established references before buying. They are pragmatists (analytic, conformist, manage risks, motivated by present problems, pursue what is probable).
- *Technology's late majority*: They share all the concerns of the early majority but are much less comfortable with the technology, so tend to wait until the technology is an established standard before buying; they seek a high level of support and always buy from established companies.
- *Technology's laggards*: They tend not to want anything to do with new technology. They will buy a technology product only when it is buried inside another product (e.g. microprocessors in cars); they are generally considered not worth pursuing by technology marketing firms.

support' and so on, which plays to the later adopters' need for support and desire for conformity).* Thus, Moore suggests that whereas innovators and early adopters make their adoption decision on the product, most people do so on the basis of the *augmented* product.

The widely cited lists of adopter characteristics (which as Boxes 5.1 and 5.2 illustrate are somewhat stereotypical and value-laden, and which are popular with the marketing industry) have rarely been empirically tested in prospective studies outside the commercial market. We found no prospective studies of any hypothesised characteristics of adopter categories in the organisational setting. Arguably, many of these categories are little more than the result of deterministic research designs. Similar criticisms can be made of the concept of fixed adopter characteristics as have been made of the concept of fixed attributes of the innovation: in reality, decisions about adopting complex innovations (and especially innovations whose adoption involves groups, teams and organisations) are influenced to a large extent by contextual judgement – most crucially, on whether the innovation is of any advantage or use to a particular individual in a particular circumstance. As Wejnert[41] observes (page 303):

*This notion of the augmented product aligns with the notion of linkage and outreach support discussed in Section 9.6 (page 191).

> [W]hether an innovation is considered for adoption by an individual actor is strongly determined by compatibility between the characteristics of an innovation and the needs of an actor.

It is beyond the scope of this book to explore the psychological antecedents of the adoption decision in any detail (these are covered in the psychological literature – see, for example, Furnham[309]), but Box 5.3 shows some worth considering. The empirical studies on adoption set out in Section 5.2 address various psychological antecedents, which are discussed in the text. Whereas personality traits are by definition highly resistant to change, perceptions and motivation can often be influenced by external factors. For example, if an individual perceives a high degree of risk around an innovation he or she will be reluctant to adopt it, but when the apparent familiarity of a new idea is increased, for instance by media information and the opinion of experts, the perception of risk by an adopter is substantially reduced, facilitating adoptive behaviour.[41]

Early work on adopter categories led unwittingly to value judgements about adoption decisions (early adoption is 'good'), but in reality such decisions are influenced to a large extent by situational factors. Perceptions, motivation, values, goals, particular skills (or lack of them) and learning style may all be crucial to the individual adoption decision. Individuals undoubtedly differ by personality traits (e.g. tolerance of uncertainty) likely to influence adoption decisions, and also by such factors as socio-economic status and social networks, but there is no evidence that such characteristics *determine* the rate of adoption, and we should distance ourselves from simplistic explanations of complex phenomena in terms of 'adopter traits'.

Box 5.3 Psychological antecedents of the adoption decision.

- Personality traits (e.g. tolerance of ambiguity)
- Prior knowledge, experience, beliefs, attitudes and perceptions
- Particular concerns about the innovation (see Fig. 5.3)
- Motivation and goals
- Cultural practices and values (generalised, enduring beliefs about the personal and social desirability of modes of conduct or 'end-states' of existence[237])
- Skills
- Learning style

We found a small number of empirical studies that looked at the adoption patterns of health service innovations by individuals. These were mostly concerned with the adoption of evidence-based practice by clinicians (especially the awareness of, and use of, research findings by nurses[310–312]). These studies suggest that psychological antecedents are indeed important determinants of adoption, and that different antecedents have a bearing on different adoption decisions in different contexts. We have not described these studies in detail for three reasons: first, this literature was marginal to our own research question about adoption in organisations; second, most studies were small, parochial (e.g. within a single hospital) and probably of limited transferability; and third, the psychological scales used to measure such characteristics as 'positive attitude to research', 'belief in the value of research', 'organisational support' and so on had not been independently validated. We suspect that the literature on cognitive psychology, adult education, and professional behaviour change will provide important insights into individual adoption decisions, and in our recommendations for further research (Section 11.3, page 225), we suggest more work in this area.

A conceptual model linking the individual's decision to adopt an innovation with wider organisational variables such as training and management support has been proposed by Frambach and Schillewaert.[313] We have adapted their model slightly in Fig. 5.2.

5.2 Adoption as a process: background literature

Before considering the adoption process, it should be noted explicitly that adoption of innovations is, of course, a form of change. An innovation (see definition, page 000) is – or at least, requires – a

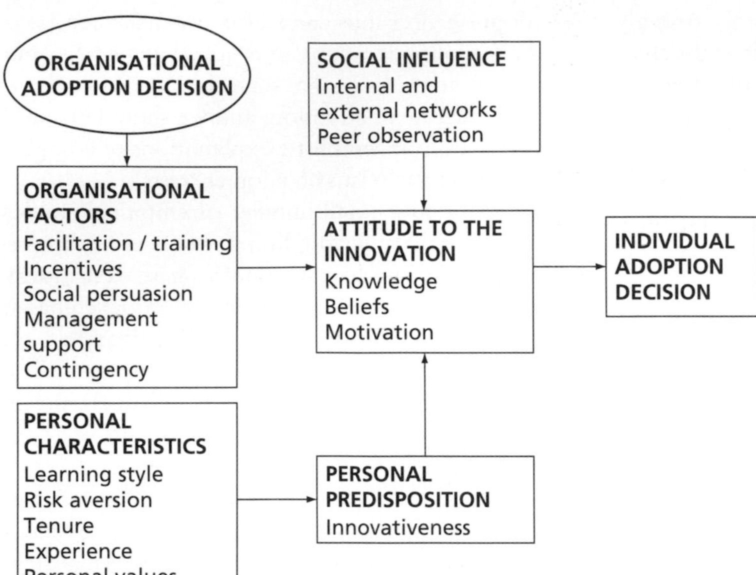

Fig. 5.2 Conceptual model linking organisational and individual adoption decisions (adapted from Frambach and Schillewaert[313]) (for an explanation of 'contingency', see page 105).

change, and resistance to adoption is a particular form of resistance to change. Unsurprisingly, the research literature on adoption (especially in organisations) overlaps conceptually and sometimes empirically with that on change in general – a territory that we defined for purely practical purposes as outside the remit of this review. Nevertheless, those familiar with change management literature will see many parallels between the concepts set out in this section and models of both individual and organisational change (and resistance to change). In some places, we have included selected references to key texts from beyond the innovations literature with which the reader may be familiar.

Although 'adoption' is often treated as an event, research by the early rural sociologists demonstrated that it is usually a lengthy process comprising sequential stages (Box 5.4). Different strategies are generally recommended for individuals at different stages in the adoption process. For example, as discussed in Section 3.5 (page 56) there is considerable empirical evidence that the mass media are particularly effective in creating awareness whereas interpersonal influence is needed at the persuasion stage.

Like many conceptual models developed to explain the adoption of simple innovations like hybrid corn, the 'stages of adoption' model did not prove directly transferable to more complex, organisation-focused and technology-based innovations. The weakness of the model was first demonstrated in educational sociology, when researchers studying the adoption of classroom technologies by teachers recognised that many

Box 5.4 Stages of adoption (first demonstrated by Ryan and Goes[189]).*

(1) Knowledge (awareness of the innovation).
(2) Persuasion (attempting to form favourable or unfavourable attitudes to the innovation).
(3) Decision (engaging in activities that will lead to a choice to either adopt or reject the innovation).
(4) Implementation (putting the innovation to use) or rejection.
(5) Confirmation (seeking reinforcement of the decision by observation of its impact).

*Compare this with Prochaska and DiClemente's[314] transtheoretical model for individual behaviour change (such as giving up smoking), in which the stages are pre-contemplation, contemplation, implementation and maintenance.

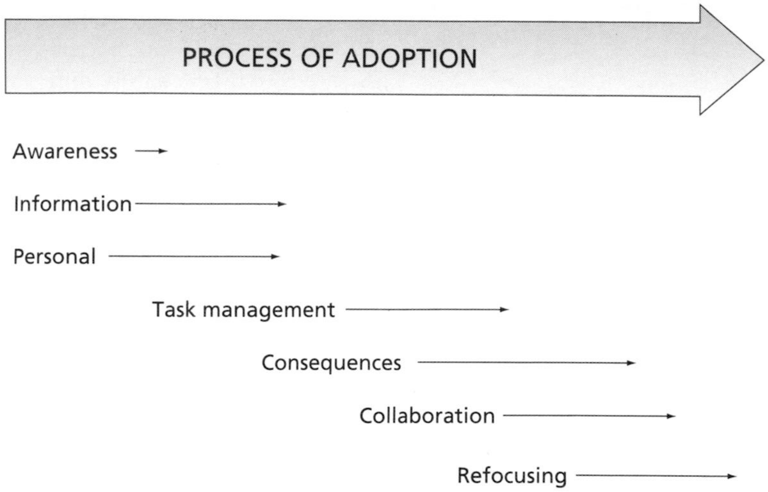

Fig. 5.3 Hall and Hord's[46] concerns-based adoption model, showing changing concerns during the process of adoption of a technology.

(probably most) technologies were not adopted to anywhere like their full potential.*

Educational researchers initially couched the problem in terms of a knowledge gap: teachers needed to be supplied with more knowledge about innovations (this approach has uncanny parallels with early writing on implementing EBM, as Section 3.9, page 64, discusses). But as the psychological basis of the adoption of complex innovations became better understood, more sophisticated models were developed, most notably Hall and Hord's[46,318] CBAM.

Hall and Hord[46] defined concerns as

> [T]he composite representation of the feelings, preoccupation, thought, and consideration given to a particular issue or task. Depending on their personal make-up, knowledge, and experience, each person perceives and mentally contends with a given issue differentially; thus there are different kinds of concerns.

Their model is shown in Fig. 5.3 and its key features summarised in Box 5.5. Whilst this model was specifically developed in relation to the adoption of innovations, it has a number of close parallels in the general literature on organisational change. See, for example, Connor's[319] model of stages of commitment to change (page 148).

One further dimension of the adoption process is the contingency of the adoption decision. Again, educational sociology was the first research tradition to demonstrate that the choices open to an individual in an organisational context are constrained in various ways – being either collective (everyone in a particular group must decide to adopt or not), authoritative (the individual is told to adopt), or contingent (the individual cannot choose to adopt the innovation until the organisation has sanctioned it).[3] But as the empirical studies in Section 5.3 show,† adoption decisions within organisations can affect individuals in different ways and occur at different stages in the overall assimilation of the innovation within the organisation, and we have not found the collective/authoritative/contingent classification to be widely used in practice.

We identified one interesting paper that addressed the psychological antecedents of *non-adoption*.[47] In an honest and reflective analysis

*For a contemporary example, see the literature on the adoption of Web-based teaching[315–317], but similar slow pace of adoption and low overall coverage has been described for a wide range of technology-based teaching innovations.

†See in particular Meyer and Goes,[38] discussed in Section 5.3.

Box 5.5 Concerns-based adoption model of Hall and Hord.[46,318]

- Adoption is a process rather than an event, and is associated in any individual with a particular pattern of motivations, perceptions, attitudes and feelings.
- Change entails an unfolding of experience and a gradual development of skill and sophistication in the use of an innovation. An individual's concerns tend to develop in a fairly predictable, developmental manner.
- The concerns of non-users of a particular technology generally centre on *awareness* (they do not know that it exists); *information* (they want to know what it does and how to use it); and *personal* (self-concerns – i.e. how adoption would affect them personally).
- Low users (i.e. those who have only recently begun to use the technology, or who use it infrequently) remain concerned about information and self. As use increases, concerns shift to *task management* (how to fit the technology into daily work).
- Experienced users tend to lose these early concerns and become increasingly concerned with *consequences* (intended and unintended impact); *collaboration* (sharing and creating knowledge about the technology with other users); and *refocusing* (adapting the technology to better fit individual and local needs).

of what might be considered a failed project (a large randomised trial comparing a computerised decision support system for end-of-life decisions with conventional decision-making, whose methods and findings are described in detail elsewhere[320]), Lynn *et al.* suggest some reasons why the innovation was not adopted by health professionals and service users and whose impact proved 'completely ineffectual'. They challenge their own initial assumption that the decision to use the innovation would be made on rational grounds. Rather, they suggest, there are established (but unexpressed and largely subconscious) expected patterns of behaviour for both health professionals and relatives in the context of a dying patient – patterns that Lynn *et al.* call 'heuristics' (rules of thumb) or 'default options' (what is usually done). A doctor will tend to follow the heuristic 'I must provide the best treatment for the patient', while a nurse follows a similar but subtly different heuristic ('I must care for the patient') and the relative a different one still ('I must do what any good daughter would do in these circumstances'). In the authors' words:

> When individuals and organisations fulfil identities, they follow rules or procedures that they see as appropriate to the situation in which they find themselves. Neither preferences as they are normally conceived nor expectations of future consequences enter directly into the calculus.[47]

Lynn *et al.* also observed that adoption of the decision support system rested on a number of additional incorrect assumptions: that patients' preferences are stable and expressible (in fact, they are unstable and large inexpressible); that decision opportunities would be recognised in which professional and patient could approach the technology (in fact, this was rarely the case); and that patients would be willing to take responsibility for making a choice (in fact, many were not). In summary, the reflective analysis by Lynn *et al.* provides an important challenge to the assumption that we can explain the psychological antecedents to adoption entirely in terms of rational motives. Although the authors do not make explicit links with the literature on sense-making (Section 3.13, page 70), their findings could be explained using this theoretical model.

5.3 Assimilation of innovations in organisations

If adoption in individuals is a complex process, adoption of an innovation by an organisation is necessarily more complex still. Indeed, the term 'adoption' is probably misleading, and we prefer Meyer and Goes' term 'assimilation' (see Box 5.6) because it better reflects the complex adjustments that are often needed in the organisational setting. There is almost invariably a formal decision-making process at the organisational level, an evaluation phase or phases, and planned and sustained efforts at implementation. In other words,

Box 5.6 Decision-making stages in the assimilation of medical innovations (scale developed by Meyer and Goes using a grounded theory approach).

Knowledge-awareness stage
(1) *Apprehension*: individuals learn of the innovation's existence.
(2) *Consideration*: individuals consider the innovation's suitability for their organisation.
(3) *Discussion*: individuals engage in conversations concerning adoption.

Evaluation-choice stage
(4) *Acquisition proposal*: it is formally proposed to purchase the equipment that embodies the innovation.
(5) *Medical–fiscal evaluation*: medical and financial costs and benefits are weighed up
(6) *Political–strategic evaluation*: political and strategic costs and benefits are weighed up.

Adoption-implementation stage
(7) *Trial*: the equipment is purchased but still under trial evaluation.
(8) *Acceptance*: the equipment becomes well accepted and frequently used.
(9) *Expansion*: the equipment is expanded or upgraded.

successful individual adoption is but one component of the assimilation of complex innovations in organisations. We found six high-quality empirical studies (and no systematic reviews) that focused on the process of adoption or assimilation of service innovations in organisations or wider systems. These are listed in Table A.8 (Appendix 4, page 260).

Meyer and Goes analysed the results of an extensive 6-year study (whose main fieldwork had been published previously[321–323]) into the assimilation of innovations in 25 community hospitals in the USA.[38] Their theoretical model of the assimilation process drew on Zaltman *et al.*,[227] who proposed the key stages of matching an innovation to an opportunity, appraising the costs and benefits, adopting or rejecting it, and making sure it becomes accepted as routine.

The innovations were selected to meet three conditions
(1) they were at an early stage in the diffusion process;
(2) they were embodied in mechanical equipment; and
(3) they were too costly and complex for individual physicians to adopt.

The research design had been a multi-method case study involving extensive observation, examination of contemporaneous documents, questionnaires and over 350 interviews with staff at all levels (206 physicians, 70 administrators, 46 board members and 33 nurses). In this ambitious project they developed a detailed instrument to measure innovation assimilation and tested three main hypotheses in relation to this dependent variable:
(1) Particular attributes of the innovation (specifically, the degree of medical risk of the associated procedure, the level of skill needed to use the equipment for a medical procedure, and observability*) would be independently associated with assimilation.
(2) Particular features of the organisation (what we have termed 'the inner context' – specifically, its size, complexity† and market strategy, as well as leadership variables of tenure, level of education and recency of education) and its wider environment (what we have termed 'the outer context' – specifically, the level of urbanisation, affluence and extent of state health insurance) would be independently associated with assimilation.
(3) *Interactions* between the innovation and the organisation (specifically, the compatibility between the innovation and the medical skill mix‡ and the level of advocacy provided by the CEO¶)

*Somewhat unusually, observability was defined in this study as the degree to which the results of using the innovation are visible to organisational members and external constituents.
†Defined in this study as the availability of distinct medical services – i.e. more akin to diversification in some other studies.
‡This was calculated as a composite index for physicians, referring physicians and indirect beneficiaries.
¶CEO advocacy was measured as a composite of their (a) support for the innovation and (b) decision-making influence. This aspect of the study is discussed further in Section 7.3 (page 140).

would add additional predictive value to the independent variables outlined above.

Meyer and Goes claim to have used a grounded theory approach to build new conceptual categories, but this is not verifiable from the information provided in the paper. The basis of their analysis appears to have been the conversion of categories and themes (independently coded by two researchers) to numerical scales (e.g. assessment of the stage of assimilation on the nine-point scale shown in Box 5.6). These numerical values were fed into both linear and multivariate regression analyses.

The results of the Meyer and Goes study broadly confirmed all three hypotheses. A hospital's assimilation of a new medical technology was found to be highly dependent on the attributes of the innovation (risk: $r = -0.65$; skill: $r = -0.44$; observability: $r = 0.35$). The organisational and leadership antecedents measured had only a very weak independent impact on assimilation, but environmental attributes (urbanisation: $r = 0.23$, and affluence: $r = -0.22$) were independently associated with assimilation (see Chapter 7). When hierarchical regression was used, the independent variables together accounted for 59% of the variance in adoption ($r = 0.77$). Of particular note is the fact that the composite variables developed to measure innovation–organisation compatibility and CEO advocacy added significantly to the final model (increase in $r^2 = 0.11$), suggesting that these factors may influence assimilation by interacting with innovation attributes.

The raw results of the Meyer and Goes study are impressive in terms of strength of association but otherwise largely unsurprising, and confirm much that was known already about attributes of innovations (see Chapter 4, page 83) and organisational context (see Chapter 7, page 134). Indeed, it would be very worrying if assimilation of large pieces of medical equipment were out of step with the patterns of medical specialisation within a hospital, of if the CEO's blessing made no difference to major expenditure decisions. It was probably also predictable that leadership per se had no effect on assimilation unless the leader in question supported the innovation, and that conversely, supporting the innovation had less impact if an individual was not in a position of strategic leadership.*

It is, however, perhaps surprising that despite the admirable efforts made by the authors of this extensive study to measure innovation–context interaction, this set of variables added relatively little to the independent attributes of the innovations (risk, skill and observability), which together accounted for 37% of the variance in organisational adoption. Our own interpretation of this is that the interaction between attributes is an elusive phenomenon to capture, and the measures used may have lacked sensitivity – but we must also acknowledge an important message from this paper: complex and risky innovations that require specialist skill and expertise are not easily adopted into organisations whatever the antecedent capacity.

In a very different context, Gladwin *et al.*[45] undertook a single case study of the adoption of a health management information system (introduced as part of national policy) in a low-income African country using in-depth ethnographic methods. The original hypothesis was that 'organisational fit'† would explain the rate and extent of diffusion of this high-technology innovation. The innovation was introduced with what was described as a 'cascade model of training' (training the trainers to use externally developed instructional materials). The researcher collected extensive field notes and contemporaneous documents, which were analysed for themes. The findings were striking (but in retrospect probably unsurprising) – the innovation was not readily adopted despite a top-down 'push', and technological issues dominated as barriers at all stages of the adoption process. Individuals of all professional groups and at all levels continued to seek 'how-to' knowledge throughout the study.

*See Section 7.6 (page 148) for more empirical work on the impact of leadership on adoption in organisations.
†See Section 4.5 (page 97), which argues that in an organisational setting, the compatibility of an innovation is centrally concerned with 'organisational fit' – i.e. the innovation's compatibility with organisational values, goals and ways of working.

Additional findings of note in the Gladwin study were:

• The innovation was difficult to define (adding weight to Denis *et al.*'s construct of the 'soft periphery', discussed below and illustrated in Fig. 5.4, page 112).

• The innovation did not stand alone but (as is commonly the case with technological innovations) came in a cluster with other new ideas, e.g. a foreign classification of disease.

• Whereas the developers of the new system viewed it as a technical innovation needing implementation, the intended users viewed the initiative in terms of a major issue of organisational change (thus, the purveyors of the innovation saw a 'technology' with a 'knowledge gap' that might be filled through 'training'; the intended users saw only a drive to change established systems and ways of working*).

• Considerable redefining of the innovation took place at local level.

• Training and support to use the innovation was considered inadequate on several counts, but in particular, it did not always address the practicalities of its use.

• There were multiple power hierarchies, which constrained adoption at key decision bottlenecks.

• The developer of the innovation lacked faith in its usefulness.

• Staff roles were confused (e.g. individuals classified as 'managers' were in reality only administrators).

• There were inadequate tools to monitor and evaluate the adoption and implementation process.

• Local implementers focused on small (incremental) changes and shied away from big (radical) ones (hence, we might conclude, there was a lack of strategic leadership).

The Gladwin study confirmed many of the principles of introducing high-technology innovations that are dependent on tacit, uncodified knowledge. The 'hard' elements of the technology were easily transferable, but the 'soft' elements (tacit, uncodified knowledge) were not, so people did not really get to grips with how to use it. But whilst this was the most obvious barrier to smooth adoption, the process was also stymied by the gamut of practical, organisational, interpersonal, micropolitical, economic and educational constraints that make up the managing change agenda.†

Champagne *et al.*[64] explored how the congruence – or compatibility – of individuals' goals with those of the organisation affected the likely implementation of the innovation and the extent of change following the decision to adopt it. They aimed to evaluate the impact of introducing sessional fee remuneration for GPs in 27 long-term care hospitals in Quebec during the period 1985–90 on the practice on physicians and on their integration into the care team and into the organisation, and also the process of implementation of this new method of payment. The study combined multiple case studies with embedded units of analysis and a correlational study design. The authors hypothesised that the probability of success would be increased if innovation receives the support of actors who control the bases of power in the organisation (the political model). This support was hypothesised to be a function of:

(1) the centrality of the innovation in relation to the actor's goals and

(2) the congruence between the policy objectives associated with the innovation and the actor's goals.

This political model for the analysis of organisational change received strong support, and the authors concluded that the implementation of sessional fees remuneration was essentially a political process whose probability of success was increased if it received the support of actors who controlled the bases of power in the organisation.‡

As part of a large Canadian government-funded programme on diffusion of innovations in health care, Denis *et al.* used an in-depth ('ethnographic') case study approach to study the adoption of four

*See Section 3.11 (page 68) on knowledge-based approaches to diffusion, which offers a theoretical explanation of why such an approach is unlikely to work.

†The implementation process is discussed further in Chapter 9 (page 175).

‡The Champagne *et al.* study is also discussed in Section 7.3 (page 140) in relation to the organisational determinants of innovativeness.

innovations selected for their evidence base and rate of adoption:
(1) low molecular weight heparin (LMWH) for deep venous thrombosis (good evidence, rapidly adopted: 'success');
(2) laparoscopic cholecystectomy (risk–benefit ratio equivocal, rapidly adopted before the emergence of evidence on which specific groups would benefit overall, leading to high initial complication rates: 'overadoption');
(3) multiple-use dialysis filters (good evidence, slowly adopted: 'prudence'); and
(4) assertive multi-disciplinary community treatment (ACT) for severely psychotic patients (risk–benefit ratio equivocal, slowly adopted: 'underadoption').

The authors used a formal, in-depth cross-case analysis, essentially building a rich picture of each case from an extensive collection of qualitative and quantitative data, and analysing the differences between them in terms of an interpretation of this rich picture.*

'Success' (the rapid adoption of LMWH) was attributed to it because it is a relatively well-defined innovation (although there were still some problems with this), has clear and unambiguous evidence,† has multiple channels of diffusion (clinicians interested in practising according to best evidence plus administrators who saw financial benefit from unblocking beds) and is aligned with prevailing values. 'Overadoption' (of laparoscopic cholecystectomy) was attributed to professional fashions along with market pressures on private-practice surgeons to be seen to be using the 'latest techniques'; and to the fact that whereas the benefits of the procedure (shorter hospital stay, smaller scar) were readily observable, the risks (damage to internal organs, need for re-operation) were less immediately visible.

'Prudence' (the slow adoption of multiple-use dialysis filters despite a good evidence base) was attributed to risks and benefits being context-dependent – since re-use requires manual or chemical cleaning of the filters for which there may or may not be overall savings; and to concerns about hidden risks (e.g. of rare but fatal infection). 'Underadoption' (of the assertive community psychiatric treatment) was attributed to the complexity and ambiguity of the evidence (and in particular to lack of detailed operational data on how exactly to run the project on the ground); the values and commitment of key stakeholders (in particular the lead consultant psychiatrist); the fuzzy boundaries of the innovation (see below); the pre-existence of similar (effectively, competing but different) local initiatives such as voluntary 'care in the community' programmes; and political and ideological resistance to an initiative, which although 'evidence-based' aroused strong political and ideological opposition.

Based on their interpretive data, Denis *et al.* developed a new theoretical model about the adoption of complex health care interventions, with three key elements (see Fig. 5.4). First, a complex innovation is not a 'thing' with fixed boundaries but comprises a 'hard core' of its irreducible elements (e.g. in the case of laparoscopic surgery, the operation itself) plus a 'soft periphery' of the structures and systems that need to be in place to support it. The latter include technologies, skill mix of staff, training and supervision needs and so on. For example, they say in relation to ACT for severely psychotic patients (page 70):

> ... extensive randomized controlled trials had been undertaken to test a complex package of measures with well-supported results. Yet the role of each of the components of the package was not theoretically or empirically clear. While some argued that the only way to ensure reliable effects was to implement the entire package, others selected from the package those elements that appeared most critical to them and could claim that they were following the principles of assertive community treatment. The boundaries of the treatment were to some extent negotiable, leaving both opposing ideological groups the scope to argue for their favoured treatment. The stakes

*For a useful introductory text on interpretation of in-depth case studies see Yin.[172]

†Compare this with the classical 'attributes of innovations' in Section 4.1 (page 83), which include relative advantage and low complexity.

were high, especially for the medical and hospital establishment, leading to attempts to solidify the legitimacy of their approach through calls for government and professional body guidelines.[33]

Second, the risks and benefits of a complex innovation are not distributed evenly in an organisation or system.* Rather, some actors will benefit and others experience unintended or unavoidable consequences. The more the risks and benefits of the innovation map to the interests, values and power of the actors in the adopting system, the easier it will be to build coalitions for spread.

Third, the actors in the adopting system appear to be motivated not only by interests (e.g. financial) but also by values (e.g. 'academic' doctors feel the need to align with evidence from research trials, while many others are more swayed by norms of practice at what they perceived to be prestigious and trend-setting institutions, e.g. 'They're doing it at the Mayo clinic').

Finally, echoing the conclusion of Meyer and Goes,[38] Denis and colleagues noted that the adoption process in organisations is not a one-off, all-or-nothing event but a complex (and adaptive) process. They observed that all innovations are by definition risky (since they are new and untried in the adopting system). All involve an element of learning and often require some period of 'trial and error' – which potentially puts patients at risk. (For example, in the case of laparoscopic surgery, the push to adopt the innovation in order to keep market share may have led to the procedure being overadopted.) Adopting and implementing one innovation alters the system by changing the capabilities, interests, values and power distribution of the adopting system, hence making it more or less likely to adopt future innovations. For example, implementing LMWH in community clinics required the development of communication systems and protocols between these clinics and the hospitals, which would potentially support implementation of other 'shared care' initiatives.† There was some evidence that the implementation of assertive community psychiatric treatment tended to energise and pull together a previously disparate primary mental health care team.

Fitzgerald *et al.*,[32] in their detailed qualitative study of the diffusion of eight innovations in the NHS (explained further in Section 6.2, page 118, in relation to opinion leadership), explored the role of certain forms of knowledge (such as evidence and science) in the process of adoption and diffusion and found that 'robust, scientific evidence is not, of itself, sufficient to ensure diffusion' (page 1437). Indeed, there was no direct association between the robustness of the scientific evidence and the speed of diffusion of the eight innovations. Rather, their in-depth case studies clearly and elegantly demonstrated the ambiguous, contested and socially constructed nature of new scientific knowledge; the highly interactive nature of the diffusion process; and the conspicuous *lack* of evidence of a single adoption decision.‡

The authors observed that 'the process of establishing the credibility of evidence is interpretative and negotiated' and that this process is particularly complex in professional organisations such as health care where much 'knowledge' is ambiguous and contested. Their conclusion in relation to adopters and adoption was that 'crucially, one needs to see adopters not as passive receptors of influence or ideas, but as active participants' – i.e. people who negotiate and *construct* what Rogers might call the 'relative advantage' of the innovation.¶

Timmons undertook an ethnographic study of the implementation of a new computerised care management system by ward nurses in three UK

*See Section 3.7, page 60, for discussion of essentially this point in relation to relative advantage.

†This suggestion aligns closely with what we have called 'organisational capacity building', 'system readiness' and 'linkage activities' – all of which are discussed in detail in Chapter 9 (page 175).

‡This theme is covered in more detail in Section 9.6, page 191.

¶See Section 3.11 (page 68) for a theoretical discussion on the fluid nature of knowledge. Like Fitzgerald *et al.*, we believe this concept is particularly apposite for the subject matter of this review – innovations in service delivery and organisation.

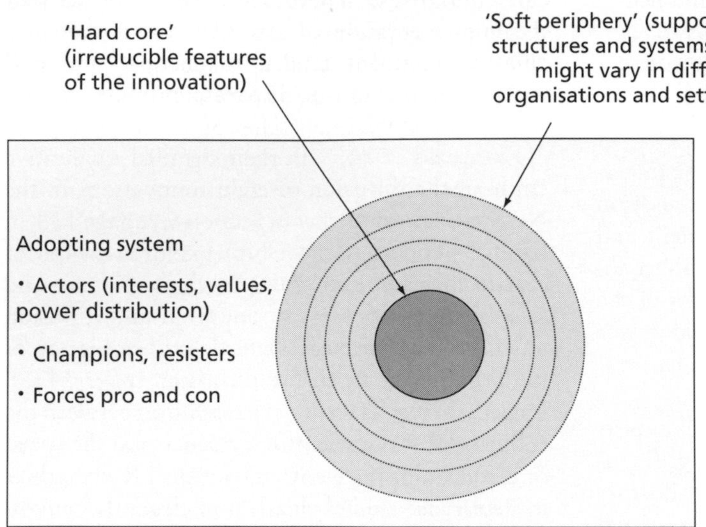

Fig. 5.4 Fuzzy boundaries of complex innovations in service delivery and organisation (based on Denis *et al.*[33]).

hospitals. She conducted in-depth interviews and observed the use (and non-use) of the system by direct observation. She found that resistance to using the new system was widespread amongst the nurses. It occurred through a number of mechanisms: reasoned argument (this was rare); allowing one's password to expire; non-reporting of technical faults; 'moaning'; and 'working round' the system (e.g. leaving data entry for the night shift). Conversely, resistance was dramatically reduced (and adoption greatly increased) when fear of litigation became an issue.

The reasons given by the nurses for their resistance to the innovation included the time needed to enter the data, which was linked with their description of the task as low status ('paperwork'); to be 'caught up on' when times were quiet; and a perceived theory–practice gap (the system did not accurately reflect what they did and how they did it). Timmons, drawing on knowledge management literature, concluded that the acceptability of a technology-based system depends on the meaning of that system to individuals and professional groups, and that this meaning is socially constructed. Actions are susceptible to differing interpretations, e.g. 'resisting the new system' versus 'putting patients first'. She also concluded that there is a political dimension to the implementation of technology-based systems, and power is unevenly distributed (e.g. managers have the power to introduce the system; professionals have the power to resist using it).

The findings of this study could be interpreted in terms of the attributes of the innovation – e.g. in terms of its relative advantage, complexity, compatibility, innovation–values fit and so on. But Timmons' methodology and interpretation moves the focus of analysis from the innovation to its contested *meaning* within the organisation, and to the power relations that lead to particular actions (and inactions) towards the innovation. This framework thus allows a rare exploration of the phenomenon of *non*-adoption. In Section 10.5 (page 208) we discuss another in-depth study by Sicotte *et al.*, which raises many of the same issues and which also describes an initiative to get nurses to use computers that spectacularly failed.[324,325]

Eveland, drawing on Hall and Hord,[46] summarises the adoption of technology-based innovations in organisations thus:

> It is self-evident that putting technology into place in an organisation is not matter of a single decision, but rather of a series – usually a long one – of linked decisions and non-decisions. People make these choices, and

> these choices condition future choices. While the researcher may identify one particular choice as a focal point of 'adoption' he only fools himself; he believes that choice has the same meaning to the user as it does to him. A concept of the leverage exerted by some decisions over other decisions is critical to making intelligent choices about where one might intervene creatively in the process to enhance the likelihood of consequences or desires.[50]

On the basis of most of the studies reviewed in this section, the 'staged' model of organisational adoption proposed (and to some extent validated) by Meyer and Goes earlier in this section (see Box 5.6, page 107) does not appear to be universally applicable. Van de Ven *et al.*[18] have suggested that these 'stages' should be reframed as 'key observations' (initiation, development and implementation or termination) but they are not strictly sequential, nor – importantly – is the assimilation process unidirectional. They propose that the initiation phase is characterised by the generation of ideas, followed by 'shocks' (triggers that propel the organisation into action), and resource plans to ensure that the innovation can be developed. The development phase is characterised by a large number of processes in which real efforts are made to transform the idea into something concrete, punctuated by 'setbacks' and 'surprises' that can lead to innovations being put on the shelf or aborted. In the development phase, the organisation may go through restructuring to accommodate the innovation.

The difference between the Van de Ven model and the Meyer and Goes (following Zaltman) model is that in the former, a key feature is the movement back and forth between events as an innovation unfolds within an organisation. Ideas may go through an initial consideration period before being shelved for months or years. Shocks may make particular innovations redundant – or especially urgent. Restructuring may require new resource plans. Micropolitical tensions and forces within the organisation will become critical. According to Van de Ven *et al.*, the adoption of simple innovations approximates the 'staged' model, but as innovations become larger, more novel (for the organisation) and more complex, a more organic model of adoption must be used. Such a model is certainly more useful for explaining the findings in the studies by Gladwin, Champagne *et al.*, Denis *et al.*, Fitzgerald *et al.* and Timmons described in this section.

In conclusion, the various empirical studies reviewed in this chapter, and particularly the in-depth qualitative work on the process of adoption, have demonstrated that people are not passive recipients of innovations. The widely cited characteristics of 'early adopters' (higher social status, high educational attainment, cosmopolitanism and so on) have some empirical basis but explain little or none of the differences between individuals in their adoption of organisational innovations. To a greater or lesser extent (and differently in different contexts), individuals seek innovations out, experiment with them, evaluate them, find (or fail to find) meaning in them, develop feelings (positive or negative) about them, challenge them, worry about them, complain about them, 'work round' them, talk to others about them, develop know-how about them, modify them to fit particular tasks, and attempt to improve or redesign them – often (and most successfully) through dialogue with other users. Furthermore, except in a few circumstances, organisations should not be thought of as rational decision-making machines that move sequentially through an ordered process of awareness–evaluation–adoption–implementation. Rather, the adoption process should be recognised as complex, iterative, organic and untidy.

This chapter links closely with Chapter 9 (page 175), in which we consider in more detail the intraorganisational processes involved in implementing an innovation and establishing it as part of 'business as usual'. Chapter 6 concerns the phenomenon of social influence that is critical to the individual adoption decision, and Chapter 7 (page 135) and Chapter 8 (page 157), as well as considering structural determinants of organisational innovation, also address aspects of the complex social processes within and between organisations in which the meaning of an innovation is constructed and innovations are refined and reinvented.

Chapter 6
Diffusion and dissemination

Key points

1. Most innovations spread primarily via interpersonal influence. The 'channels' through which such influence flows are the social networks that link individual members of a social group. The wider literature on diffusion of innovations provides a wealth of information on different social influence roles. But the specific literature exploring such roles in the context of health service delivery and organisation is relatively sparse and of variable quality.

2. Some individuals (opinion leaders) have more social influence than others, but attempts to systematically harness the influence of opinion leaders have generally met with only modest success.

3. Despite clear conceptual distinctions between them, the terms 'opinion leader', 'change agent', 'champion' and 'boundary spanner' are used inconsistently and sometimes synonymously in the literature, making comparisons between studies difficult.

4. When programme champions play an active role in the development, spread and implementation of innovations, these processes are generally more effective.

5. When organisational boundary spanners are present and are able to facilitate information flow between organisations, innovations generally diffuse more effectively.

6. When the opinion leaders, champions and boundary spanners are homophilous with intended users, for example when opinion leaders for clinicians arise from amongst the clinicians themselves, diffusion is generally more effective.

7. Critical to the success of an external change agent is effective communication, client orientation and empathy.

8. Where innovations have been produced by formal developmental research, their spread tends to be via vertical dissemination networks and can to some extent be planned strategically. Where innovations arise spontaneously (often through problem-solving aimed at meeting local needs), spread occurs mainly by informal diffusion within horizontal peer networks. The second type of spread cannot be centrally planned or controlled but central agencies may play a facilitative and enabling role, which will be discussed in subsequent chapters.

6.1 Communication and influence through interpersonal networks

Interpersonal networks: background literature

The main findings from wider research into communication of innovations by interpersonal channels and especially through social networks, discussed in detail in Chapter 3, are summarised in Table 6.1.

Valente,[4] one of the most eminent researchers on social networks, defines them as 'the pattern of friendship, advice, communication or support which exists among members of a social system'. People belong to the same groups because they have things in common, and Rogers[3] (drawing on earlier work by sociologists) has argued that a key determinant of the success of communication in a social network is *homophily* – defined as 'the extent to which two or more individuals who interact are similar in certain attributes, such as beliefs, education, social status and the like'

Table 6.1 Summary of findings from different research traditions addressing interpersonal communication and social networks.

Research tradition	*Section*	*Main findings*	*Source for summary of empirical research*
Communication studies	3.4, page 55	Communication is more effective where the source and receiver share common meanings, beliefs and mutual understandings.	MacGuire 1978[202]
Social network analysis (from rural and medical sociology)	3.2, page 51, and 3.3, page 53	Innovations spread through social networks. The embeddedness of an individual in a particular social network is an important determinant of how readily they will adopt.	Rogers and Shoemaker 1972,[177] Valente 1995,[98] Rogers 1995[3]
Marketing and economics	3.5, page 56	Mass media are important for creating awareness but interpersonal channels are vastly more influential in promoting adoption of innovations. Marketing requires careful tailoring of message, medium and messenger to particular audiences.	MacGuire 1978[202]
Health promotion	3.8, page 62	A key success factor in health promotion campaigns is the identification and recruitment of individuals from within the target community to act as messengers and change agents.	Macdonald 2002[201]; see also Rogers[3] for a wealth of additional examples from developing countries

(1995, page 18). In other words, the extent to which experiences, values and norms are shared among the members of a social network enhances the diffusion of information and promotes adoption. Rogers[3] has further observed (page 287) that homophily and communication networks reinforce each other: 'The more communication there is between members of a dyad, the more likely they are to become homophilous.'

It is thus well established that the degree of similarity among group members will affect the ease and spread with which the diffusion of an innovation takes place.[299] Clinicians are a relatively homophilous group (compared, say, with a mixed group of clinicians, managers, service users and so on). Therefore, as a general rule, innovations generated within a particular community of clinicians will diffuse more effectively than those coming from without.

Another consistent finding from the wider literature is the notion that high social status (however defined) is a requirement for social influence. In her systematic review of the sociological literature on diffusion of innovations, Wejnert[41] concludes (page 304):

> An actor's high social position significantly modulates the likelihood of adoption within culturally homogenous groups ... The predictive power of an individual actor's status on adoption of an innovation varies positively with the prominence of the actor's position in a network.

Social networks influence the diffusion of innovations mainly because they form the channels through which interpersonal communication takes place, but they also have an additional benefit: they increase the 'adoptability' of an innovation by increasing its observability* (since membership of a social group enables actors to become familiar with the outcome of an innovation[5,326–329]). Learning through such observation lowers the perceived risk associated with adoption by eliminating novelty or uncertainty of outcome.[161,330–333] Rogers warns against a simplistic linear notion of communication of innovations in which the idea is transferred in one direction from the person who has adopted it to someone who has not. Rather, he suggests, communication amongst homophilous members of a social system is a two-way process of negotiation through which the meaning (and hence the advantage) of the innovation is socially constructed – a process he refers to as the 'convergence' model.

One final important finding from the wider literature is that when actors are introduced to something that they are not familiar with as a group, the degree of homophily may change. For example, GPs may be considered a homophilous group in terms of their clinical knowledge, professional values, social ties and so on. But when a new information technology is introduced, their homophily as clinicians becomes overshadowed by their heterophily as IT consumers, and the degree of interpersonal communication and mutual support is likely to be much less than occurs around clinical or professional issues. We have been unable to find specific empirical studies from the health services literature to confirm this suggestion, but see Rogers'[3] book for a more general discussion on homophily as a fluid rather than fixed characteristic of a dyad or social group.

Adler *et al.* suggest that because of the powerful effect of homophily, all the roles discussed in Sections 6.2–6.4 (opinion leader, champion, boundary spanner and so on) will be more effective if these individuals arise (or are recruited) from within a particular profession and social network. They also discuss the role of professional organisations in enhancing the social networks of professionals and thereby spreading innovations between homophilous groups of clinicians. They note that such organisations vary in their capacity to ensure effective diffusion, since this capacity is a function of their role in society (technical, lobbying, etc.), as well as their internal strategy (strength), structure (centralised more effective in diffusion), culture (e.g. promote change, sharing), training programmes (for the new innovation), and credentialing systems (how far they 'regulate' for diffusion).[43]

Interpersonal networks and diffusion of innovations: empirical studies

We found no systematic reviews and only two primary research studies that met our inclusion criteria and that looked specifically at interpersonal influence (as opposed to opinion leadership, which is covered in Section 6.2) within social networks of health professionals. These studies are summarised in Table A.9 (page 262) in Appendix 4. Two important early studies of social networks – that of Coleman *et al.*[5] and that of Becker *et al.*[52,192] – are discussed further in Section 6.2 (page 118).

Fennell and Warnecke[36] looked at the diffusion of cancer patient management strategies between networks of clinicians. They studied seven separate cancer networks using formal network analysis as described in Section 3.3 (page 53). Their detailed historical case studies confirm that homophily between clinicians was an independent factor influencing the spread of management strategies. However, the main focus of this extensive study was the impact of organisation-level influences and the wider environment, so it is covered in more detail in Section 8.2 (page 163).

West *et al.*[51] studied the social networks of two groups of elite health professionals, clinical directors of medicine and directors of nursing, in English hospitals. They conducted semi-structured interviews from a random sample of 50 in each group recruited from a national directory. They set out to test five hypotheses:

*See Sections 4.1 (page 83) and 4.2 (page 87) on innovation attributes.

• The social networks of the two groups would differ in characteristic ways – and these differences would be determined by norms of professional socialisation, organisational structure, and occupational position.
• The networks of directors of nursing would be more hierarchical (i.e. they would be more likely to name juniors than seniors or peers as the individuals with whom they discussed important professional matters).
• The networks of directors of nursing would be less dense (i.e. each nurse director interviewed would name fewer professional ties to other individuals).
• The networks of directors of nursing would be more centralised (i.e. those actors at the top of the hierarchy would be more central than those lower down – particular individuals near the top of the hierarchy would consistently be named as the person with whom others discuss professional matters), whereas those of directors of medicine would be more decentralised (i.e. there would be less difference in the centrality of the actors at different levels of the hierarchy).
• Directors of nursing would have higher actor information centrality scores than directors of medicine (i.e. they would be named as the person who passed on a particular item of information or as someone through whom that item needed to pass).

The response rate was not given but a total of 100 clinical directors were interviewed. The authors used a standard interview schedule for network analysis and calculated scores for network density, group degree centralisation, and actor information centrality* separately for the directors of nursing and medicine, which were subjected to formal statistical tests of significance.

All the initial hypotheses were broadly confirmed. Directors of medicine were found to have significantly denser, more cohesive, and more horizontal social networks, and to be members of significantly more professional associations. They were significantly less likely to discuss professional matters with juniors and more likely to discuss them with peers. West *et al.* comment that their most striking finding was the very different structure of the social networks of senior nurses and doctors. Directors of medicine were generally embedded in a richly interconnected network, in which most actors knew several others in the same network and often described their relationships as 'close'; the authors suggest the term 'clique' for this general structure. In contrast, directors of nursing had significantly less dense and more vertical networks, in which most actors generally had no links with each other except through a third party (the central actor – typically the director of nursing); they describe such a network as a 'hierarchy'.

In their discussion, West *et al.* suggest advantages for both types of network. The dense, decentralised, non-hierarchical networks typical of senior doctors exhibit a high degree of homophily and lend themselves to powerful interpersonal influence on the adoption process. The disadvantage of such a structure (as with any clique) is that its members have few external ties and hence are not particularly open to innovations coming from outside the clique. On the other hand, the less dense networks of directors of nursing (weaker ties *within* the network) mean that these individuals have stronger ties *outside* the network, and hence – as shown by Granovetter[196] and Burt[195] – are better placed to capture new ideas from outside. Furthermore, because of the more hierarchical nature of the nurses' network, directors of nursing do not merely receive or transmit information – they have considerable power to endorse it, control its flow, and direct it strategically to particular subsidiaries. Directors of medicine, on the other hand, have relatively weak power to 'manage' or 'endorse' information because their social network (which owes its structure partly to the different professional norms of doctors) is egalitarian and made up of individuals who see their decision-making as highly autonomous.[51,†]

*See the appendix in the article by West *et al.*[51] for a definition of these terms.

†See Section 6.6 (page 131), which includes a table comparing centralised (vertical) spread with decentralised (horizontal) spread, and which suggests that whereas the former is well suited to spreading the findings of formal research, the latter is more suited to spreading innovations that arise spontaneously in practice.

In summary, the empirical literature on social networks of health professionals is extremely sparse, and we found no comparable studies at all on the social networks of health service managers (although Valente[98] has looked at the networks of managers in general). The studies support the findings from the wider literature on the social networks of professionals – that the structure of the network (which is powerfully shaped by both organisational structure and professional norms) crucially influences the *channels* of communication of innovations; that homophily (i.e. shared experiences, perspectives, norms and values) is associated with *high-quality* communication and powerful interpersonal *influence*; and that external (weak) ties allow *new innovations* to be identified and captured from outside the network. However, in view of the small number and limited scope of the studies in health service organisations, these findings should not be seen as definitive.

6.2 Opinion leaders

Opinion leaders: background literature

Opinion leaders have been defined by Locock *et al.*[53] as 'those perceived as having particular influence on the beliefs and actions of their colleagues in any direction, whether "positive" (in the eyes of those trying to achieve change) or "negative" '. This definition differs critically from that used by others (including the authors of the only systematic review relevant to this study[54]), which is 'health professionals nominated by their colleagues as educationally influential'. We concur with Locock *et al.* that since opinion leadership can occur in either direction, it makes sense for the definition of an opinion leader to reflect that. Nevertheless, it is important to note that key studies have used inconsistent definitions.*

It is often assumed that opinion leaders are key actors in the diffusion of medical and information technologies, and considerable effort is sometimes put into identifying them and attempting to convince them to become early adopters of particular innovations.[299] Whilst most health professionals and managers have heard of the term 'opinion leader' (indeed, it could be said to have become a colloquialism), we were surprised at how few empirical studies there were in the literature on opinion leadership.†

The notion that someone is 'an opinion leader' implies that opinion leadership is an inherent, fixed trait of the individual and that it is separate and separable from the innovation and the context. In fact, there is evidence that someone may be an opinion leader on one issue but not on other issues (what Rogers[3] calls 'monomorphic' opinion leadership), and also that certain individuals are opinion leaders on a very wide range of issues ('polymorphic' opinion leadership). Interestingly, Rogers does not recognise (or, at least, does not refer to) the concept of the 'champion' (discussed in Section 6.3, page 126), but there is some overlap between the latter and the notion of monomorphic (innovation-specific) opinion leadership.

Rogers, reviewing a vast range of studies across the different sociological sub-disciplines, identifies four main methods used to measure opinion leadership (Box 6.1).

These different methods have different strengths and limitations. Sociometric methods can provide detailed quantitative information (which can be further quantified by using a roster questionnaire – i.e. the respondent is presented with a list of all potential actors in the network and asked to indicate for each of them how often they communicate and what about). But the technique, although relatively straightforward, is laborious and requires a large number of respondents to locate a small number of opinion leaders.‡

*Indeed, despite their conceptual distinctiveness as illustrated by the definitions cited in this chapter, in practice the terms 'opinion leader', 'change agent', 'champion' and 'boundary spanner' are used inconsistently and sometimes synonymously in the literature, making comparisons between studies difficult.

†For example, a search of the Medline database from 1966 to mid 2003 identified only 15 papers using this term in the title or abstract.

‡One cannot really imagine busy doctors patiently cooperating with such an approach in the same way as the Iowa corn farmers might have done in the 1930s.

Box 6.1 Methods for measuring opinion leadership (summarised from Rogers[3]).

(1) *Sociometric.* Based on the number of times an individual is nominated as someone from whom the actor has sought (or might seek) information about a particular innovation.
(2) *Ratings of key informants.* Individuals who know the social network well are asked to name those individuals who have particular influence on others.
(3) *Self designation.* Respondents are asked to indicate the tendency for others to regard them as influential.
(4) *Observation.* The researcher observes first-hand who seeks information from whom.

Rankings by key informants are much quicker to obtain, but may be less valid, especially if the 'key informant' lacks an in-depth knowledge of the workings of the network. Anecdotally, we were told that the pharmaceutical industry uses an approach somewhere between these two extremes to identify the opinion leaders in doctors targeted for pharmaceutical marketing, but we were unable to confirm this. Self-designation is probably accurate for some individuals (by definition those with insight into their own place in the social network), but much less accurate for others. Observation is only suited to a small system and loses validity in situations where people know they are being observed.

The four general characteristics of opinion leaders established from empirical studies in the wider sociological literature are shown in Box 6.2. The contingent nature of the 'innovativeness' factor is important. We should not think of opinion leaders as the people with the bright new ideas or even the people who are most receptive to new ideas. Rather, we should think of them as individuals who reflect – and enact – the broad norms of their social system and who thereby command the respect of their peers. If innovation is a 'norm', opinion leaders will be more innovative than most, but if not, they won't.*

As Rogers[3] (page 295) comments, 'a common error made by change agents is that they select opinion leaders who are too innovative' – and who are hence too heterophilous to influence their peers. He offers some examples from educational sociology of 'opinion leader organisations' (well-resourced 'laboratory schools' with good facilities and talented students) that had been set up to develop and model innovations. But the laboratory schools were perceived as 'too different' by

Box 6.2 General characteristics of opinion leaders from empirical studies reviewed by Rogers.[3]

- *External communication.* Opinion leaders have greater exposure to mass media, more links with the external world ('greater cosmopolitanism') and greater exposure to change agents than their followers.
- *Accessibility.* Opinion leaders have greater social participation than their followers – e.g. attendance at face-to-face meetings, density of interpersonal networks.
- *Socio-economic status.* Opinion leaders have higher socio-economic status than their followers.*
- *Innovativeness.* Overall, opinion leaders are more innovative than their followers – but this generalisation is qualified by social norms: in a social system that views innovation negatively (i.e. a system that is inherently highly resistant to change), opinion leaders are not especially innovative.

*Rogers[3] (page 294) quotes Tarde[182] (1903) who observed: 'Invention can start from the lowest ranks of the people, but its extension depends upon the existence of some lofty social elevation'.

*A review of opinion leader characteristics by Chan and Misra[334] from an advertising perspective makes fascinating reading, but their extensive list of characteristics (which in addition to those mentioned includes level of knowledge about the product, a favourable view of the product, willingness and skills to communicate that view to others, venturesomeness, gregariousness and 'public individuation' – i.e. the extent to which one feels different from others and is prepared to show it) is probably not directly transferable to the non-commercial sector.

the average school, and innovations spectacularly failed to diffuse.

A final seminal paper on opinion leadership was Burt's network analysis of the adoption of immunisation by members of a primitive rural community in El Salvador. He mapped 21 separate 'cliques' (individuals who knew and influenced one another) and on the basis of a sophisticated statistical analysis concluded that there were two distinct social networks in this community: one for awareness and another for influence.[6] Perhaps unsurprisingly, individuals identified by their peers as having 'communication prestige' (i.e. valued as a source of information) were characterised by high socioeconomic status and access to the mass media (e.g. a radio). Those identified as having 'influence prestige' (i.e. as someone to copy) were characterised only by high socio-economic status. The notion of different types of opinion leader is discussed below in relation to empirical work in health services.

Opinion leaders: empirical studies in the health service literature

We found one systematic review of randomised trials, two additional randomised trials, three network analyses and two in-depth case studies that explored the role of opinion leaders and met our inclusion criteria. These are summarised in Tables A.10 (page 263) and A.11 (page 265) in Appendix 4. We describe them in approximately historical order and divide them into three traditions: the sociometric studies on opinion leadership in early medical sociology; the intervention trials of opinion leaders in EBM; and a series of in-depth, qualitative studies of 'sense-making' by contemporary social scientists.

The landmark study in which opinion leadership was first demonstrated in the health care field was the work by Coleman *et al.* on prescribing of tetracycline (summarised in Table 6.2 and discussed for its historical significance in Section 3.3, page 53).* Researchers used a sociometric approach to identify the opinion leaders – i.e. they counted the number of times an individual was nominated as a network partner, and correlated this with time to adopt the innovation.[4] The findings of Coleman *et al.* in relation to opinion leadership are summarised in Box 6.3†.

Another early study was that of Becker.[52,192] This author traced the diffusion paths of two ser-

Box 6.3 Characteristics of opinion leaders demonstrated by early medical sociology studies by Coleman *et al.*[5,335,336]

- Opinion leaders had particularly wide social networks (e.g. they were more likely to be named by other doctors as a 'best friend' or as 'someone with whom I discuss my patients' or as a source of information*).
- They had more extensive and broader information sources, and thus were likely to learn of an innovation earlier (both from interpersonal communication and mass media).
- They tended to adopt the innovation slightly earlier than most, but were generally not themselves innovators or early adopters.
- They had high social status and technical competence.
- Once these opinion leaders adopted the innovation, the S-curve reached critical inflection and rapidly 'took off'.†

*In the language of social network theory, discussed in Section 3.3 (page 53), these citations constitute 'sociometric nominations' and are the main unit of analysis of social network researchers.

†Subsequent research has shown the role of opinion leaders to be more complex. In particular, there is an important link to the prevailing norms of the social system, in that when that system is oriented to change, opinion leaders are quite innovative; but when the system's norms are opposed to change, the behaviour of the leaders also reflects this norm.[3]

*Strictly speaking the Coleman *et al.* study was not a study of innovation in service delivery and organisation, since the innovation was a simple health technology (tetracycline), but we have included it because of its seminal status and its methodological importance.

†These landmark studies are not included merely for historical interest: although they were not without limitations, their rigorous methodology allows them to still stand today as two of the few examples of 'quality' sociometric studies in the medical literature.

vice innovations (measles immunisation and diabetes screening) among directors of local health departments in three states in the USA during the late 1960s. This study should be interpreted in the light of prevailing demographic trends and disease patterns of the 1960s (when, for example, diabetes was less common and perceived as less serious than measles), and in the light of the wider context of US health care at the time (in which 'office physicians' in private practice viewed screening as their territory, and the role of public health departments was still primarily the control of infectious diseases). The study addressed the 'attitudes, motivations, and information sources of pioneer adopters of [these] different innovations'. It was based on a fairly simple survey instrument from which sociometric analyses were derived. The authors demonstrated a high correlation between time of adoption of the innovations and both relative centrality (opinion leadership) in the group's communication networks and several rankings of most-valued source of information.

The study by Becker *et al.* was probably the first to demonstrate empirically that there is an interaction between opinion leadership and the nature of an innovation. The innovation that was at the time perceived to have 'high potential' (measles immunisation) was adopted earlier by opinion leaders who increased its rate of diffusion; the innovation classified at the time as having 'low potential' (diabetes screening) was more likely to be adopted earlier by marginal individuals, which if anything tended to decrease its level of

Table 6.2 Two types of opinion leader identified by Locock *et al.*,[53] analysed in terms of key constructs in the diffusion of innovations literature.

	'Expert' opinion leader	*'Peer' opinion leader*
Location in social network	Generally in high-status position, typically an academic with national or international reputation or a senior consultant	An 'ordinary' member of the social group, e.g. a local GP without special status
Homophily	Heterophilous with followers	Homophilous with followers
Main role	Their endorsement reduces uncertainty about the strength of evidence (i.e. improves its perceived relative advantage)	Their endorsement reduces uncertainty about the 'implementability' of the innovation and provides a 'worked example' for others to follow
Mechanism of influence	Formal academic authority (know-what)	Informal 'tacit' authority (know-how)
Key characteristics	Respected by virtue of higher knowledge – their endorsement is what defines the innovation as 'evidence based': able to explain the evidence to others; able to respond convincingly to challenges and debate	'Shop-floor' credibility: able to lead the adaptation of innovations to fit local priorities and circumstances
Main stage of influence	Early in the project (Hall and Hord's 'awareness' and 'information' stage*)	Late in the project (Hall and Hord's 'task management' stage)
Typical descriptions and metaphors	'Academic expert': 'someone who knows what he or she is talking about'	'One of us': 'understands the realities of clinical practice'; 'if he can do it perhaps I can', 'can make it work *here*'

*See Section 5.2 (page 103).

adoption). Specifically, the public health officials taking the lead in the adoption of measles immunisation were young, urban, liberal and cosmopolitan (thus meeting the 'person specification' for an effective opinion leader), while the pioneers in the adoption of diabetes screening were old, rural, conservative and parochial.[52,192] This study thus elegantly (and perhaps unwittingly) demonstrated the difference between an early adopter (who is open to new ideas and practices but is not necessarily copied) and an opinion leader (who may or may not adopt early but when he or she does adopt is influential over others).

These two studies – which were published in the mainstream medical literature as well as the sociological literature – probably sowed the seed of the idea of opinion leadership in the minds of doctors and directly or indirectly spawned the eight primary studies reviewed by O'Brien's systematic review, which are summarised in Table A.11 (page 265) in Appendix 4. Seven of the eight trials covered in that review measured opinion leadership through a somewhat obscure questionnaire published as a conference proceeding and purporting to measure 'communication, humanism, and knowledge'.[337]* The overall methodological quality of some trials appeared to be poor. For example, only two had clear evidence of concealment of randomisation; only two had blinded assessment of outcome; and at least two had unit of analysis errors, i.e. randomisation was by one unit (e.g. hospital or ward) while analysis of data was by another unit (e.g. individual).

Six of the seven trials in this systematic review that measured health professional practice demonstrated some improvement for at least one predefined outcome measure, but the absolute differences were small and in only two of these trials[338,339] were the results statistically significant and clinically important. Furthermore, since many trials used multiple outcome variables even 'significant differences' may have been spurious. In three trials that measured patient outcomes, only one achieved an impact upon practice that was considered to be of practical importance (improving the rate of vaginal birth after previous Caesarean section[338]).

The authors of the systematic review concluded that 'using' local opinion leaders results in mixed effects on professional practice, and that 'it is not always clear what local opinion leaders do'. They called for further research to determine whether and how opinion leaders can be identified and the circumstances in which they are likely to influence the practice of their peers.

We found two additional empirical studies of opinion leaders as an intervention in randomised trials: the use by Searle *et al.*[340] of a senior gynaecologist as opinion leader in an educational intervention to reduce unnecessary gynaecological procedures and the large group randomised trial of quality improvement initiatives in US hospitals by Berner *et al.*[341] (in which hospitals were randomised to no intervention, a conventional quality improvement intervention, or the same quality improvement intervention with a local physician opinion leader attached). Identification of opinion leaders was done by peer nomination and not independently verified, and the process of opinion leader influence was not explored in depth. Both studies demonstrated modest effects on some but not all predefined clinical outcomes, and both concluded that the direction of influence of the opinion leader was generally positive, but that the strength of influence was small.

The O'Brien systematic review (which closely reflected the 'clinical trial' approach favoured by empirical researchers within their own tradition) viewed opinion leaders as a discrete 'intervention' that (implicitly) could be manipulated by the change agency to influence an 'outcome'; and furthermore, that the impact of opinion leaders could be isolated from other variables sufficiently cleanly to be evaluated against the experience of a control group treated identically in all other respects. As explained in Section 3.9 (page 64), this was until recently the standard approach of the EBM movement, whose 'hierarchy of evidence' would have led to the rejection of non-experimental study designs to explore opinion leadership (see, for example, the work of Locock *et al.*[53] and Fitzgerald *et al.*[32]).

We prefer to take a more pluralist view, and believe that whilst controlled trials have an im-

*We were unable to obtain a copy of the study, which is out of print.

portant place in assessing the direction and magnitude of a complex intervention, they are a blunt instrument for measuring the *process* of complex effects, and furthermore, that inherent to the 'trial' design are a number of questionable epistemological assumptions (such as the separability of opinion leadership from other variables and the idea that it can be manipulated by external agencies without being fundamentally changed). Locock *et al.*,[53] drawing on in-depth case study work by others on the management of change, express this difficulty thus:

> If doctors subsume the influence of opinion leaders within their definition of their own clinical experience, this has implications for researchers trying to isolate and measure the effect of opinion leader influence.

The final research stream relevant to opinion leadership in service delivery and organisation comprises two recent studies into the implementation of evidence-based practice that have taken a qualitative, 'whole-systems' perspective.

Dopson *et al.*[342] conducted in-depth, multimethod case studies of two government-funded initiatives: the Promoting Action on Clinical Effectiveness (PACE) Programme and the Welsh Clinical Effectiveness Initiative National Demonstration Projects,[343] which between them funded 22 separate 'evidence-into-practice' initiatives via a competitive bidding process. Their brief was specifically to explore, using qualitative methods, attempts by organisations to change clinical practice, and thereby gain a greater understanding of the complexity of the factors affecting implementation. They were asked to ground their analysis in the perceptions of those conducting the projects, and to avoid measuring quantitative 'outcomes' for any of the projects (a task that was allocated to a separate research team).

The team used semi-structured (mainly telephone) interviews (263 in total) supplemented by a written questionnaire (sent to 488 front-line clinicians) and documentary analysis. From these, they produced 22 case studies, which were reported in a series of evaluation reports. They assessed 'success' both in terms of achieving the clinical goals identified in the specific project (e.g. improving the management of leg ulcers) and also in terms of more general organisational learning. They summarise their main findings thus:

> Three factors stood out as particularly influential [in the success or otherwise of the project]: the strength and clarity of the evidence which the project sought to implement; the committed support of key opinion leaders; and the extent of wider organisational commitment to evidence-based practice.[53]

'Strength of evidence' is a construct that probably maps directly to relative advantage (see Section 4.1, page 83), and 'extent of wider organisational commitment' is related to what we have called 'organisational readiness' (see Section 9.3, page 180); we therefore consider only opinion leadership in this section.

Locock *et al.* found the question 'who were the opinion leaders in this project' a remarkably difficult one to answer. Indeed, individuals identified as enthusiastic supporters of the innovation by one informant were dismissed by others as ambivalent. None of the 22 projects had gone through a systematic process at the outset to identify opinion leaders or harness their influence. As the authors comment:

> The opinion leaders generally emerged at a more informal, opportunistic and implicit level, and there was considerable blurring of roles between the opinion leaders and those running the project.[53]

One key finding of this extensive study was that there appear to be different sorts of opinion leaders, and that these have different influences at different stages of the project. Specifically, the authors distinguished between 'expert' and 'peer' opinion leaders, as shown in Table 6.2. To construct Table 6.2, we took data from the study by Locock *et al.* and linked them to diffusion concepts such as relative advantage and stages of adoption discussed elsewhere in this book. The expert–peer distinction approximates Burt's[6] earlier finding in a more primitive community (and using very different research methods) that opinion leaders might have 'communication prestige' or 'influence prestige'.

Another important finding by Locock *et al.* was the mixed influence of opinion leaders. Opinion leaders were readily identifiable in several projects that had had negative influence on followers. These included single-issue campaigners who were seen to have attempted to 'hijack' the project for their own ulterior ends; key stakeholders who adopted a stance of 'active indifference' (as one informant said, '[if seen as an opinion leader by others] you can cause a lot of damage by just being neutral'); and the ambiguous behaviour of those supposedly leading the project (e.g. hospital consultants endorsing guidelines for GPs on the one hand while on the other hand refusing to use the same guidelines themselves).

In summary, this project demonstrated that opinion leadership is a highly complex process. Factors identified as pivotal to the success of the projects and discussed further in the study by Locock *et al.* include:

- ambivalence towards the innovation by the main opinion leaders;
- failure to engage the 'right' opinion leaders;
- the presence of 'rival' opinion leaders who were neutral or hostile to the innovation;
- dissonance between the views of 'expert' and 'peer' opinion leaders;
- restricted credibility or appeal of certain opinion leaders;
- opinion leaders whose enthusiasm had exhausted their credibility; and
- lack of any appropriate opinion leaders.

The finding that some opinion leaders were valued for their specialised knowledge (and hence their *heterophily*) is perhaps surprising given the wealth of evidence on the importance of homophily. However, it accords with common sense and serves as a warning against constructing an oversimplistic model of opinion leadership – which, in reality, is a complex phenomenon. This finding aligns with that of Fennell and Warnecke[36] that in addition to their special place within the group, opinion leaders have linkages outside the group to sources of information regarded as important to the group's activities – a finding that is perhaps only true of 'expert' opinion leaders.

One further point to note is that the various 'opinion leader-specific' problems interacted closely with more general issues, most notably poor project management and lack of resources:

> A project which is in administrative difficulties will clearly find it hard to make good use of opinion leaders' time and skills; local clinicians may respect their views but become frustrated by administrative delays. The opinion leaders themselves may not wish to be associated with a poorly run project, or one based on contested evidence.[53]

In a separate large study that took a similar perspective and used similar methods, Fitzgerald *et al.*[32] conducted qualitative case studies of the diffusion of eight innovations in the NHS during the period 1996–9. Three of these were innovations in service delivery and organisation: the use of a computer support system for anticoagulation, the introduction of new service delivery systems for care of women in childbirth and the direct employment of physiotherapists in GP practices. The purpose of the study was to explore (using a comparative case study design) three aspects of the diffusion of innovations into organisations:

(1) knowledge bases (the roles of certain forms of knowledge;
(2) the nature of adoption decisions and
(3) the influence of differing contexts on the diffusion process.

The case studies were selected in relation to three criteria to give a maximum-variety sample:

(1) strong or weak scientific evidence on their efficacy;
(2) uni- or multiprofessional; and
(3) primary or secondary care.

Thus, for example, they had one case study of an innovation that was strongly evidence-based, multiprofessional and secondary care (computerised decision support for anticoagulation), one that had a weak evidence base and was uniprofessional in primary care (use of HRT to prevent osteoporosis) and so on.

Fitzgerald *et al.* broke their case studies into two stages: in stage 1, they analysed the diffusion of each innovation across a geographical region, and in stage 2, they undertook a micro-analysis of each innovation in one specific setting. Altogether they undertook 232 interviews (144 in stage 1 and 88 in stage 2). They used in-depth qualitative methods to analyse their data.

The authors found that there was no simple uniform pattern of diffusion either by sector (primary or secondary care) or by any other single variable. Rather, the extent of diffusion was determined by the *interaction* between a number of key variables, including credibility of the evidence, organisational and environmental context ('the local situation in which a clinician operates appears to be a potent mediator of everyday experience') and interorganisational networks ('networks are one of the key determinants of whether an innovation is successfully diffused into use').* The critical importance of credibility of the evidence concords with Rogers'[3] notion of relative advantage and the finding of several other research groups[29,298] that evaluation of this attribute occurs first, and if unfavourable, other attributes are not considered (see Section 4.2, page 87). They also found that opinion leaders played an 'active and influential role in the diffusion of innovations' (page 1441–42).

In their analysis, Fitzgerald *et al.* distinguished between three types of opinion leader:

- A node or focal point for information and a model of behaviour, who may act as a link between the worlds of academic research and practice (see 'boundary spanners').
- An 'expert' opinion leader with local credibility.
- A strategic, 'political' opinion leader with combined management and political skills.

This threefold taxonomy is similar but not identical to the taxonomy produced independently by Locock *et al.*, into 'peer' and 'expert' opinion leader (see Table 6.3). Whilst the binary classification is appealing for its simplicity, the notion of Fitzgerald *et al.* regarding a 'boundary-spanning' opinion leader with links to the world of the expert and the world of the practitioner deserves further exploration.

The authors use the example of innovations in service delivery in maternity care to illustrate how it is unlikely that adoption of an organisational innovation will occur without a basis of trust between groups, and that depending on prevailing opinion about the value of the innovation, networks can either engage people in the diffusion process or they can halt the process.

In summary, the findings of Fitzgerald *et al.* align closely with those of Locock *et al.* – opinion leadership is multifaceted, complex and different in different circumstances, but few successful projects to implement innovations in organisations have managed without the input of identifiable opinion leaders. Reflecting on the mismatch between the conclusions from qualitative work and that of the Cochrane review,[54] Ferlie *et al.*[12] comment (page 37):

> It is interesting that the conclusions of this overview are more supportive of the role played by the clinical opinion leader than the Cochrane review of RCT-based studies. This raises the intriguing possibility – if confirmed in other case studies – that findings may be in part dependent on methods. It will be interesting to see whether other teams of organisational behaviour researchers also find it useful to band together to produce other such overviews.

The suggestion that different researchers using different research designs might obtain 'different results' might make some scientists uneasy, but it accords with the notion that the different research traditions all contribute to the rich picture in a cross-disciplinary (and trans-paradigmatic) overview. The results may be different but they are not incommensurable. Indeed, they are readily explained by the overall interpretation that opinion leadership is a complex phenomenon that interacts with a host of other factors including the nature of the evidence, the resources available to the project, competing demands and priorities and so on. If opinion leadership is studied as part of this wider interaction, and especially if the input of the research team exerts some formative influence on those interactions, it is surely predictable that significant effects will often be detected. If, on the other hand, opinion leadership is isolated as a single 'variable' and all contextual elements 'controlled for', it is equally predictable that a smaller effect will generally be demonstrated.

*Interorganisational networks are discussed further in Chapter 7 (page 134).

6.3 Champions and advocates

Champions and advocates: background literature

As Section 6.2 showed, opinion leaders have a following but may or may not support an innovation. Individuals who dedicate themselves to supporting, marketing, and 'driving through' an innovation are collectively known as champions – a term probably first coined by Schon,[56] who conducted a study of radical military innovations* and described the champion's role in these stirring terms:

> No ordinary involvement with a new idea provides the energy required to cope with the indifference and resistance that major technical change provokes. ... champions of new inventions display persistence and courage of heroic qualities. ... The new idea either finds a champion or dies.

Schon's[56] fieldwork led him to develop four principles of product championship:

- At its inception, a new idea in an organisation generally encounters sharp resistance.
- Overcoming this resistance requires vigorous promotion.
- Supporters of the idea work primarily through informal channels within the organisation.
- Typically, one person emerges as the champion of the idea.

The axiom that an innovation requires active and energetic efforts by particular individuals to 'keep it alive' and create a robust coalition for change is a recurring theme in the literature (e.g. Van de Ven,[123] Strang and Soule,[124] Rogers[3] and Adler *et al.*[43]). In short:

> ... [the] probability of success will be low unless [people] can find a sympathetic and respected individual from a high-status profession to act as a champion.[43]

As with adoption (and resistance to adoption) of innovations, the mainstream change management literature has many comparable concepts and there is a wealth of empirical evidence on 'change champions', which is probably highly relevant to this section, but which we excluded from the scope of our review. Taking only the literature on innovation champions, the empirical evidence to support the pivotal influence of such roles is relatively weak. In the introduction to a systematic study of the work of champions, Markham[55] observed:

> The image of the project champion fighting corporate inertia, rallying support, and leading a project to success makes for a great story, but that story may not reveal the true nature of the champion's role. All those off-tom tales about champions fail to provide hard evidence of the techniques that champions use, the activities they, perform, and the effects that champions have on project success'.

One of the most widely cited reviews of champions is that by Maidique,[344] who lists a multiplicity of synonyms for the term used in organisational literature including 'internal entrepreneurs', 'sponsors', 'Maxwell demons' and so on. He also cites (page 61) a 1964 study by Collins *et al.*[345] of the personality profiles of 150 champions in US industry (all of whom, if the title is anything to go by, were men), which concluded that:

> [T]he entrepreneurial personality, in short, is characterised by an unwillingness to submit to authority, an inability to work with it, and a consequent need to escape from it.

This sweeping conclusion, which marks out the champion as inherently maverick, has not been independently verified in subsequent work. In his review, Maidique also describes a large, systematic study, using a detailed survey instrument, of 43 pairs of innovations in the chemical and manufacturing industry. The researchers tested, and their results supported, the hypothesis that there are four different 'champion' roles (Box 6.4).

The taxonomy presented in Box 6.4 includes a specific role for an individual who does little but propagate enthusiasm (and, importantly, who is prepared to risk informal status and reputation

---

*Since the health-service-specific literature is particularly sparse on this topic area, we have included several studies from the wider literature in this section.

Box 6.4 Four different 'champion' roles described by Maidique[344] and based on a large empirical study in manufacturing firms (see Box 6.5 for alternative taxonomy).

(1) *Technical innovator.* The person who designed or developed the product from the technical side.
(2) *Business innovator.* The person within the managerial structure who was responsible for the innovation's 'overall progress'.
(3) *Product champion.* Any individual who made a decisive contribution to the innovation by 'actively and enthusiastically promoting its progress through critical stages'.
(4) *Chief executive.* The 'head of the executive structure' of the innovating organisation, but not necessarily the CEO or managing director.

over the innovation). It also suggests that three additional – more formal – roles are also required: an individual who can justify and explain the technical and scientific dimensions of the innovation; a middle manager responsible for project management; and support or advocacy from top management. The issue of top management support for innovations is discussed further in Section 7.6 (page 148).

Maidique presents a number of more detailed taxonomies of the champion's role relating to different organisational structures, but concludes that the overall empirical evidence for any of these is weak. In summary, his overview makes interesting reading but its relevance is mainly historical and its transferability questionable.

In their systematic review of innovation implementation in industrial process (see Section 9.1, page 176), Meyers *et al.*[91] use the terms 'patriarch' or 'godfather' to describe the strategic-level champion (e.g. the CEO) whose input to the innovation's success is generally an initial critical input to the adoption decision followed by episodic support and 'protecting the innovation from nay-sayers'; and 'evangelist' to describe the operation-level champion on whose shoulders implementation responsibilities generally rest.

Markham conducted a survey of 53 champions of innovation projects in four large firms as well as of team members from those projects. He focused specifically on the influence that champions had on other people to support their projects, rather than their direct impact on the projects. He found that the one variable that significantly increased others' willingness to participate in the project was if the champions enjoyed 'positive personal relationships' with those individuals; the choice of influence tactics (e.g. collaborative or confrontative) was not independently associated with success as a champion.[55]

A more recent empirical study addressed the cross-cultural transferability of the champion's role. Shane *et al.*[58,346] surveyed over 4000 individuals in 68 countries, and (perhaps unsurprisingly) showed that people had different preferences for how champions should work depending on prevailing cultural norms. In particular:

> [T]he more power distant a society is the more people prefer champions to focus on gaining the support of those in authority before other actions are taken on an innovation rather than on building a broad base of support among organisation members for new ideas.[58]

Thus, we should question the notion of the champion always and necessarily work horizontally through informal channels. In a more hierarchical and formal society, the champion's modus operandi may be quite different. Based on an extensive review of the literature, Shane suggests a different taxonomy for champions (Box 6.5). These roles are sequential (although overlapping) in time: in the early ('ideas') stages of an innovation, the innovator needs time out from regular duties and permission to 'break the rules' – hence the need for a 'maverick' who creates space and resources for this to happen. In the initiation stage, the transformational leader is needed to mobilise resources and provide information to the development team. In the implementation stage, the buffer role ensures that the innovation is efficiently mainstreamed taking due account of other priorities and constraints, and in the incorporation stage, the main champion role is one of making connections between the various individuals and teams in the organisation who all have an interest in the innovation.

The study by Shane demonstrated that the different champion roles are more culturally acceptable in

Box 6.5 Four different 'champion' roles described by Shane[58] and based on a survey of over 4000 individuals in 68 countries.

(1) *Organisational maverick*. Provides the innovators with autonomy from the rules, procedures and systems of the organisation so they can establish creative solutions to existing problems.
(2) *Transformational leader*. Persuades other members of the organisation to provide support for the innovation.
(3) *Organisational buffer*. Creates a loose monitoring system to ensure that innovators make proper use of organisational resources, while still allowing them to act creatively.
(4) *Network facilitator*. Defends innovators from interference from the organisational hierarchy by developing cross-functional coalitions between managers in different functional areas who support the innovation.

some societies than in others (most notably, the maverick role has low legitimacy in 'uncertainty-avoiding' societies). He concludes that certain societies are *inherently* resistant to organisational innovation for cultural reasons.[58] Whilst his survey findings are interesting, the drawing of such bold conclusions on the basis of a closed, quantitative survey might be challenged. Nevertheless, this study does caution against assuming the transferability of organisational research undertaken in different settings, especially that relating to social roles and influence. (It is worth reflecting in passing that the evidence base for much of our own report comes from North America – a very different society from the UK. Caveat emptor.)

One final 'champion' role to add to the menu above is Royer's notion of the 'exit champion'. He describes what he calls 'two chilling case studies' of over-championed projects that became company disasters. He concludes that to avoid the scenario where staff time and organisational resources are continually poured into an innovation idea that is going nowhere, several principles should be followed: assembling project teams not entirely composed of like-minded people; putting in place – and sticking to – well-defined review processes; and developing the role of the 'exit champion' – an individual who can 'push an irrationally exuberant organisation to admit when enough is enough'.[347] Again, his recommendations, while appealing, are largely speculative.

The empirical findings set out above, which were based on rigorous studies in the non-healthcare sector, some of which are now several decades old, may or may not be relevant to health service innovations in the twenty-first century, but they provide a conceptual framework against which the more health-service-specific and recent literature on champions (which as noted earlier is particularly sparse) might be compared.

Champions and advocates: empirical studies in health services research

We found no systematic reviews, no controlled trials, four survey-based studies and one multiple case study that explored the role of champions in implementing innovations in health service delivery and organisations. These are summarised in Table A.12 (page 267) in Appendix 4.

Only one study looked at 'executive champions'. Meyer and Goes (1988) hypothesised that 'innovations would be more likely to be assimilated into organisations in which the chief executives were influential proponents'.* The study measured advocacy as a composite of the extent to which the CEO
(1) personally supported the innovation and
(2) exerted personal influence during the decision-making processes.

The results showed a modest but statistically significant benefit of CEO advocacy on level of assimilation. However, introducing various other attributes of leadership into the model yielded no significant increment in predictive power after environmental and organisational factors had been taken into account.

It is hard to envisage a major innovation in service delivery and organisation being achieved without the support of the CEO, but Meyer and Goes' study aligns with the wider literature – there

*See Sections 5.3 (page 106) and 7.3 (page 140) for further discussion.

is surprisingly little evidence that CEO advocacy is a major independent variable. The study by Carter *et al.*[348] of the introduction of software innovations into the US aerospace and defence industries suggests a possible explanation. They found that advocacy by middle management had a small positive effect on adoption, but advocacy by technical staff and top management had no effect either way. However, a secondary analysis of their data showed that 'broad-based advocacy' (i.e. by individuals at all levels in the management hierarchy) was significantly associated with adoption. If this finding is generalisable to the health service context, it might explain why CEO advocacy alone has little independent impact.

Backer and Rogers'[57] case study of the adoption of work-site AIDS programmes confirmed their prediction that a clearly identifiable champion was necessary (but not sufficient) for the innovation to be adopted. However, their study contains insufficient methodological detail to show that the researchers were not merely confirming their preconceptions.

Two further studies, O'Loughlin *et al.*[349] and Riley,[215] considered (among other variables) the role of 'clinical champions' in the dissemination of health promotion programmes (in Maidique's taxonomy shown in Box 6.4, page 127, this might be the true 'product champion' role). Both found a positive impact, and these studies are discussed further in Section 9.7 (page 195).

One study focused on what might be called 'middle management' (Maidique's 'business management') champions. In evaluating the implementation of a structured infrastructure for school health programmes in USA, Valois and Hoyle hypothesised that an identifiable individual from within the staff team whose role centred on 'program champion, liaison and facilitation' would be critical to the success of the implementation process. Their study confirmed this hypothesis (the other variables that proved significant in the final model were administrative support and buy-in, effective team coordination and an index of staff health).[350] Little information was given on how staff in this middle management 'champion' role actually operated, and their impact was difficult to quantify as the statistical analysis used non-standard methods.

In summary, the literature on champions (as distinct from opinion leaders) in implementing innovations in health service delivery and organisation is sparse, but the few empirical studies identified strongly support the importance of such a role.

6.4 Boundary spanners

As discussed by Kaluzny,[304] Rogers[3] and others, boundary spanners – people with significant ties across organisational and other boundaries – influence the internal decisions within their organisation and also represent the organisation to the external environment. As information processors, boundary spanners receive, filter and control the flow of information from the environment into the organisation. The organisation is dependent upon them for information about the environment, including those aspects most critical to the organisation's survival and growth.

Information-processing theorists have argued that firms with extensive boundary-spanning capacity and environmental sensory systems are more open to change, more likely to detect another firm's actions and more likely to respond (and respond quickly) to these actions. The general hypothesis is that when boundary spanners are present and are able to facilitate information flow across boundaries, innovations will diffuse more effectively.

Boundary spanning (linking the organisation to the outside world) is closely linked to cosmopolitanism (having one's own links with the outside world), which was identified by Rogers as one of the four key attributes of an effective opinion leader (see Table 6.1). As Kimberly and Evanisko[59] state:

> Although there have been some exceptions ..., researchers generally have found that cosmopolitanism is associated with higher receptivity to innovation ... [cosmopolitanism] measures the extent to which [key individuals] have contacts with professional colleagues outside the immediate work setting. The rationale ... is that cosmopolitans would be more likely to be

exposed to new developments in the field. (page 696)

Tushman[60] documented and explored the nature of special boundary roles in the wider organisational literature as a means for innovating organisations to deal with the necessity of cross-boundary communication. On the basis of his review, he offered some practical suggestions:

- Those interested in managing innovation should explicitly recognise the importance of key individuals in the system's communication network.
- Managers should actively encourage the development of boundary roles (by recognising and rewarding boundary-spanning activity, by easing access to external information and professional literature, and by facilitating extensive communication networks through job assignments).
- Managers should be sensitive to the impact of task characteristics on boundary roles; different task areas may require boundary roles with particular backgrounds and characteristics.

The notion of boundary spanning is linked to that of knowledge management and knowledge manipulation (discussed in Section 3.13, page 70).

Whilst the role of boundary spanner is frequently alluded to in health service literature, empirical studies exploring this role are extremely sparse, and we found no studies that set out to explore such a role and that met our inclusion criteria. Occasionally, we identified an in-depth evaluation of a complex intervention project that retrospectively identified a particular key role, which we or others might classify as that of a boundary spanner. Such studies are discussed in Section 9.4 (page 186). In addition, there is the closely related notion of 'linkage' (effectively boundary-spanning activity that is not necessarily attached to an individual), which is increasingly seen as critical to interorganisational working, and which is covered in Section 9.6 (page 191).

6.5 Change agents

Rogers[3] defines a change agent (page 335) as 'an individual who influences clients' innovation decisions in a direction deemed desirable by a change agency'. Implicit in this definition is the idea that the change agent's goals are aligned more closely with those of a third party agency than with the organisation that he or she is attempting to change (indeed, such individuals may be employed by, or contracted by, such agencies). Whilst there is a wealth of empirical research into the role of change agents in general (Rogers,[3] for example, devotes 35 pages to these studies), the literature on the change agent's role in disseminating innovations in health service delivery and organisation is once again sparse, and we found no studies meeting our inclusion criteria that set out prospectively to explore this role.

Rogers' overview of the wider literature on change agents is summarised in Box 6.6. The original change agents were the experts employed in the US agricultural extension model in the mid twentieth century, whose brief was to persuade farmers to adopt innovations developed in agricultural research centres. Whilst there is now a very broad literature on change agents, the overall conclusions from this literature is still fairly heavily focused on promoting individual adoption rather than addressing the more complex issue of organisational change. The sequence of activities required of the change agent (which, incidentally, closely reflect the mainstream literature on organisational change) is shown in Box 6.6.

The critical success factors in the change agent role are shown in Box 6.7. Particularly important is *communication* – which Rogers defines as the sharing of information to create mutual understanding – and empathy with the client's predicament and perspective. One factor conspicuously absent from the list in Box 6.7 is any prescriptive recommendation for change tactics, confirming Markham's work on champions (see above), which showed that the quality of the interpersonal relationship was independently associated with influence, but the type of tactics (collaborative or confrontative) was not.

6.6 The process of spread

Whereas the vast majority of diffusion research has addressed formally developed innovations

Box 6.6 Stages in the change agent role (taken from Rogers'[3] summary of empirical studies from sociology and communication studies).

(1) Develop a need for change.
(2) Establish an information-exchange relationship.
(3) Diagnose problems.
(4) Create an intent to change in the client.
(5) Translate the intent into action.
(6) Stabilise adoption and prevent discontinuance.
(7) Achieve closure/termination.

(e.g. technologies or products developed in formal research programmes) for which the main mechanism of spread is centrally driven and controlled (dissemination), most innovations in health service delivery and organisation occur as 'good ideas' at the coal face that spread informally and in a largely uncontrolled way (diffusion). Rogers[3] writes (page 365):

> In recent decades I gradually became aware of diffusion systems that did not operate at all like centralized diffusion systems. Instead of coming out of formal R&D systems, innovation often bubbled up from the operational levels of a system, with the inventing done by certain lead users. Then the new ideas spread horizontally via peer networks, with a high degree of reinvention occurring as the innovations are modified by users to fit their particular conditions. Such decentralized diffusion systems are usually not run by technical experts. Instead, decision making in the diffusion system is widely shared, with adopters making many decisions. In many cases, adopters served as their own change agents'.

The different characteristics of centralised and decentralised diffusion systems are summarised in Table 6.3. In situations where it is appropriate to use central, planned approaches, the principles of (social) marketing theory are highly relevant. These are summarised in Box 6.8 and discussed in more detail in Section 3.5 (page 56).

For an elegant example of how the principles of social marketing were used to analyse the reasons for impact (or failure of impact) of over 150 different HIV prevention programmes in two countries (USA and Thailand), see the comparative case study by Rao and Svenkerud.[351] Using in-depth qualitative interviews with programme officials,

Box 6.7 Critical success factors in the change agent role (taken from Rogers'[3] summary of empirical studies from sociology and communication studies).

(1) *Effort*. The successful change agent puts considerable effort into contacting clients.
(2) *Client orientation*. The successful change agent (who has an inherent role conflict because of working between two systems) orients himself or herself towards the client rather than towards the change agency.
(3) *Compatibility with client's needs and resources*. The change agent's success depends on how compatible the dissemination programme is with the client's needs and resources (i.e. the successful change agent can adapt or repackage the innovation so it can be presented as an affordable solution to the client's perceived problem).
(4) *Empathy*. The successful change agent can put himself or herself in the client's position and achieve a high degree of rapport.
(5) *Homophily*. The successful change agent has similar socio-economic status, professional background, educational level, and common social networks to his or her clients.*
(6) *Credibility*. The successful change agent (and the information he or she conveys about the innovation) is seen as credible in the client's eyes.
(7) *Use of opinion leaders*. The successful change agent works through opinion leaders.
(8) *Demonstrations*. The successful change agent conducts demonstrations of innovations to increase their visibility and observability to clients.
(9) *Client ability to evaluate*. The change agent's success depends on the ability of the client to evaluate the innovation.

*See Rogers (page 346–352) for a discussion on the 'homophily phenomenon', in which change agents have a natural tendency to focus their efforts on innovators and early adopters because they tend to share more characteristics with them, whereas their input is arguably most needed for the late adopters and laggards.[3]

Table 6.3 Centralised versus decentralised networks for spread.[3]

Characteristic	*Centralised network*	*Decentralised network*
Nature of spread	Planned and targeted (dissemination)	Unplanned, spontaneous (diffusion)
Degree of centralisation	High – most decisions are made by government administrators and technical subject experts	Low – wide sharing of power and control amongst members of the diffusion system
Direction of spread	Vertical dissemination from centre to periphery and to top management	Horizontal diffusion through peer networks
Who decides what innovations to spread?	Experts, on the basis of formal, objective evaluation	Users, on the basis of informal, subjective evaluation
Driver for spread	Innovation centred; technology push	Problem centred; user pull
Extent of reinvention by individual users	Low	High

Box 6.8 Elements of a successful social marketing campaign, which should be applied when spread is centrally driven (compiled from various sources).[3,210,211]

(1) *Client orientation* – as a minimum, defining who one's consumers or clients are and finding out their perceived needs and preferences. More sophisticated (and effective) approaches involve building close relationships with consumers and engaging them actively at every stage in the project.
(2) *Exchange theory* – the notion that the intended recipient of the marketing message is being asked to exchange one thing (a particular attitude or behaviour) for another (a different attitude or behaviour): this trade-off must be presented as worthwhile.
(3) *Audience segmentation and analysis* – determining, and taking into account, the demographic, psychological and behavioural characteristics of particular target groups.
(4) *Formative evaluation research* – i.e. research undertaken before full implementation of the innovation.
(5) *The marketing mix* – i.e. how the innovation is to be marketed in terms of language, style, symbolism and so on. This includes attention to timing – a message that arrives too early or late in the decision-making process will fail to have an impact.
(6) *Cost* – both financial and human costs for the intended audience should balance the perceived benefits.
(7) *Channel analysis* – the specification and understanding of communication and distribution systems as they relate to distinct target groups.
(8) *Process tracking* – the detailed integration and monitoring of all aspects of the programme against predefined goals and milestones.

they extracted information on the original goals and evaluated each programme against its declared goals. They also gained rich qualitative information about the process of programme dissemination and implementation, which they analysed formally for themes. The results suggested that four critical success factors accounted for most of the successful programmes (and the same factors also explained a number of failures):
(1) homophily between change agent and client;
(2) use of peer opinion leaders from within the target community;
(3) audience segmentation (with different approaches tailored to the different segments); and
(4) careful assessment of the actor's stage in the innovation-decision process.*

*We have included a brief mention of the Rao study because (a) we classified it as of methodologically high quality and (b) although its own focus was an intervention aimed at service users rather than a change in health care systems, it has a potentially transferable methodology for evaluating programmes aimed at disseminating and implementing innovations in service delivery and organisation.

Section 5.1 (page 100) considered different marketing strategies for different individual adopter categories, and there is scope for additional research into 'audience segmentation' of organisations and parts of organisations so that the marketing message might be better tailored to them.

The dissemination of good ideas is a rapidly growing industry. As Strang and Soule[124] comment (page 286):

> . . . the fashion setters who construct and disseminate new practices deserve renewed attention. . . . Study of the media, consultants, and professional communities permits attention to cultural work and forms of agency that adopter-centric research overlooks. The impact of vibrant diffusion industries on the political and the business scene has hardly begun to be tapped.

It should be noted, however, that formal, planned dissemination (or which marketing is an important element) only applies – or at least, has only been empirically demonstrated to apply – to innovations that have been produced by formal research and disseminated via planned, centrally driven strategies (see Box 6.8). The role of a central change agency (such as the Modernisation Agency) in the more informal, decentralised model of spread is more ambiguous. Strang and Soule[124] go so far as to say:

> Much recent organisational analysis treats the state and the professions as change agents that spread new practices and facilitate particular lines of innovative action. State policy instruments range from coercive mandates to cheerleading and often form a complex balance of the two.

However, there is arguably much that central agencies can do in the way of creating and enabling appropriate *contexts* for informal spread (say, between organisational boundary spanners) in the same way as Kanter[17] has argued for creating a context for innovation within organisations. Section 8.2 (page 163) presents some emerging work on intentional spread strategies aimed at promoting transfer of best practice (collaboratives, Beacons and so on), in which the subjects of research have been the various organisations and linkages involved. The role of central change agencies in facilitating and enabling the informal spread of innovations via such linkages has rarely if ever been addressed as a central theme in this research stream, and this deficiency should certainly be addressed.

Chapter 7
The inner context

Key points

1. This chapter considers the inner (organisational) context as it influences the adoption, spread and sustainability of innovations. 'Inner context' comprises both the 'hard' medium of visible organisational structure and the 'soft' medium of culture and ways of working, both of which vary enormously between organisations. Certain system antecedents, discussed in detail in this chapter, will tend to make the organisation more innovative (i.e. more open to innovations in general). In addition, as discussed in 'Summary Overview', an organisation may be more or less prepared to assimilate a particular innovation (system readiness, discussed in Section 9.3, page 180).

2. Empirical research on organisational studies has sought to identify the key antecedents of organisational innovativeness. We included a total of 18 studies (three related meta-analyses from outside the health care context, and 15 additional primary studies, most of which were set within a health care context). The various determinants and moderators were defined and measured in different ways by different researchers, which makes it impossible to draw definitive or prescriptive conclusions.

3. Bearing these methodological caveats in mind, five broad determinants have been consistently found to have a positive and significant association with innovativeness: (a) structural complexity, measured as specialisation (number of specialties) or functional differentiation (number of departmental units); (b) organisational size (related to structural complexity but also acts as a proxy for slack resources); (c) leadership; (d) support for knowledge manipulation activities; and (e) receptive context (defined on page 151 and including leadership and vision, good managerial relations, supportive organisational culture, coherent local policies based on high-quality data, clear goals and priorities and effective links with other organisations).

4. The associations between these key determinants and organisational innovativeness are moderated by other variables, which affect the strength (but not the direction) of the association. For example, the association between organisational complexity and innovativeness is strengthened when there is either environmental uncertainty, when the innovations concerned are of a technical or product-based nature, or when the adoption and implementation process takes place within a service organisation.

7.1 The inner context: background literature

As discussed in detail in Section 3.10 (page 66), several key traditions in diffusion research focused on organisations rather than individuals.[63,352] As well as their specific structural features (size, complexity, etc.), organisations have particular political, social, cultural, technological and economic characteristics. Abelson (2001, as cited by Fitzgerald *et al.* 2002[32]) separates context into outer, societal 'predisposing' influences; inner institutional 'enabling' influences and 'precipitating' political influences. This section addresses the inner context whilst Chapter 8 (page 157) discusses the outer context including broader political influences.

'Inner context' can be thought of as the medium through which any organisational innovation must pass in order for it to be assimilated and routinised, which affects the rate and direction of adoption.[27,352] It includes both the 'hard' medium of the visible and measurable organisational structures and the 'soft' medium of culture and ways of working. These media, of course, vary enormously between organisations and impact on implementation and routinisation both directly (e.g. via the organisation's structures and goals) and indirectly (via an influence on actors and on the innovation itself).[43]

We found three meta-analyses[14–16] and 15 primary studies[32,38,63–65,68,71,74,76,81,229,352–355] related to organisational context and innovation adoption that met our inclusion criteria. Details of all these studies are provided in Tables A.13–A.15 (pages 269–274) in Appendix 4 and discussed in the text below.

We have distilled from these studies the key factors that have been found to influence the adoption and implementation of an innovation in an organisational context. We have focused in particular on empirically demonstrated mediators (factors through which an independent variable has an impact) and moderators (factors which, if present, alter the impact of an independent variable). These are summarised at the end of this chapter. In Section 10.1 (page 199), we add them to our overall model of critical influences on diffusion of innovations in health service organisations and apply them to four brief case studies of innovations in the UK NHS.

One important weakness of much of the literature covered in this chapter is the implicit assumption that the determinants of innovation can be treated as variables whose impact can be isolated and independently quantified. For example, the empirical studies on organisational size (Sections 7.2, page 135, and 7.4, page 141) implicitly assume that there is a 'size effect' that is worth measuring and that is to some extent generalisable. More recent theoretical work[77] and the more in-depth qualitative studies reviewed in this chapter[32,64,75,356] suggest that in reality the different determinants of organisational innovativeness interact in a complex way with one another. This 'interlocking interactions' perspective should be borne in mind when interpreting the studies described below.

7.2 Organisational determinants of innovativeness: meta-analyses

In the 1990s Damanpour[14–16] conducted three meta-analyses, all addressing the assimilation of innovations in organisations ('organisational innovativeness') as the dependent variable, and considering different organisational properties ('determinants') that might enhance or hinder the tendency to adopt (Table A.13, page 269, in Appendix 4). The primary studies included in these meta-analyses were not limited to the health care sector. In none of the meta-analyses was the search strategy comprehensive, but in all cases it was explicit and identified a large and varied sample of papers.*

Organisational determinants and moderators: the 1991 meta-analysis

The first published meta-analysis[14] (the 1991 study) tested the hypothesised relationships between 14 organisational determinants (various structural, process, resource and cultural variables) and the rate of adoption of multiple innovations (taken as a measure of organisational innovativeness). These determinants are defined in Table 7.1, which also shows the overall results. Inclusion criteria for this study were:

(1) the rate of adoption of innovations or organisational innovativeness was the ultimate dependent variable;

(2) the unit of analysis was the organisation;

(3) when a numerical score for organisational innovativeness was used, the score was based on at least two innovations; and

*The literature on organisational innovation is vast and widely dispersed throughout several different traditions. In such situations the goal of comprehensive coverage is realistically unattainable and researchers generally need to be satisfied with acquiring 'sufficient' primary studies. With quantitative designs, 'sufficient' will be measured in statistical terms while in qualitative studies the notion of 'theoretical saturation of themes' is now becoming accepted.

Table 7.1 Impact of organisational determinants on innovativeness (from Damanpour's[14] 1991 meta-analysis).

Potential determinants	*Definition*	*Association found with organisational innovativeness*
Administrative intensity	Indicator of administrative overhead	Positive, significant
Centralisation	Extent to which decision-making autonomy is dispersed or concentrated in an organisation	Negative, significant
Complexity	'Specialisation', 'functional differentiation' and 'professionalism' (see below) represent the complexity of an organisation; an overall indicator of complexity was sometimes used in studies where these three components were not present in the studies reviewed	Inconsistently defined (see previous column)
External communication	Degree of organisation members involvement and participation in extraorganisational professional activities	Positive, significant
Formalisation	Reflects emphasis on following rules and procedures in conducting organisational activities	No significant association
Functional differentiation	Extent to which divided into different units	Positive, significant
Internal communication	Extent of communication amongst organisational units	Positive, significant
Managerial attitude towards change	Extent to which managers or members of the dominant coalition are in favour of change	Positive, significant
Managerial tenure	The length of service and experience that managers have within an organisation	No significant association
Professionalism	Professional knowledge of organisational members	Positive, significant
Slack resources	Reflects the resources an organisation has beyond what it minimally requires to maintain operations	Positive, significant
Specialisation	Number of specialties in an organisation	Positive, significant
Technical knowledge resources	Reflects an organisations technical resources and technical potential	Positive, significant
Vertical differentiation	The number of levels in an organisation's hierarchy	No significant association

(4) the study was published in a scholarly journal or book.

Damanpour identified 23 empirical studies that met the inclusion criteria for meta-analysis. Three of the primary studies identified by our own search were published prior to 1991 and included in this meta-analysis, so we have not discussed them further. Two relevant studies included in our own review were published before 1991 but not reviewed by Damanpour. Twenty of the 23 studies in the Damanpour meta-analysis (of which one was in the health care field) were not otherwise identified by our searches.*

The nature and direction of association between the hypothesised determinants and organisational innovativeness is shown in Table 7.1. Although actual figures for strength of association were provided in the meta-analysis, we have deliberately not provided detailed statistical information since we question the transferability of quantitative estimates derived mainly from primary studies that would not themselves have met our own inclusion criteria (since they were mostly from outside the health care field). The study found a statistically significant ($p < 0.05$) association for ten of the determinants and organisational innovation; nine of these (Table 7.1) were positive associations and one (centralisation) was negative. No associations were found between formalisation, managerial tenure and vertical differentiation and organisational innovativeness. Statistically, the strongest determinants of innovation were specialisation, functional differentiation and external communication.

No formal tests of statistical heterogeneity were reported, but the direction and magnitude of association demonstrated for each determinant was strikingly similar across studies. For example, the association between specialisation and innovativeness was based on 20 correlations, which resulted in a mean correlation of 0.394 with an observed variance of 0.0546. In other words, specialisation appeared to be correlated with innovativeness to approximately the same degree in all or most of the primary studies.

Damanpour[14] was thus able to challenge the commonly held view that the general patterns of relationships between organisational determinants and innovation are not stable or predictable (page 582):

> The findings of this study suggest that the effects of determinants on organisational innovation are not necessarily unstable across different studies ... the present findings do not indicate the instability of innovation research results that Downs and Mohr (1976) proposed and many writings on organisational innovation have taken for granted.

However, Damanpour's subsequent meta-analyses, discussed below, did not support the same degree of confidence in the stability of structural determinants of innovativeness.

As well as considering organisational determinants, Damanpour explored which *dimensions* of innovation effectively moderate the relationship between innovation and its determinants. He included seven moderators in four categories (Table 7.2).

When these moderators were applied across the organisational determinants, in all except eight of 80 instances the *direction* of the relationship between the independent variables and organisational innovativeness remained as expected. This finding suggests that the distinct influence of moderator subgroups on determinant–innovation relationships affect the *strength* of associations but not their direction. Damanpour concluded that:

> In evaluating the moderating power of various moderators, I found that the associations between organisational variables and innovativeness are not distinguished significantly by any of the three types of innovation. Instead, the type of organisation and the scope of innovation more distinctively separate the determinants–innovation relations.

In other words, as Table 7.2 shows, some organisations (for-profit, and geared towards large numbers of innovations) are in general more successful innovators than others, whatever the par-

* This was partly because our inclusion criteria were different (a major difference being that we focused on studies relevant to health services) and partly because we covered different databases and pursued different review articles.

Table 7.2 Impact of moderator categories on innovativeness (from Damanpour's[14] 1991 meta-analysis).

Dimension of innovation (categories)	*Moderators*	*Association found with organisational innovativeness*
Type of innovation	Administrative or technical; product or process; radical or incremental	No
Stage of adoption	Initiation or implementation	No
Type of organisation	Manufacturing or service; for-profit or not-for-profit	Yes – effective moderators
Scope of innovation	Low (less than 5 innovations) or high (more than 5 innovations: comprehensive group of innovations related to various parts of an organisation)	Yes – effective moderator

ticular nature of the innovation or the stage of the innovation process.

Organisational size: the 1992 meta-analysis

The second of Damanpour's meta-analyses to be published was a preliminary exploration of the relationship between organisational size and innovation. The scope and findings of the study are summarised in Table A.13 (page 269) in Appendix 4. Inclusion criteria were same as in the 1991 study with one addition: in the case of several publications from one database, only one publication was included.

Overall, the 20 primary sources considered by Damanpour provided 36 independent estimates of the relationship between organisational size and innovation. Large size emerged as a significant independent predictor of innovativeness. When the moderating effects of the measure of size and several dimensions of innovation were considered, the mean correlations for all subgroups were also positive. Incorporating selected moderating factors into the analysis showed that:

- Size was more positively related to innovation in manufacturing and profit-making organisations than in service and non-profit-making organisations.
- The association between size and innovation is stronger when a non-personnel or a log transformation measure of size is used than when a personnel or a raw measure of size is used.*
- Types of innovation do not have a considerable moderating effect on the relationship between size and innovation.
- Size is more strongly related to the implementation than to the initiation of innovations in organisations.

Overall, there seems little doubt that large organisations are, in general, better placed to hear about, adopt and implement innovations than smaller ones, but it is also highly likely that size itself is not the *direct* variable of interest. In the commercial sector, large organisations tend to be the most commercially successful ones, but this may not be true of service organisations. Increasing size tends to come with increasing specialisation, increasing differentiation and perhaps increasing professionalism† – in other words, size is an indirect (and arguably fairly blunt) measure of organisational complexity. As we see in the next subsection, Damanpour went on to explore organisational size as one element of organisational complexity.

Organisational size and complexity: the 1996 meta-analysis

Damanpour[16] published a third meta-analysis in 1996, which sought to develop and test theories that explain the relationship between organisational complexity and innovation. The scope and findings of this are summarised in Table A.13

*In other words, when size is measured by (say) turnover or profits rather than by number of employees, it has a greater correlation with innovativeness.

†See Table 7.2 (above) for definitions of these determinants.

(page 269) in Appendix 4. The inclusion criteria were the same as in the 1991 meta-analysis (described above) with the additional observation that when several publications were based on one data-set, only one publication was included. Damanpour adopted two separate indicators of organisational complexity:
(1) structural complexity and
(2) organisational size (see previous paragraph for an explanation of this link).

His search yielded 21 relevant studies that related structural complexity or size to organisational innovation (27 separate comparisons correlated structural complexity, and a further 36 comparisons correlated organisational size with the dependent variable of organisational innovativeness).

Two indicators of structural complexity were employed in the studies: functional differentiation (measured by the total number of units below the CEO) and occupational differentiation or role specialisation (measured by the number of occupational specialties or job titles). Organisational size was based either on a personnel (number of employees) or on a non-personnel (physical capacity, input or output volume or financial resources) indicator. Organisational innovation was typically measured by the rate of adoption of innovations, operationalised as the number of innovations adopted within a given period of time.

The mean correlations, weighted by sample size, between structural complexity and innovativeness and between size and innovativeness were 0.382 ($p < 0.001$) and 0.346 ($p < 0.001$), respectively (in other words, *in general* both complexity and size were significant determinants of innovativeness). Damanpour concluded that both structural complexity and organisational size are positively related to organisational innovativeness and explain about 15% and 12%, respectively, of variation in it.

However, there was significant variance in the correlations reported in the individual studies (e.g. the range of correlation for structural complexity–innovation and size–innovation were −0.09 to 0.71 and −0.04 to 0.76, respectively). In other words, *in some studies*, the correlation was far higher and in others there was no correlation at all. This contrasts, incidentally, with Damanpour's earlier conclusion (see page 136) that the relationship between structural determinants and innovativeness are highly stable across studies.

In his 1996 article, Damanpour also considered the impact of 14 'contingency factors' on the association between structural complexity and innovativeness, and between organisational size and innovativeness. These factors were categorised into three groups:
(1) commonly cited contingency factors (environmental uncertainty, organisational size);
(2) industrial sectors (manufacturing, service, for-profit and not-for-profit); and
(3) dimensions of innovation, including types of innovation (administrative, technical, product, process, radical and incremental) and stages of innovation adoption (initiation and implementation).

The impact of these factors are summarised in Table 7.3.

Using a stepwise multiple regression analysis Damanpour found that across all relevant studies, seven contingency factors had a statistically significant impact on the association between structural complexity and innovativeness, and six had an impact on the association between organisational size and innovativeness. Four contingency factors were common to both indicators: environmental uncertainty, use of service organisations, focus on technical innovations, and focus on product innovations.

To summarise, the three Damanpour meta-analyses strongly support the notion that organisational size and complexity (i.e. specialisation, functional differentiation and professional knowledge) are both *associated* with innovativeness. However, this relationship is moderated by various factors. It tends to be significantly stronger in the for-profit sector than the not for-profit sector and marginally stronger in the manufacturing sector than in the service sector. The overall magnitude of the effect should be noted, however (the contribution to overall innovativeness score is of the order of 15%). Furthermore, the primary studies reviewed by Damanpour do not show that size *determines* innovativeness, and there is certainly no evidence thus far that manipulating the size of an organisation per se (e.g. by providing incentives for small GP practices to merge into group practices, as was done in the UK in the 1960s), or tinkering with its structure,

Table 7.3 Contingency factors whose impact on the association between organisational complexity and innovativeness was tested in the Damanpour[16] 1996 meta-analysis.

		Significant impact on the association between:	
Contingency factor	*Definition or categories*	*Structural complexity and innovativeness*	*Organisational size and innovativeness*
Innovation-adoption factors			
Type of innovation	Administrative	Negative	Negative
	Technical	Positive	Not significant
	Product	Positive	Positive
	Process	Not significant	Not significant
	Radical	Positive	Positive
	Incremental	Not significant	Not significant
Stage of adoption	Initiation	Negative	Negative
	Implementation	Positive	Not significant
Inner context factors			
Size		Negative	NA
Sector	Manufacturing	Positive	Positive
	Service	Positive	Positive
	For-profit	Not significant	Positive
	Not-for-profit	Not significant	Positive
Outer context factors			
Environmental uncertainty		Positive	Positive

will *make* that organisation more innovative. Chapter 8 (page 157) discusses the few empirical studies in which modifications to organisational structure, notably the setting up of multi-disciplinary teams, were studied prospectively in relation to the implementation of particular service innovations.

A number of empirical studies have been published since the Damanpour meta-analyses, many relating specifically to health care organisations, which also address the link between organisational factors and innovativeness. We discuss these in Sections 7.3–7.8.

7.3 Organisational determinants of innovativeness: overview of primary studies in the service sector*

On the basis of the Damanpour findings reported above, and also from our early exploratory readings of the literature, we chose to examine in more detail a number of dimensions of the 'inner context' that appear to be critical in shaping the medium through which innovations must travel in order to be assimilated and routinised within organisations. We have restricted our coverage of primary studies to those with an important message for health care organisations. In practice, this meant that we applied a somewhat flexible set of inclusion criteria depending on how rich the literature was in particular areas. Where there were many relevant primary studies of health care organisations, we restricted our analysis to these;

*To avoid double counting, we have not generally reiterated findings from early studies that were considered by Damanpour in the three meta-analyses reported in the previous section. However, we have gone into additional detail in the case of studies where they were especially relevant to this review.

where there were not, we included other service sector studies and occasionally (where the study was particularly original or of particularly high quality or had a transferable idea for further work), we included studies from the industrial or commercial sector.

On the basis of the empirical studies available, we have divided organisational determinants of innovativeness into three dimensions (Sections 7.4–7.6):

(1) size of organisation (and the association of this with organisational slack; below);
(2) structural complexity (page 146); and
(3) leadership and loci of decision-making (page 148).

Two additional organisational antecedents are considered:

(1) organisational climate and receptive context (Section 7.7, page 150); and
(2) initiatives to enable and support knowledge manipulation (Section 7.8, page 154).

The contribution of the different empirical studies reviewed in this chapter to these five themes is summarised in Table 7.4, which gives an approximate indication of the changes in focus of organisational research since the mid-1970s.

Table 7.4 does not represent a comprehensive list of the determinants of organisational innovativeness. Rather, it represents the determinants that have been most widely studied and hence those on which evidence is available. Conspicuously absent from most empirical work, for example, is the important issue of internal politics (e.g. doctor–manager power balances), identified as one of several critical influences in a single qualitative study[64] (see page 144).* We were surprised to find so few studies that considered the impact of power balances on innovation in the health care sector. The main characteristics and findings of the studies listed in Table 7.4 are summarised in Table A.14 (page 271) in Appendix 4.

Whereas the antecedents addressed in this chapter reflect the general capacity of the organisation to spread and sustain any innovation, there are also some innovation-specific factors, notably motivation and commitment – which we have included within 'system readiness' (i.e. readiness for a particular innovation rather than receptivity to innovation in general; discussed in Section 9.3, page 180. Clearly, an organisation might be capable of generating and capturing innovations but may decide – perhaps for very good reasons – not to take up a particular innovation at a particular time.

7.4 Empirical studies on organisational size

The size of an organisation was not initially considered by Damanpour[14] as an independent determinant of innovativeness, but as described above, he subsequently identified size as a major determinant (accounting for around 12% of the variation in innovativeness), and explored its impact in detail. We found seven primary studies (write-ups in eight papers) that met our inclusion criteria and that explored how the size of an organisation impacts the adoption of innovations.[38,59,63–65,68,73,76] Each of these studies tested the relationship between a range of independent variables and the adoption of specific innovations over a period of time. The overall organisational context for all the studies was a professional bureaucracy (six took place within hospitals in the USA, Canada or Europe, and one was in an academic institution).

Five of the seven primary studies[38,59,63,68,73,76] concluded that size had a positive (and statistically significant) association with the adoption of innovations, and two of these studies identified the organisation's size and complexity (see below) as the most significant variables. One study did not find any overall relationship,[65] and one found a negative relationship.[64] These studies are reviewed briefly below.

Baldridge and Burnham[63] examined organisational innovations and changes in the education

*Our own team, in an evaluation of five projects to implement complex service innovations in primary health care, found that power relations (especially between a project steering group and the main project worker) were critical to successful implementation, but that they were extremely difficult to explore systematically and raised ethical issues for the research team.[87]

Table 7.4 Determinants of innovation explored in empirical studies of 'inner context' of health care organisations (discussed in Sections 7.4–7.8).

Author/date	*Size (Section 7.4, page 141)*	*Structural complexity (Section 7.5, page 146)*	*Leadership and decision-making (Section 7.6, page 148)*	*Climate and receptive context (Section 7.7, page 150)*	*Supporting knowledge manipulation (Section 7.8, page 154)*	*Others*
Baldridge and Burnham 1975[63]	•	•	•			Characteristics of individual adopters
Kimberly and Evanisko 1981[59]	•	•	•			Characteristics of individual adopters
Meyer and Goes 1988[38]	•	•	•			Urbanisation, 'championship'
Champagne *et al.* 1991[64]	•	•	•			Political influences, urbanisation
Burns and Wholey 1993[65]	•	•				Interorganisational influences
Dufault *et al.* 1995[66]					•	
Patel 1996[67]					•	
Goes and Park 1997[68]	•	•				
Anderson and West 1998[69]				•		
Barnsley *et al.* 1998[61]					•	
Wilson *et al.* 1999[74]				•		
Dopson, Fitzgerald *et al.* 2002[32,75]		•		•	•	
Nystrom *et al.* 2002[76]	•		•	•		Risk orientation, external orientation
Rashman and Hartley 2002[72]				•	•	
Newton *et al.* 2003[71]				•		
Gosling *et al.* 2003[70]				•		

sector.* On the basis of findings from previous literature, they proposed three hypotheses:

- Certain individuals (educated, cosmopolitan, high socio-economic status) are likely to adopt innovations; therefore, organisations with a high percentage of such individuals are likely to adopt more innovations.
- High organisational complexity and large size will promote adoption of innovation because these determinants permit specialised expertise to be concentrated in subunits, and because there will arise within these units critical masses of problems that demand solutions.
- Heterogeneous or changing environments are likely to promote the adoption of innovations

*Unlike many studies before and since, Baldridge and Burnham's empirical work in the educational sector was explicitly hypothesis-driven, and led to an important change in the direction of research in this field. We have therefore included their work in our analysis.

because organisations are subject to varied pressure from outside (see Section 8.3, page 170, for coverage of this aspect of the study).

They conducted semi-structured interviews with district superintendents and school principals in 20 randomly selected schools in seven districts in San Francisco (1967–8) and sent a questionnaire to 264 Illinois school districts in 1969–70. They sought to examine organisational innovations and changes:
(1) with relatively unclear technologies;
(2) with long-range pay-offs;
(3) that were adopted by organisations; and
(4) that were difficult to evaluate.

Baldridge and Burnham made the important discovery that individual adopter characteristics (such as gender, age, cosmopolitanism, education), which as Chapter 5 (page 100) showed have strong predictive value for *individual* adoption, did not make these individuals better able to achieve organisational change, although administrative positions and roles did seem to have an impact on the involvement of an individual in the innovation process. Their findings did, however, strongly support the hypothesis that organisational size and complexity are associated with increased adoption of educational innovation. The moderating effect of the external environment in the Baldridge and Burnham study is discussed in Chapter 8 (page 157).

These authors concluded that individual adopter characteristics are poor predictors of assimilation of innovations within organisations;* that a large, complex organisation with a heterogeneous environment is more likely to adopt innovations than a small, simple organisation with a relatively stable, homogenous environment; and that environmental change did not significantly influence the adoption of innovations by the school districts. Theirs was thus a 'milestone' paper that challenged previous assumptions that innovative individuals can make their organisations more innovative, which prompted a new stream of research of looking at the organisation itself.

Kimberly and Evanisko[59] sought to examine the combined effects of individual, organisational and contextual variables on the hospital adoption of two types of innovation (technological and administrative). The independent variables addressed in this study are summarised in Box 7.1. These authors also considered characteristics of the individual as an organisational member (job tenure and the nature of organisational involvement of leaders).

Five of the 12 variables tested (of which four were classified by the authors as 'organisational' and the fifth was organisational age) were found to explain a significant proportion of unique variance in adoption behaviour for innovations in medical technologies: size of hospital, degree of centralisation, specialisation, functional differentiation and age of hospital. Two variables had a significant independent impact on adoption of administrative innovations: size of hospital and cosmopolitanism of the hospital administrator.

The authors concluded (page 709) that 'organisational level variables – and size in particular – are indisputably better predictors of both types of innovation than either individual or contextual

Box 7.1 Determinants of organisational innovativeness studied by Kimberly and Evanisko,[59] showing those significantly (and positively) associated with adoption of technological innovations (T) and administrative innovations (A).

Individual (characteristics of individual people in positions of authority):
- Job tenure
- Cosmopolitanism (A)
- Educational background
- Nature of organisational involvement of leaders

Organisational ('inner context')
- Centralisation (T)
- Specialisation (T)
- Size (T) (A)
- Functional differentiation (T)
- External integration

Contextual ('outer context')
- Competition
- Size of city
- Age of hospital (T)

*This finding confirmed that of a previous large (and widely cited) empirical study by Hage and Aitken in social welfare agencies.[355]

level variables'.[59] An important finding in relation to our own research question was that adoption of the two different types of innovations was differently influenced by the variables tested. In particular, these variables were much better predictors of the adoption of technological innovations than of administrative innovations. The authors concluded that adoption of technological innovation (and to a lesser extent, that of administrative innovations) tends to be most prevalent in organisations that are large, specialised, functionally differentiated and decentralised.

Meyer and Goes[38] (along with other researchers) examined the assimilation of 12 medical innovations into community hospitals.* Their results supported those of Kimberly and Evanisko[59] to the extent that the innovations were more likely to be adopted by larger hospitals with relatively complex structures. In both analyses, organisation-level variables afforded the best predictions of innovativeness, environmental variables explained about half as much variance as the organisation-level variables, and leadership variables proved to have less explanatory power than the other sets. However, these authors noted that whilst organisational attributes like size and complexity may mark an organisation out as innovative, they will not necessarily predict the adoption of particular innovations – a point we return to in Section 9.3 (page 180).

The study by Champagne *et al.*[64] of fee structures for physicians was one of the two studies we identified that did not find that large size had an effect on adoption of innovations in health care organisations. The factors hypothesised to affect the adoption of the innovation were

(1) Political: successful adoption is more likely if the innovation receives the support of leaders who control the bases of power in the organisation. This support is a function of
   (a) the centrality of the innovation in relation to the actor's goals and
   (b) the congruence between the policy objectives associated with the innovation and the actors' goals.

(2) Organisational:
   (a) structural complexity, formalisation and professionalism and
   (b) the degree of attention paid to the innovation by organisational leaders.

(3) Urbanisation (distance of the organisation from a large urban centre, discussed in Section 8.3, page 170).

'Political' influences were measured by an interesting combination of factors:

(1) the actors' cosmopolitan–local orientation;
(2) the actors' locus of control (a psychological construct that measures whether individuals generally believe things to be under their personal control or whether they explain events in terms of chance or external circumstances); and
(3) the actors' degree of satisfaction with the organisation's performance.

The leadership elements of this study are discussed below.

High levels of implementation of this innovation (sessional fee remuneration for GPs in long-term care hospitals) was found to be positively associated with

(1) a high degree of satisfaction by the GP leaders with the organisation's performance;
(2) an urban environment; and
(3) a small number of beds.

The extent of change following the introduction of sessional payments was also negatively and strongly associated with the level of professionalism and the cosmopolitan orientation of managers.

This somewhat unusual study raises more methodological questions than it answers about how to measure 'political power bases' in health service organisations, and certainly whets the appetite for further research into the nature and impact of such power bases – in particular, the interaction between doctors and managers when the innovation potentially affects the income of the former. The authors acknowledge (page 105) that 'the small negative relationship between organisational size (structural complexity) and level of implementation remains to be explained'.

The study by Champagne *et al.* looked at a very specific and (in comparison with the other studies covered here) unusual innovation. In the terminology of systematic review, this study might be

*This work was also covered in Section 5.3 (page 106) in relation to the adoption process.

said to be heterogeneous in important respects in comparison with the rest of the sample, and hence its divergent findings are perhaps not surprising. There are certainly good common-sense reasons why its quantitative results should not simply be summed with the other results.

Burns and Wholey studied the introduction of an administrative innovation (unit matrix management*) into 1375 non-federal general hospitals in the USA.[65] Hospitals were included if they had moderate or large size (over 300 beds) or teaching programmes in 1961, 1966, 1972 or 1978. At the time of the study, 346 hospitals had adopted some version of unit management and 901 hospitals had not. Using an organisational survey instrument, Burns and Wholey tested the impact of

(1) 'Technical factors' – what we have called organisational characteristics:
 (a) organisational diversification and scale and
 (b) slack resources and capabilities.
(2) 'Non-technical factors' – what we have called 'outer context' factors†:
 (a) network embeddedness and
 (b) normative institutional pressures.

The authors found significant effects for two (outpatient and teaching diversity) of the three measures of organisational diversity but found no evidence that organisational scale or slack resources led, overall, to hospitals being more likely to adopt unit management structures. However, in the early periods of assimilation, teaching diversity and size did exert positive effects on adoption, as did prestige. They also found that hospitals more centrally placed in their inter-institutional networks, and the degree of pressure perceived from interorganisational norms ('cumulative pressure to adopt') was significantly related to adoption of the innovation. These last two factors are discussed further in Section 8.1 (page 157).

It is perhaps not surprising that the Burns and Wholey study found significant effects for two of the three measures of organisational diversification (supporting the general notion that concentrating knowledge within subunits leads to greater ability to support innovation), but it is surprising that they found no overall effect of organisational size or slack resources (note, however, that very small hospitals were excluded from the sample). An additional important finding was that owing to 'organisation-level social influence', the prestige of a hospital influences not only its own decision to adopt but also the decisions of neighbouring hospitals.

Goes and Park[68] undertook a large 10-year longitudinal study of adoption of both technical and administrative innovations in 356 Californian hospitals. Although they focused mainly on the influence of interorganisational links on organisation-level innovation (and hence, this large landmark study is discussed in more detail in Section 8.1, page 157), they also tested the effect of hospital size, and found that larger hospitals were consistently more innovative than smaller hospitals. The results highlighted a confounding variable that could partly explain the consistent relationship between size and innovativeness shown in other studies: hospitals with more and deeper links to other hospitals (which Goes and Park found to be strongly related to innovativeness for both technologies and administrative changes) were also more likely to be large.

Castle[73] examined a number of organisational and market characteristics associated with the adoption of two groups of innovations – special care units and subacute care units – in 13 162 nursing homes in the USA during the period 1992–7. The market characteristics are discussed in Section 8.3 (page 170). Four organisational factors were explored: organisational size (number of beds), whether the homes were for-profit or not-for-profit, whether the homes were members of a larger chain and the rate of private-patient occupancy. Using two national routine datasets, Castle found that three of the four organisational factors increased the likelihood of early innovation adoption. The factors with statistically significant associations with early adoption in this large study were organisational size ($p < 0.01$), chain membership ($p < 0.01$) and high levels of private pay residents ($p < 0.001$).

Nystrom *et al.*[76] explored adoption of medical imaging technologies in US hospitals. Using a

*Matrix management is defined as 'laying one or more forms of departmentalisation on top of an existing form' (e.g. liaison roles to provide coordination across functional departments).

†See Chapter 8 (page 157).

postal questionnaire, they tested the hypothesis that organisational size (measured as a logarithmic transformation of number of beds) and organisational slack (a composite of financial resources, skilled labour, managerial talent, and extent to which funds have already been committed for capital projects) are positively related with innovativeness (a composite measure of the radicalness of innovations adopted, the extent of benefits they provide and the number of innovations adopted over time). They also hypothesised that risk orientation (defined as top management's attitude towards change) and external orientation (defined in terms of boundary-spanning roles and achievement orientation) would moderate the influence of organisational size and organisational age.

The study found that both organisational size and slack resources had significant positive influences on innovativeness. They also suggested that the significant interaction they found between size and risk orientation means that the overall positive relationship between size and innovativeness is even stronger in those organisations with a climate favouring risk-taking, providing additional support to the findings of the studies, described above, showing that organisational size is directly and positively related to innovation adoption.

In summary, as previously demonstrated by Damanpour (see Section 7.2, page 135), one of the most commonly observed findings about organisational innovation is the positive correlation with large size. Organisational theorists continue to debate *why* size is generally associated with innovativeness. As discussed in Section 7.3, one explanation is that larger size increases the likelihood that other predictors of innovation will be present, including the availability of financial and human resources (organisational slack) and differentiation or specialisation. Quinn[358] has even argued that large, successful companies stay innovative because efficient differentiation enables subunits to 'behave like small entrepreneurial ventures' (i.e. work semi-autonomously, thereby being freed of bureaucratic constraints) while at the same time enjoying the benefits (e.g. buffering of cash flow) offered by a larger company.

Of the two studies in our sample that failed to demonstrate a significant positive relation between size and innovativeness, one had a high degree of heterogeneity with the rest of the sample (i.e. it measured adoption of a very different innovation),[64] and the other excluded very small organisations from its sampling frame.[65] It is also true, however, that large organisational size may make the adoption of some innovations (especially administrative ones) virtually essential, so the effect of size will itself be moderated by the nature of the innovation.

7.5 Empirical studies on structural complexity

As discussed in Section 7.2 (page 135), two of the determinants found by Damanpour's[14] earliest meta-analysis to have significant (indeed, the strongest) positive associations with organisational innovation were specialisation and functional differentiation. For Damanpour,[16] taken together with professionalism (which incidentally was not found to have a significant association with innovation), these three determinants represented 'complexity'. His 1996 meta-analysis found that structural complexity was positively related to organisational innovation and explained about 15% of variation in it.

We found eight primary studies that explored the relationship between the adoption of an innovation and some measure of the level of structural complexity within the adopting organisation(s).[32,38,59,63–65,68] All except one of these (in a school[63]) were in health care organisations, six in primary care and two in secondary care.

In the early 1970s, drawing on a previous study in social welfare agencies by Hage and Aiken,[355] Baldridge and Burnham hypothesised an association between functional differentiation (division into subunits with different roles) and innovativeness. The reasons for this likely association are twofold. First, a functionally differentiated organisation creates multiple interest groups and multiple demands for technological innovations. Second, the problems of coordination and control are exacerbated when organisations are formally divided into larger numbers of functional units; hence, administrative innovations are also adopted more readily (or at least, are more obviously necessary). They measured 'heterogeneity of the organisational environment' using a combination of measures of socio-economic status and ethnic mix. They found that schools with such an environment were significantly more likely to adopt innovations than those with more homogenous environments.[63]

The variables explored in Kimberly and Evanisko's 1981 study of the adoption of technological and administrative innovations in health care are set out in Box 7.1 (page 143). They also addressed the hypothesis that functional differentiation leads to increased adoption of innovations. The results suggested that whilst adoption of technological innovation was significantly more prevalent in organisations that are large, specialised, functionally differentiated and decentralised, complexity did not seem to be a predictor of adoption of administrative innovations.

Meyer and Goes[38] measured structural complexity in the 25 US community hospitals they followed in terms of the assimilation of 24 technical innovations. As these services required either separate structural subunits or specialised staff members, they took the number of these available in a hospital as a reflection of horizontal differentiation (the most common operational definition of complexity). Overall, the study found that innovations were more likely to be assimilated into hospitals that

(1) served urban rather than rural environments and

(2) exhibited relatively large size, complex structure and aggressive market strategies.

Champagne *et al.*[64] examined how structural complexity affected the implementation of sessional fee remuneration for general practitioners in long-term care hospitals. They found that the level of implementation was negatively associated with structural complexity and commented that previous studies by other authors had had equivocal findings in relation to this variable.

Burns and Wholey[65] investigated the impact of organisational diversity on the adoption of unit management in over 1300 hospitals in the USA. The authors measured 'diversity' in terms of the range of clients treated and the 'tasks' performed (teaching and research activities) and hypothesised that *'task diversity'* would be positively associated with the adoption of unit management. The results confirmed a significant positive effect of task diversity on adoption. However, the impact of teaching diversity diminished over time, suggesting that the importance of this variable is contingent on the period in the diffusion process under study (in other words, diversity may be more important in the earlier stages of adoption).

In their 1997 study on adoption of technical and administrative innovations in Californian hospitals, Goes and Park hypothesised that 'hospitals are more likely to adopt service innovations when they are structurally linked with other hospitals'. Their study was undertaken in the context of multi-hospital systems in the USA and found that innovation was more likely among hospitals using the structural link of membership in such a system ($r^2 = 0.22$, $p < 0.001$). The explanation for this effect is that such structural links bring hospitals greater awareness of and exposure to new technologies and administrative systems, greater access to know-how and learning gained by other system members, and greater access to the resources needed for innovation. These issues are described in more detail in Section 8.1 (page 157), which covers interorganisational networks.

Fitzgerald *et al.*[32] in their comparative case studies (using mainly in-depth qualitative methods) of the diffusion of eight innovations in the primary and acute care sectors, described in more detail in Section 5.3 (page 106), and in this chapter (page 153) found that 'structural complexity has an impact' (page 1443). In two of their case studies, interprofessional and interorganisational boundaries acted as 'inhibitors' to the diffusion process and these could only be overcome with 'substantial effort'.

The findings of the seven primary studies from the service sector described above thus confirm the findings of Damanpour's meta-analysis of the wider literature – that large, functionally differentiated organisations with low levels of formalisation and centralisation tend to be more innovative.*

As first suggested by Burns and Wholey,[65] there is good evidence that the impact of structural complexity on innovation is moderated by the stage of the diffusion process under study and the nature of the innovation (technological or administrative) being adopted. These moderating influences are generating considerable contemporary research interest. Adler *et al.*[43] hypothesise, for example, that whilst more structurally complex organisations may be more innovative and hence *adopt* innovations relatively early, less structurally complex organisations will be able to *diffuse* innovations more effectively (page 17).

It cannot be overemphasised that structural explanations of innovation adoption may be falsely deterministic (in other words, even when a particular structural feature is consistently *associated with* innovativeness, it does not mean it *causes* innovativeness). As long ago as 1979, Kervasdoue and Kimberly[229] had argued that in order to understand hospital innovation it is necessary to go beyond the structuralist paradigm and ask questions about socio-political, historical and cultural factors in and around organisations. These factors are discussed further in Chapter 8 (page 157).

7.6 Empirical studies on leadership and locus of decision-making

Leadership is a compelling concept in organisational literature, whose measurement has fascinated and frustrated organisational theorists for centuries.[359] We have been struck by two features of the empirical literature relating leadership to organisational innovativeness: the lack of consistent measures of this variable and the lack of theoretical discussion on how the different measures of leadership were selected for particular studies. We were not able to review the mainstream literature on leadership for this book, but as with the mainstream literature on change management, there is likely to be much that is relevant to our research question. One particular aspect of leadership – opinion leadership – is covered in detail in Section 6.2 (page 118). This section addresses formal leadership roles in organisations and their link with innovation.

Damanpour's[14] 1991 meta-analysis found a significant positive association between 'managerial attitude towards change' and organisational innovation, and a significant negative association with centralisation of decision-making. The organisational literature suggests that it has long been assumed (even in the absence of empirical evidence) that a primary antecedent of an organisation's climate for implementation is managers' support for implementation of the innovation. Van de Ven,[123] for example, comments (page 601):

> ... institutional leadership is critical in creating a cultural context that fosters innovation, and in establishing organisational strategy, structure and systems that facilitate innovation.

We found five empirical studies that directly explored the association between leadership (and the locus of decision-making) and innovation adoption and that met our inclusion criteria[38,59,63,64,76] (see Table 7.4, page 142, for brief details and Table A.14, page 271, in Appendix 4 for summary of characteristics and findings).

Although Baldridge and Burnham's study (described in detail above) focused more on opinion leadership than on organisational leadership, they observed that organisational position and role appeared to influence their impact on the adoption decisions of other actors (innovation adoption was most strongly influenced by those with power, communication linkages and with the ability to impose sanctions), a finding comparable with the somewhat tangential evidence from earlier studies that those who allocated organisational resources had greater influence on the innovation-adoption decision.[360]

In their 1981 study of innovation in US hospitals, Kimberly and Evanisko[59] studied four char-

*This finding, incidentally, is also consistent with some of the earliest organisational studies of innovation (reviewed by Strang and Soule[124]), again suggesting that such determinants are stable and to some extent predictable.

acteristics of leaders (the chief of medicine and the hospital administrator):
(1) length of job tenure;
(2) cosmopolitanism;
(3) educational background; and
(4) the nature of their organisational involvement.

Two of the variables showed a significant independent influence on the adoption of administrative innovations: adoption was positively affected when the hospital administrator was highly educated and (a particularly strong association) cosmopolitan.

None of the leadership variables measured was a significant overall predictor of the organisation's adoption of technological innovations, but the results showed some trends that might have proved significant in a larger study. Adoption of technological innovations was positively affected when the hospital administrator was highly educated, did not participate in committees dealing with matters of medical policy, was relatively heavily involved in medical activities, and had served in his or her role for a relatively long period of time. Similar effects were noted when the chief of medicine had been in a post for a relatively long period of time, and when he or she was relatively actively involved in administrative affairs.

The authors suggest that these results are at first sight somewhat counter-intuitive (i.e. the hospital administrator is a more central figure in the adoption of medical technologies than is the chief of medicine). They suggest that in organisations such as hospitals where there is a dual-authority structure, innovation is facilitated where the leaders of each are actively involved in the affairs of the other. Such activity provides an opportunity for the kind of bargaining and negotiation required when potentially conflicting interests are at stake.

In their 1988 study of adoption of large medical technologies,* Meyer and Goes hypothesised, firstly, that 'innovations would be more likely to be assimilated into organisations whose chief executives had long tenures and high levels of education', and, secondly, that 'innovations would be more likely to be assimilated into organisations in which the chief executives were influential proponents'. In order to test the second of these, the study assessed the extent to which the CEO
(1) personally supported acquisition and
(2) exerted influence during the decision-making processes.

The Meyer and Goes study is thus one of the few studies on the influence of leadership variables on organisational adoption of innovations in which the selection of measures of leadership were rigorously hypothesis-driven.

The results (as mentioned in the Section 6.3, page 126) implied that a medical innovation is particularly likely to be assimilated if it is championed by a CEO who exerts substantial influence on its behalf. However, introducing attributes of leaders yielded no additional significant increment in predictive power after environmental and organisational factors had been taken into account. In other words, this study suggests that although CEOs' demographic characteristics have no particular influence on the *overall* adoption of innovations by their organisations, CEOs nonetheless can have a substantial impact by championing the assimilation of *specific* innovations.

The study by Champagne *et al.*[64] of sessional fee introduction for GPs examined GP leaders'
(1) cosmopolitan–local orientation;
(2) locus of control; and
(3) degree of satisfaction with their organisation's performance.

They found that the level of implementation of the innovation was positively and very strongly associated with the leaders' satisfaction with the organisation's performance. The extent of change following implementation was *negatively* and strongly associated with the cosmopolitan orientation of managers. The authors suggest that a strong external orientation of the managers may reflect the displacement of their allegiance from the hospital to other organisations. In that case the managers will have a minor influence on the implementation process since they will be minimally involved in the organisation of care.

In their study of adoption of medical imaging technologies in US hospitals, Nystrom *et al.*[76] proposed 'risk orientation' as an important determin-

*Discussed in more detail in Section 5.3 (page 106).

ant of organisational innovativeness, and defined the concept as 'top management's attitude toward change'. They used a conventional postal questionnaire survey sent to 70 hospitals and seeking a range of data on structural and 'climate' variables. The study confirmed previous findings that both organisational size and slack resources have significant positive influences on innovativeness. But it also demonstrated a new finding – that both risk orientation and external orientation (see Section 7.7) interact significantly with these two established determinants to increase the radicalness of the innovations adopted, the extent of the benefits they provide and the number of innovations adopted over time.

Most studies of leadership and innovation adoption focused on particular characteristics (educational background, job tenure,[*,†] etc.) of individuals holding a formal leadership role. But the wider contribution of leaders to creating a climate that facilitates innovation adoption is inherently much more difficult to measure, and very few studies have attempted to do so. As earlier sections in this chapter have shown, whilst organisational size and structural complexity have been consistently found to encourage innovative behaviour, without the intervention of leaders these attributes have the potential to stifle innovation. In the words of Van de Ven (page 596):

> Organisational structures and systems serve to sort attention. They focus efforts in prescribed areas and blind people to other issues by influencing perceptions, values, and beliefs ... the older, larger and more successful organisations become, the more likely they are to have a large repertoire of structures and systems which discourage innovation while encouraging tinkering. ... The implication is that without the intervention of leadership, structures and systems focus the attention of organisational members to routine, not innovative activities.

*Damanpour's[14] meta-analysis did not find a significant association between 'managerial tenure' and organisational innovation.

†In a high-quality study outside the service sector, Sharma and Rai[354] found that in the context of Information Systems Departments (ISDs), job tenure of the ISD leaders was significant in discriminating between adopters and non-adopters. ISD leaders in adopter organisations had shorter tenures (4.7 years) than those in non-adopter organisations (8 years). Positional power of the ISD leaders was also found significant in differentiating adopter organisations from non-adopters.

7.7 Empirical studies on organisational climate and receptive context

The concept of organisational climate has received considerable attention from applied psychologists and organisational sociologists over the last decade. A working definition of organisational climate for our purposes might be: 'To what extent do staff in this organisation feel that it's OK to experiment with new ideas?'

Perrin argues forcefully that innovation is inevitably associated with risk and that efforts at innovation will have a failure rate. If innovation is evaluated in terms of success, and the organisation responds to failure by punishing the innovators, the prevailing climate will not support necessary risk-taking. Rather, he argues, we must acknowledge the inherent failure rate in organisational innovation, and develop an evaluation system that rewards risk-taking and learns systematically from failures.[361] Research into organisational climate has increasingly focused on the cognitive schema approach, which conceptualises climate as individuals' perceptions or cognitive schemata of their work environments, and has been operationalised through attempts to uncover individuals' sense-making of their work environment.[362,363]

Whilst organisational climate is a popular construct for researchers to measure, it is (intentionally) very focused on one aspect of the organisation's receptivity to innovation and hence may be of limited use in the practical setting. 'Receptive context'[‡] is a broader concept made up of

‡Note the difference between the general notion of organisational receptivity to change and the particular factors that make up the construct 'receptive context'. Huy has proposed that, at the individual level, receptiv-

eight factors (Bate *et al.* adapted from Pettigrew *et al.*[78,390]) and is summarised in Box 7.2.

These concepts together encompass not only the nature of 'the informal organisation'* and organisational routines† but also the receptive context for innovations and knowledge management capabilities within the organisation. This final point relates to the notion of absorptive capacity[23,265] (see definition and dimensions of this construct, page 72), which is strongly shaped by the antecedent repertoire of the organisation. The capacities in the repertoire will be those that are distributed throughout the organisation and are capable of being articulated:

> The ability to exploit external knowledge is thus a critical component of innovative capabilities. ... An organisation's absorptive capacity does not simply depend on the organisation's direct interface with the external environment. It also depends on transfer of knowledge across and within sub-units that may be quite removed from the original point of entry. Thus, to understand the sources of a firm's absorptive capacity, we focus on the structure of communication between the external environment and the organisation, as well as among the subunits of the organisation, and also on the character and distribution of expertise within the organisation.[265]

There has been growing interest in how particular types of climate and receptive context lead to (or inhibit) organisational innovation and how they can enhance the organisation's capacity to diffuse innovation. We found six empirical studies that looked at the impact of organisational climate, receptive context or absorptive capacity on the implementation of innovations in health service delivery and organisation. One of these (Rashman and Hartley's[72] evaluation of the Beacon Council Scheme) is discussed in detail in Section 8.2 (page 163) in relation to interorganisational knowledge transfer; the other five are considered below.

Anderson and West[69] developed a four-factor theory of climate for group innovation, hypothesising that four major dimensions of climate are

Box 7.2 Components of receptive context (from Bate *et al.*, after Pettigrew[78,390]).

(1) The role of intense environmental pressure in triggering periods of radical change.
(2) The availability of visionary key people in critical posts leading change.
(3) Good managerial and clinical relations.
(4) A supportive organisational culture (which is closely related to the three preceding factors).
(5) The quality and coherence of 'policy' generated at a local level (and the 'necessary' prerequisite of having data and being able to perform testing to substantiate a case).
(6) The development and management of a cooperative interorganisational network.*
(7) Simplicity and clarity of goals and priorities.
(8) The change agenda and its locale (e.g. whether there is a teaching hospital presence and the nature of the local NHS workforce).

*See Section 8.2 (page 163).

ity denotes a person's willingness to consider change, whilst at the organisational level, receptivity refers to organisation members' willingness to consider – individually and collectively – proposed changes and to recognise the legitimacy of such proposals. Receptivity as a process shapes and is shaped by the continuous sense-making and sense-giving activities conducted among various members of the organisation. Receptivity to change can be characterised by resistance to change through varying gradations of willingness to accept the proposed change, from resigned, passive acceptance to enthusiastic endorsement.[236]

*Tushman and Nadler[364] suggest that important aspects of the informal organisation are core values, norms, communications networks, critical roles, conflict resolution and problem-solving processes.

†Edmondson *et al.*,[95] drawing on previous writers, state that organisational routines refer to the respected patterns of behaviour bound by rules and customs that characterise much of an organisation's ongoing activity. Experience with known routines inhibits active seeking of alternatives but exceptional mismatches between current routines and environmental conditions can provoke change. Routines also thought to provide a source of resistance to organisational change and the process through which organisations and managers alter routines remains underexplained in the technology and organisational literatures.

predictive of innovativeness: vision, participative safety, task orientation and support for innovation. An extensive review of published measures of climate led to the development of the climate for innovation scale, which was validated within 27 management teams in 27 respective hospitals and a total sample of 155 managers. Their dependent variable was reports of innovations implemented by the management teams in 27 hospitals, and these were judged by raters on a number of dimensions including overall innovativeness, number of innovations, radicalness, magnitude, novelty and administrative effectiveness. Support for innovation emerged as the only significant predictor of overall innovation, accounting for a substantial 46% of the variance; and the only predictor of innovation novelty. Participative safety (defined as 'a single psychological contract in which the contingencies are such that involvement in decision-making is motivated and reinforced while occurring in an environment which is perceived as interpersonally non-threatening', page 240) emerged as the best predictor of the number of innovations and self-reports of innovativeness, while task orientation predicted administrative effectiveness.

Dopson *et al.*[75] undertook an extensive secondary analysis of a group of seven studies previously published by the same group of authors.[32,234,342,343,365–369] All the primary studies were comparative case studies based on in-depth qualitative methods (chiefly semi-structured interviews), and involving a total of some 1400 in-depth interviews across 49 in-depth cases.* The studies had all been based in UK health care organisations (primary and secondary care) and explored the reasons behind actors' (mostly clinicians') decisions to use (or not to use) research evidence, and what makes this information credible for utilisation. By independent criteria, the evidence itself varied in quality from 'strong' to 'weak'. The secondary overview by Dopson *et al.* involved a comparative analysis of the interactions between different variables within and across the different studies. (Methodologically, they sought to conduct an overview of a family of related studies where they were sure – unlike in a conventional systematic literature review – that they were comparing like with like. In some ways their analysis was akin to meta-ethnography,[146] but since these authors were reanalysing their own work and did not systematically seek comparable work from other authors, their overview probably should not be classed as formal secondary research.)

Their study (the findings on knowledge utilisation are described in more detail in Section 7.8, page 154) underlined the role of a receptive context for change for the effective diffusion of research evidence. They identified a number of characteristics of a receptive context including (page 45):

- A favourable history of relationships between professional and managerial groups and between professional groups.
- Sustained political and managerial support and pressure for clearly defined change at a local level.
- The creation of a supportive local organisational culture, clear goals for change, appropriate infrastructure and resources are critical.
- Effective and good quality relationships within and among local groups.
- Access to opportunities to share information and ideas within the local context.
- The introduction of organisational innovations to foster improved and effective interchanges among groups.

In their study of the adoption of imaging technologies in US hospitals, Wilson *et al.*[74] expected that US health care organisations with a greater risk-orientated climate are likely to

(1) adopt innovations that were more radical and
(2) adopt innovations that offer greater relative advantage.

They measured risk orientation by means of Litwin and Stringer's[370] risk scale from their Organisational Climate questionnaire. They found that organisations with more risk-orientated climates did indeed tend to adopt more radical innovations ($r = 0.22$; $p < 0.06$). The authors suggested that top managers serve as a bridge between their organisation and the technical environment and that their ideas and influence on organisational

*See Section 6.2 (page 118) for detailed descriptions of two of these primary studies (Locock *et al.*[53] and Fitzgerald *et al.*[32]), which were covered from the perspective of opinion leadership.

Table 7.5 Themes from an overview of qualitative studies by Dopson *et al.* on evidence utilisation in health service organisations.

Theme from empirical work	*Explanation*
The strength of evidence does not drive its diffusion	There was no evidence in any of the studies that innovations supported by stronger evidence were diffusing faster than those supported by weaker evidence.
Evidence is socially constructed	The production of knowledge is a social as well as a scientific process. There are competing bodies of evidence, which are capable of differing interpretations by different stakeholders both within the organisation and across interorganisational (professional) networks.
Evidence is differentially available to different groups within the organisation	Different groups within the organisation have different levels of access to knowledge. Nurses and the professions allied to medicine in particular may lack access to the facilities for adopting and using new knowledge.
Evidence is differentially valued by different groups within the organisation	Different professions place different value of different forms of evidence, i.e. they have different 'hierarchies' of the forms of evidence. Professions (and managers) took different views about what constituted credible evidence.
Boundaries between professions inhibit the transfer of evidence	Knowledge does not readily flow across professional boundaries. Doctors and nurses, for example, have separate networks that form the channels for distributing knowledge.
Networks within professions enhance the transfer of evidence	Clinical behaviour is shaped as much by experience and peer comparison as by scientific evidence, e.g. interprofessional networks, continuing professional development training schemes.
Research evidence competes with, and is seen as different from, other forms of evidence	The distinction between research evidence, tacit knowledge and craft skills was very apparent. Tacit knowledge was perceived to exist in a reciprocal relationship with scientific evidence.
Environmental context influences the rate and extent of evidence transfer	External context was generally a poorly understood mediator of the diffusion of innovations (e.g. government health policy/local influences for organisations and individuals).
Opinion leaders have a powerful influence on the adoption and dissemination evidence	See full details in Section 5.3.

on the importance of developing a 'learning organisation', Rashman and Hartley's study was the only study that met our inclusion criteria, which actually identified and analysed this construct. It is possible that our search strategy excluded important studies, but an alternative interpretation is that the health care sector talks about, but has so far failed systematically to research, the notion of the learning organisation.

Patel[67] in her editorial review of a number of health promotion programmes identified four main barriers to the interpretation of knowledge dissemination for adequate utilisation of knowledge. These include conditions where:

(1) there is a clash of conceptual models;
(2) there are differences in sociocultural belief systems;
(3) symbols and images are considered as having universal standards for interpretation; and
(4) human cognition and machine cognition are assumed to operate similarly.

Dufault *et al.* conducted a quasi-experimental study in order to examine whether exposing nurses to a collaborative research utilisation

Table 7.6 Facilitators of organisational learning demonstrated empirically by Barnsley *et al.*[61]

Shared vision	*Facilitative leadership*	*Communication channels*
Predisposing activities		
(a) Clarify mission, values and goals		(a) Develop communication networks that span boundaries
(b) Promote collective understanding of vision		(b) Formal and informal lines of communication
(c) Develop trust		(c) Internal and external communication links
(d) Learning as an organisational value		(d) Avoid information overload
(e) Cooperation and collaboration		(e) Tailor communication to fit the message and the audience
		(f) Institute integration-enhancing mechanisms
Enabling activities		
	(a) Provide incentives for learning	(a) Organic structure to facilitate information flow
	(b) Support risk-taking	(b) Develop shared knowledge bases
	(c) Provide opportunities to apply new knowledge and skills	(c) Cross-organisational projects
	(d) Supportive budget practices	(d) Organise patient care around clinical service lines
	(e) Cross-organisational and multi-disciplinary teams	
	(f) Decentralised decision-making	
Reinforcing activities		
	(a) Link performance review and career progression to the application of innovative knowledge and skills	
	(b) Monitor post-training performance and provide feedback	

model would influence their attitudes towards research and would change their day-to-day pain assessment practice. They identified three main factors influencing the utilisation of scientific knowledge[66]:

(1) There exists a body of validated knowledge with a high degree of predictability.

(2) The user of the new knowledge has the ability to translate and use it in response to local needs (a concept that has been operationalised and defined as 'knowledge readiness' by Snyder-Halpern[372]).

(3) The organisation and its structure promote a research climate – 'an inquiring spirit' – and encourage new forms of practice, especially collaborative practice and inquiry.*

Chapter 8 addresses the outer (environmental) context and its influence on organisational innovativeness and the important topic of interorganisational networks and other linkages that extend beyond the organisation.

*Whilst it does not specifically address the spread of innovation, the study by Bate *et al.* of knowledge management and communities of practice in the private health care sector provides additional empirical evidence on the nature of knowledge manipulation activities amongst health care organisations.[105]

Chapter 8
The outer context

Key points

1. This chapter explores why particular innovations in health service delivery and organisation might be adopted more rapidly in some social systems and environmental contexts than in others. We review the relatively few primary studies on innovation adoption that examined the impact of factors beyond the organisation.

2. In Section 8.1 (page 157), we consider interorganisational influence through informal networks. In one of Damanpour's meta-analyses, and also in six out of seven additional primary studies in the service sector, 'external communication' was a significant determinant of organisational innovativeness. It seemed particularly important when the innovation under consideration was highly complex, when routinisation rather than assimilation was the focus of research, and during the later stages of the diffusion process (i.e. when other organisations have already set a norm).

3. In Section 8.2 (page 163) we review intentional spread strategies, using two specific examples: interorganisational quality improvement collaboratives and Beacons. The relatively sparse literature on collaboratives suggests that such initiatives are popular but expensive. The gains from such initiatives appear to be (a) difficult to measure and (b) contingent on the nature of the topic chosen and the participation of motivated teams with sophisticated change skills from supportive and receptive organisations.

4. In Section 8.3 (page 170), we consider the broader environmental context within which health care organisations operate. The evidence base for the impact of environmental variables on organisational innovativeness in the health care sector is sparse and heterogeneous, with each group of researchers exploring somewhat different aspects of the 'environment' or 'changes in the environment'. The overall impact of environmental uncertainty appears to be positive in direction but small in magnitude, and there is some evidence for small positive effects from interorganisational competition and higher socioeconomic status of patients/clients.

5. In Section 8.4 (page 172) we review four empirical studies of the impact of political and policymaking streams on the innovativeness of health care organisations, which suggest that these forces can have a large impact on the decision to adopt an innovation and the success of implementation. The timing of innovation in relation to the policymaking decision cycle is critical.

8.1 Interorganisational influence through informal social networks

Background literature: interorganisational networks, norms and bandwagons

Numerous researchers from different traditions have noted that the diffusion and organisational assimilation of innovations are dependent on the wider environmental ('outer') context.[41,63,242] The early 'classical' approach to studying diffusion of innovations amongst organisations – which stressed the values of pluralism and rivalry as the best approach to promoting organisational innovation – has largely been replaced by a more structural approach suggested by Granovetter,[19,196] who drew heavily on social network theory. In this conceptual model, interorganisational links are thought to enhance the innovative capabilities of organisations by providing opportunities for shared learning, transfer of technical knowledge, legitimacy and resource exchange.

Granovetter and others[4,373] argued that weak ties were necessary for diffusion to occur across subgroups within a system because they provide access to novel information by creating bridges between otherwise disconnected individuals.[4,373] As explained in Section 3.10 (page 66), the phenomena of social networks, as well as features such as homophily, have parallels at the organisational level. Empirical studies outside the health service sector have demonstrated that similarities in size, level of specialisation, functional differentiation and agenda between organisations enhance interorganisational diffusion.[178,293,374,375]

Abrahamson and Fombrun[376] define such an interorganisational 'agenda' or macroculture as the 'the relatively idiosyncratic, organisational-related beliefs that are shared among top managers across organisations' (page 730). O'Neill *et al.*[44] outline the implications of these shared beliefs (page 104):

> Homogenous macrocultures tend to have very similar strategic agendas ... which are listings of the most important issues facing the industry. A similarity of beliefs about agendas leads to a similarity of beliefs about necessary actions to take in response to that agenda. Therefore, firms in a homogenous macroculture are likely to adopt similar strategies.

Studies undertaken mostly in the manufacturing sector have demonstrated how interorganisational agendas and norms influence the likelihood of adopting organisational innovations. Galaskiewicz and Burt,[330] for example, in a study of interorganisational contagion in corporate philanthropy showed that firms were more likely to donate to specific charities or political action committees, engage in corporate acquisitions, or make other changes in corporate strategy or governance structure if decision-makers have informal social ties to leaders of other firms engaging in similar practices. Other examples of robust empirical studies of interorganisational norm-setting (not reviewed in detail here because their focus was outside the service sector) include work by Baron *et al.*,[377] Davis[378] and Palmer *et al.*[379] A more diffuse literature on knowledge transfer, which is beyond the scope of this book, provides considerable evidence that interorganisational linkages and common governance structures facilitate the spread of particular innovations across organisations (see, for example, Tushman[60] and Darr *et al.*[380]) or promote innovation in general (see, for example, Shan *et al.*[381]). Alternatively, when the organisational and 'supra-organisational' (as, for example, in the UK National Health Service) culture is segmentalist (i.e. non-linked) in nature, innovations will not diffuse as readily as when they are 'integrative' cultures.[17]

Abrahamson and colleagues[20,21,382,383] broadened understanding of how administrative innovations are diffused or rejected within organisational groups by introducing the now widely used notions of organisational 'bandwagons' and 'fads and fashions'. He undertook a series of seminal studies exploring how administrative innovations (e.g. quality circles as a management technique) diffuse within organisational groups.[21,382,383] His later papers used mathematical modelling to explain 'bandwagons'.[20] Bandwagons are diffusion processes wherein adopters choose an innovation not because of its technical properties but because of the sheer number of adoptions that have already taken place. As more firms adopt innovations, pressure increases for other firms to adopt them. Abrahamson and Rosenkopf[244,383] demonstrated in an elegant computer simulation that success is not a prerequisite for diffusion of the innovation or change. Where bandwagons prevail, of course, interorganisational diffusion can exhibit the phenomenon of the 'blind leading the blind'.[44]

Empirical studies of interorganisational networks in health services

The importance of informal interorganisational networks for spreading innovations in health service delivery and organisation is partly explained by the general characteristics of interorganisational norms and 'fashions' discussed above, but there might also be a particular effect from the nature of the innovations. As discussed in Section 6.6 (page 131), innovations in health service delivery and organisation are generally developed informally by local innovators in response to their needs, and disseminated horizontally through peer networks or professional associations.[384] This contrasts with most innovations that have been the subject of formal research (typically technological in nature), which have tended to be centrally produced (e.g. in research programmes) and spread (marketed) vertically by planned and controlled dissemination programmes.[384]

We found nine studies – one was part of a meta-analysis[14] and eight were primary studies[32,36,59,65,68,80,81,385] – that examined the impact of informal interorganisational influence on innovation adoption and implementation and met our inclusion criteria. Their characteristics and main findings are summarised in Table A.16 (page 276) in Appendix 4.

Only one of Damanpour's[14] three meta-analyses considered external networks as a potential determinant of innovation. He found that 'external communication' (the degree of organisation members' involvement and participation in extra-organisational professional activities) was significantly and positively associated with the rate of adoption of multiple innovations (demonstrated through 14 correlations; $p = 0.055$). Indeed, in this meta-analysis 'external communication' was one of the three strongest and most significant determinants of organisational innovativeness out of 14 possible determinants studied.

In contrast, Kimberly and Evanisko's[59] study of the adoption of technological and administrative innovations in US hospitals (discussed in more detail in Section 7.4 et seq., page 141) did not find any significant association between 'external integration' and adoption of innovation. The authors expressed some surprise at this since it conflicted with the findings of previous work (including their own); they speculated on contextual reasons for the dominance of intraorganisational determinants in this particular study.

Robertson and Wind[80] investigated what they called 'organisational cosmopolitanism' in a study of adoption of radiology innovations in US hospitals in the early 1980s. Using a postal questionnaire, they measured 'cosmopolitanism' by a questionnaire study of the external contacts and activities of physicians (radiologists) and administrators in 182 US hospitals, to test their hypothesis that 'organisational innovativeness will be more pronounced under conditions in which the professional component is cosmopolitan and the bureaucratic component local, than the reverse'. Each individuals level of cosmopolitanism was measured by four factors:

(1) journal publications;
(2) attendance at professional meetings;
(3) offices held in professional associations; and
(4) journal readership.

The adoption of seven radiology innovations by the 182 organisations was then correlated against the individual cosmopolitanism scores. The hypothesis was confirmed – i.e. highly innovative hospitals were characterised by externally oriented physicians (i.e. those who have extensive professional and academic links) but 'local' administrators (i.e. those *without* such links). When both the professional and administrative participants were local, this was associated with the lowest level of hospital innovativeness. However, differences between hospitals with different cosmopolitanism scores were not impressive and the level of statistical significance was not stated.

The authors proposed two explanations for their findings. One explanation is that the professional captures and promotes the idea for an innovation and the administrator has enough power (because of his or her local orientation) to bring about the change. Alternatively, success might be 'based on an assessment of the power structure within the professional–administrator dyad'. For example, a cosmopolitan physician may find his or her bargaining power strengthened when matched with a local administrator and therefore clinical innovation is more likely, In contrast, if the administrator is also cosmopolitan the physician may have less bargaining power. The issue of doctor–manager power relationships was discussed in Section 7.4 (page 141) in relation to the study by Champagne *et al.*; we commented there that remarkably few studies have explicitly researched this important area.

Fennell and Warnecke's[36] retrospective network analysis (discussed in relation to interpersonal influence in Section 6.1, page 114) traced the diffusion of multi-disciplinary interventions and shared decision-making in seven US head and neck cancer networks. One element of the study was to explore how the wider environment influenced the formation and functioning of the channels through which the innovations diffused (findings in relation to this are discussed in Section 8.3, page 170). A further aim was to assess how the form of network interaction (interpersonal or interorganisational) related to the institutionalisation or abandonment of the innovation. The researchers observed that in relation to the *interpersonal* networks between participants in the study, no 'discernible structure' was left after the end of the initiative and it was hard to identify cancer control programmes that continued to exist after funding was withdrawn. In contrast, cancer control outreach in some form survived in all four *interorganisational* networks. The authors concluded that 'the importance of institutional and regional support for a network program is clearly evident' (page 223).[36]

Burns and Wholey (whose study is discussed in various sections of Chapter 7 in relation to intraorganisational determinants of innovativeness) also investigated the impact of organisational and network factors on the adoption of matrix management (defined on page 145) in 1247 non-federal general hospitals that had either large size (over 300 beds) or teaching programmes in 1961, 1966, 1972 and 1978.[65] In relation to 'outer context' factors, they found that although hospitals with high diversification were more likely than others to adopt matrix management, the adoption decision was only weakly determined by this factor. The prestige of a hospital was a determinant not only of its own decision to adopt but also of the decisions of neighbouring hospitals ($p < 0.01$). Furthermore, professional media and regional ($p < 0.05$) and local hospital networks ($p < 0.05$) were significant influences (page 133):

> [T]he matrix adoption models suggest organisations may implement these approaches primarily for non-technical reasons, including desires to gain prestige, to emulate larger rivals that have already adopted [innovation], and the foster the appearance of quality.... Adoption ... may reflect conformity to institutionalized norms regarding state-of-the-art management methods.[65]

Burns and Wholey's study also suggested that the effects of organisational characteristics are contingent on the period in the diffusion process studied (see also Westphal *et al.*[81]) and on a local area's contemporaneous acceptance of the innovation. The authors concluded that four factors overall significantly influenced adoption:

(1) Task diversity.
(2) The organisation's sociometric location in the interorganisational network.
(3) Dissemination of information.
(4) The cumulative force of adoption in interorganisational networks.

The notion that the 'prestige' of a hospital is a key determinant of whether other hospitals follow its norms has some grounding in other empirical work. Di Maggio and Powell[242] have suggested that organisational fields that include a large professionally trained labour force (such as health care) will be driven primarily by status competition: organisational prestige and resources are key elements in attracting professionals and this process encourages homogenisation as organisations seek to ensure that they can provide the same benefits and services as their competitors.

In their 10-year (1981–1990) longitudinal study, also covered in Chapter 7 in relation to intraorganisational determinants of innovation, Goes and Park[68] examined the growth of interorganisational links in 388 Californian acute care hospitals and the influence of these links on organisation-level innovation. Interorganisational links were defined in this study as 'enduring transactions, flows, and linkages that occur among or between an organisation, and one or more organisations in its environment'. The general proposition was that organisation-level innovative capability and adoption of innovations is enhanced by the development of interorganisational links. To test this, the diffusion of 15 innovations – including six technical innovations (e.g. laser surgery) and nine administrative innovations (e.g. home hospice care) – were tracked over the study period.

Goes and Park's findings confirmed that structural, institutional and resource-based interorganisational links can provide efficient conduits for exchanges of technological and service capabilities and knowledge between hospitals, can enhance hospital leaders' understanding of environmental trends and can bestow legitimacy on the pursuit of innovations. The results also indicate that hospitals exhibiting multiple and extensive interorganisational links were more likely to be large and that large hospitals were consistently more innovative than small hospitals.

Westphal *et al.*,[81] in a longitudinal study of total quality management (TQM) programmes introduced by 2712 general medical surgical hospitals in the US over the period 1985–93 and examined institutional and network effects on innovation adoption. The authors hypothesised that social network ties either facilitate customisation of TQM ('an administrative innovation in the hospital environment') in response to internal efficiency needs or promote conformity in response to external legitimacy pressures, depending on the stage of institutionalisation and the attendant motivation for adoption.

The results provided strong support for the theoretical framework proposed by the authors – and others – on the adoption of administrative innovations:

> [E]arly adopters of organisational innovation are commonly driven by a desire to improve performance. But new practices can become ... infused with value beyond the technical requirements of the task at hand. As innovation spreads, a threshold is reached beyond which adoption provides legitimacy rather than improves performance.[242] (page 148)

Thus Westphal *et al.* found that, in comparison to early adopters, later adopters of TQM programmes conformed more closely to the normative pattern of quality practices introduced by other adopting hospitals. The findings are consistent with the view that early adopters, motivated by the technical efficiency gains from adoption, are more likely to customise quality practices to their organisation's unique needs and capabilities. In contrast, later adopters, experiencing normative pressure to adopt 'legitimate' quality practices, appear more likely to mimic the normative model or definition of innovation adoption implemented in other hospitals.*

Copying others because they are seen as norm-setters is known as normative influence, and should be distinguished from mimetic influence (copying others because they are seen to have a solution to a particular problem that the organisation is currently facing) and coercive influence (copying others because of the influence of an organisation on which one is dependent).[386] In the normative components of cue-taking, the collective example of other adopters legitimates an innovation and increases pressure on other organisations to follow suit whether or not the innovation is actually seen as solving a problem.[65]

Johnston and Linton[385] used network analysis to study the effect of interorganisational networks on the adoption of environmentally 'clean' process technology by 83 North American electronics firms. We have included this study even though it does not meet our inclusion criteria (as it is not based in the service sector) because it was a high-quality study that adopted a non-standard and

*As an interesting historical comparison, a similar conclusion to that of Westphal *et al.*[81] was reached by Tolbert and Sucker[353] who investigated the diffusion and institutionalisation of change in formal organisation structure through a longitudinal quantitative study of the adoption of civil service systems by American city governments during the period 1880–1935. They found that internal organisational factors predicted the adoption of civil service procedures at the beginning of the diffusion process but did not predict adoption once the process was well underway. The authors concluded that as an increasing number of organisations adopt a program or policy, it becomes progressively institutionalised or widely understood to be a necessary component of rationalised organisational structure. In other words, as a reform measure is increasingly taken for granted because of social legitimation, organisations will begin to adopt it as a 'social fact', regardless of any particular organisational characteristics. Hence, the ability of organisational variables to differentiate between adopters and non-adopters should progressively decline.

highly innovative approach to mapping network effects. The study focused specifically on the individual in the organisation responsible for *implementing* the technology and traced the networks of that individual (a technique they call 'egocentric mapping'), rather than scoping out 'one amorphous network' and the links between everyone within it. The authors hypothesised that:

- Social networks (local, intra-firm; inter-firm and public) will assist implementation.
- The more local the network the more influence it will have on implementation.
- The greater the complexity of the implementation the greater the significance will be the network to success.
- Within each type of network three different elements of the relationship are important (frequency of contact, perceived importance of contact, perceived reciprocity of contact – i.e. the perception that communication occurs in both directions rather than just from sender to receiver).

The analysis revealed that the two types of social networks (inter-firm and public) were significantly associated (both $p < 0.05$) with successful implementation of the innovation, but that – very surprisingly – networks of publicly accessible sources of information and expertise had a *negative* relationship to success, a finding that warns against any simplistic and linear explanation of the impact of networks. Within inter-firm networks, for implementation of complex innovations, reciprocity of contact had a hugely significant association with implementation ($p < 0.01$). As the authors hypothesised, the greater the complexity of the implementation, the greater the significance of the network to success. The authors note (page 474) that 'the significance of inter-firm networks to achieving results with highly complex implementations is in step with the growing literature about the importance of inter-organisational cooperation as the facilitating environment for information exchange about innovation'.

This finding, even though from a non-service sector study, has a potentially important message for the health care sector both in terms of study methodology (the network analysis was particularly rich and creative) and in terms of a hypothesis that should be tested further in the health care setting (that interorganisational networks are especially critical for innovations with high implementation complexity).

Whilst most of this subsection concerns interorganisational networks and normative pressures operating at the organisational level, the role of the individual boundary spanner is also critical. Fitzgerald *et al.* studied the processes of diffusion of innovations into health care organisations in the UK during the period 1995–9 by means of eight comparative case studies – five technological and three organisational (the use of a computer support system for anti-coagulation, the introduction of new service delivery systems for care of women in childbirth and the direct employment of physiotherapists in GP practices.). Although they reported briefly that the boundary-spanning networks of individual professionals were 'one of the key determinants' of successful diffusion, they did not elaborate on the process of networking. This study is discussed in more detail in Section 5.3 (page 106) in relation to sense-making activities.

As Rogers[3] demonstrated, information obtained from close peers located in social and organisational networks has more weight than information obtained from objective sources, such as from the media or from scientific evaluations of an innovation. The study by Fitzgerald *et al.* lends further support to this argument. The hypothesis is that individual actors adopt innovations with mainly private, personal, individual consequences and consequently network connectedness (and high levels of homophily) facilitates interpersonal interactions in the adoption of scientific methods in professional specialties.[98,161] As Scott (cited in Burns and Wholey[65]) noted:

> [B]eing embedded in a network of social relations can bring one news of innovations, support for adoption, helpful hints regarding implementation, and social support encouraging change. Such processes clearly operate among professionals across organisations.

In their overview of mostly manufacturing studies, Swan and Newell[384] found that networks of professional organisations was the single most influential variable in determining the adoption of new technology by firms (accounting for 18% of the variance). We were surprised not to find more empirical studies in the health service literature that addressed the role of professional associations and networks in spreading innovations between organisations.

In summary, the studies reviewed above highlight the important but relatively under-researched role of informal interorganisational linkages in diffusing innovations in health care organisations (and some interesting examples from outside this sector). Section 8.2 considers the more planned and formal end of the networking spectrum – initiatives under the general umbrella 'intentional spread strategies' and including multi-organisational structured quality improvement collaboratives (often referred to by the noun 'Collaboratives', see below) and Beacons (page 168).

8.2 Interorganisational influence through intentional spread strategies

Multi-organisational improvement collaboratives

Given the clear findings from organisation and management research of the benefits of interorganisational networking, it is not surprising that formal, planned initiatives to promote such networking have arisen, particularly in the public service sector (where competition between organisations is less likely to threaten collaboration). Most such initiatives have been geared to quality improvement rather than to the diffusion of innovations per se, and hence were not revealed in our formal search strategy. Furthermore, the brief for this review (reflected in the definitions we set in Section 1.3, page 25) was predicated on the notion that there is a discrete 'innovation' to be spread that is *discontinuous with previous practice*. Hence, an initiative based on the idea of emergent and continuous quality improvement is not strictly within our scope. Nevertheless, we considered that research into the effectiveness of Collaboratives for the spread of ideas would have important 'bottom line' messages for this review, especially since this work was commissioned at the request of the NHS Modernisation Agency, which has led the introduction of this model in the UK. We therefore cover them briefly in this section.

A Collaborative – strictly, a multi-organisational structured improvement collaborative – is an initiative that 'brings together groups of practitioners from different healthcare organisations to work in a structured way to improve one aspect of the quality of their service'.[40] Øvretveit *et al.* suggest that it can be thought of as a 'temporary learning organisation' (see Section 3.13, page 70). The defining characteristics are listed in Box 8.1.

Participants in a quality collaborative work together over a number of months, sharing ideas and knowledge, setting specific goals, measuring progress, sharing techniques for organisational change and implementing rapid-cycle, iterative tests of change. Learning sessions are the major events of a Collaborative: these are 2-day events where members of the multi-disciplinary project teams from each health care organisation gather to share experiences and learn from clinical and change experts and their colleagues. The time between learning sessions is called an action period, in which participants work within their own organisations towards major, 'breakthrough' improvement, focusing on their internal organisational agenda and priorities for changes and improvements whilst remaining in continuous contact with other Collaborative participants.

The most widely researched collaborative model is probably the 'Breakthrough' model developed by the US IHI* under Professor Don Berwick and colleagues[387,388] (see www.qualityhealthcare.com). A less sophisticated (and less expensive) model involves interorganisational benchmarking through virtual collaboration.[389] The UK government, in its white paper, *The NHS Plan*, placed the IHI Breakthrough model at the centre of its modernisation agenda, which

*IHI is a not-for-profit organisation that supports collaborative health care improvement programmes on an international basis using evidence-based improvement principles.

Box 8.1 Characteristics of health care quality improvement collaboratives (reproduced with permission from Øvretveit *et al.*[40])

- Participation of a number of multiprofessional teams with a commitment to improving services within a specific subject area and to sharing with others how they made their improvements, each from an organisation which supports these aims.
- A focused clinical or administrative subject,e.g. reducing Caesarean sections or wait times and delays or improving asthma care.
- Evidence of large variations in care, or of gaps between best and current practice.
- Participants learn from experts about the evidence for improvement, about change concepts and practical changes that have worked at other sites, and about quality improvement methods.
- Participants use a change testing method to plan, implement, and evaluate many small changes in quick succession,e.g. in the Institute for Healthcare Improvement (IHI) model, the rapid-cycle improvement method.
- Teams set measurable targets and collect data to track their performance.
- Participants meet at least twice, usually more, for 1–3 days to learn the methods, report their changes and results, share experiences and consider how to spread their innovations to other services.
- Between meetings participants continue to exchange ideas and collaborative organisers provide extra support, sometimes through visiting facilitators, emails and conference calls.

would be based on a 'new system of devolved responsibility' that would 'help local clinicians and managers redesign local services around the needs and convenience of patients'.[1] Collaboratives led by the UK Modernisation Agency have been evaluated in cancer services,[103] mental health,[104] orthopaedic services[390] and many others. These initiatives are generally popular with participants and lead to visible improvements in services, but they are known to be costly (e.g. the ongoing UK Cancer Collaborative is said to have cost £5 million as of mid 2002[391]).

Current published evidence for the effectiveness of the collaborative approach consists mainly of descriptions and commentary pieces from proponents of this model.[392–395] But as the references to the previous paragraph (most of which are to internal reports) illustrate, there is far more known about quality collaboratives than has so far appeared in mainstream academic journals. Much of the work has been undertaken as internal evaluation (based largely on self-reported data) rather than research per se. Independent evaluations are becoming more common but have so far been published mostly in the grey literature as internal reports.[103,104,390] Some excellent practical guidance and process reports can be downloaded or ordered from the websites listed above, and a number of large-scale, hypothesis-driven evaluations are still ongoing.* For practical reasons, therefore, we have confined our own review to empirical studies published in peer-reviewed journals, which therefore represent only a fraction of potentially relevant evidence.

Øvretveit *et al.* identified four (as yet largely unanswered) research questions about collaboratives, as compared with traditional quality improvement initiatives:

(1) Do they spread improvements in practice *more quickly*?

(2) Are the resulting improvements *larger in magnitude*?

(3) Do the results *last longer*?

(4) Are the ideas spread *more widely*?

An overarching fifth question relates to cost-effectiveness – are any gains achieved at acceptable cost?[40] Whilst all these quantitative questions are indeed important, there is another, qualitative, research dimension on the nature of the changes and the process by which they are achieved (the 'how' rather than 'how much' or 'how far' of diffusion, assimilation and routinisation). Furthermore, as Bate and Robert[113] argue, there is a palpable tension between a summative, outcomes-oriented approach based on predefined and largely quanti-

*Note in particular that a large-scale multi-site study led by RAND (with the University of California, Berkeley) of a series of quality improvement Collaboratives directed towards improving chronic illness care, which are based on the IHI approach, is currently ongoing in the USA.

tative success criteria and a more formative, developmental approach (say, using an action research framework) in which 'success criteria' would necessarily be negotiable and changeable.

We found five empirical research papers (described in six studies) on Collaboratives that had been published in peer-reviewed journals.[82–86,396] These studies are summarised in Table A.17 (page 278) in Appendix 4. Only one of these was explicitly a study of cost-effectiveness,[85] although we are aware that economic evaluations have been included in 'grey literature' reports.

One of the very first collaborative improvement groups – the Northern New England Cardiovascular Disease Study Group (NECVDSG) – compiled in-hospital mortality data from 15 095 coronary artery bypass grafting procedures and, after the focused intervention period, the group tracked a further 6488 consecutive cases and reported a 24% reduction in in-hospital mortality rate ($p = 0.001$).[82] Another study by Flamm *et al.*[83] documented the use of the IHI Breakthrough model in reducing Caesarean section rates in US hospitals. The published report describes the principles of the model and reports that a small fraction of the participating units (15%) achieved reduction in Caesarean section rates of 30% or more. One-third of the units, however, achieved little or no change.

In another early application of the IHI Breakthrough model, Leape *et al.*[84] describe the participation of 40 US hospitals in an initiative to reduce adverse drug events. This Collaborative made extensive use of the rapid-cycle test-of-change technique, in which a focused, explicit and measurable change in practice is identified and data are gathered quickly to demonstrate whether an effect occurs. Over 700 such cycles were attempted by the participating units, and 70% of all changes were described as successful against locally set criteria. The authors concluded:

> Success in making significant changes was associated with strong leadership, effective processes, and appropriate choice of intervention. Successful teams were able to define, clearly state, and relentlessly pursue their aims, and then chose practical interventions and moved early into changing a process. They did not spend months collecting data before beginning a change. Changes that were most successful were those that attempted to change processes, not people.[84]

Horbar *et al.*[86] and Rogowski *et al.*[85] report on the clinical and economic impact of a neonatal intensive care unit (NICU) collaborative in the USA. This was a before-and-after study in ten NICUs that aimed to assess whether collaborative quality improvement efforts could change patient-relevant outcomes in neonatal intensive care. Between 1994 and 1996 the rate of infection with coagulase-negative staphylococci decreased from 22.0% to 16.6% ($p = 0.007$) at the six project NICUs and the rate of (undesirable) supplemental oxygen at 36 weeks adjusted gestational age decreased from 43.5% to 31.5% ($p = 0.03$) at the four NICUs in a chronic lung disease group. The changes observed at the project NICUs for these outcomes were significantly larger ($p = 0.026$ and $p = 0.14$) than those observed at the 66 comparison NICUs over the 4-year period from 1994 to 1997.[86] Between 1994 and 1996 the median treatment cost per infant with birth weight 501–1500 g at the six project NICUs in the infection group decreased from $57 606 to $46 674; at the four chronic lung disease hospitals, for infants with birth weights 501–1000 g, it decreased from $85 959 to $77 250. Treatment costs at hospitals in the control group rose over the same period ($p < 0.0001$ and $p = 0.7980$).[85]

The authors of these two studies concluded that not only did multi-disciplinary collaborative quality improvement have the potential to improve the outcomes of neonatal intensive care but also that 'cost savings may be achieved as a result'. They also emphasised the important role of 'active participation in structured multi-disciplinary, cross-institutional collaborative learning' in bringing about improvements in clinical outcomes.

In a recent article, Green and Plsek describe a more refined version of the original 'Breakthrough' collaborative model, in which 'Wave 1' teams (the success stories from the first wave of intentional spread activities) are purposively brought together with 'Wave 2' teams and provided with opportunities for informal networking. In this way, ideas, tacit knowledge and general enthusiasm for the process can be transmitted.[396] Like most of the publications on this approach, this article documents successful change initiatives from most (17 out of 26) of the participating teams, but the study did not include an independent evaluation.

As indicated previously, the reader who is interested in health care quality improvement collaboratives will find additional studies in the 'grey literature', but it was beyond our remit to cover such studies in this report.*

Øvretveit *et al.*[40] have published a useful overview of the lessons from research into quality collaboratives (the accompanying editorial by Leatherman[391] is also recommended). The Øvretveit article was co-authored by leading researchers into collaborative initiatives in the USA, UK and Sweden, based on two face-to-face meetings between the teams whose aim was to draw generalisable lessons from their different experiences and identify areas for future research. According to these authors, the rationale for collaboratives is partly economies of scale in finding and processing the evidence for what works and presenting it succinctly to busy clinicians and managers. In traditional (intraorganisational) quality improvement, the team first has to identify a problem, seek out all the relevant evidence on effectiveness and cost-effectiveness of different strategies, and only then begin to implement the evidence. In a collaborative, the evidence is packaged and presented at regular meetings, and experts (in the clinical topic area, change management, quality improvement and data analysis) are made available to discuss how it might be operationalised in different settings.

*Bate *et al.*, for example, recently independently evaluated a UK NHS Collaborative based on the IHI Breakthrough model, which focused on total hip replacement surgery and reported an average reduction in length of stay of 1.0 day (12.2%) across 28 participating hospitals – compared with a 0.1 day (1.6%) reduction in four 'control' hospitals. Seventeen (61%) of the participating hospitals recorded a statistically significant reduction.[390]

These authors have argued that the 'lead phase' of any quality improvement initiative should in theory be much shorter in the collaborative model because the evidence is already supplied.[40] In practice, there has been no randomised trial of quality improvement initiatives that include an element of structured interorganisational collaboration versus comparable quality improvement initiatives without the collaborative element, although two studies that used contemporaneous controls showed a faster uptake of innovation in the collaborative groups.[86]

A rival theoretical hypothesis is that if the function of the collaborative is expressed in terms of collective sense-making,[137] transmission of tacit knowledge[397] and personalisation of knowledge[398] (see Section 3.13, page 70) rather than 'provision of evidence and expertise', the impact of the collaborative will be evenly distributed throughout the quality improvement period rather than simply shortening the run-in period. Indeed, it might have its most significant effects in the mid and late stages as the processes of collective sense-making and knowledge transfer gain momentum. The empirical work published in academic journals to date has not specifically tested this hypothesis, nor has it given much insight into the process of change, since it has focused mainly on documenting and quantifying the overall changes. The overview of Øvretveit *et al.*,[40] whilst in some respects 'anecdotal', taps into the know-how of change agents and researchers who have led or evaluated collaborative initiatives, and provides one of the best sources of qualitative information on the reasons for successes or failures. These are summarised in Box 8.2.

As indicated in Box 8.2, the six key characteristics of successful topic areas for collaborative quality improvement identified by Øvretveit *et al.* have remarkable similarities to the six attributes of innovations identified by the early sociologists and summarised in Chapter 4 (page 83). The need for motivated and goal-oriented participants aligns with the evidence on adopters and adoption outlined in Chapter 5, and the need for credible and knowledgeable experts links with the evidence on diffusion and dissemination set out in Chapter 6. Given the evidence reviewed in

Chapter 7 on the inner context, it is perhaps unsurprising that organisations with an appropriate culture and climate, congruent strategic goals, generic quality improvement skills and top management support produce better outcomes from collaborative initiatives than those without.

The recommendations in Box 8.2 on implementation link both with mainstream literature on change management and also with our specific empirical findings on implementation and sustainability of innovations set out in Chapter 9. The Øvretveit article made few specific suggestions about the actual *process* of knowledge exchange in collaboratives, but there are clear overlaps with the theoretical literature on knowledge manipulation, which is summarised in Section 3.13. Drawing on the literature on knowledge construction, sense-making and communities of practice from the private sector, Bate and Robert[105] have recommended that the work of quality collaboratives and comparable models is more explicitly grounded in these theoretical concepts.

Box 8.2 Factors associated with success of health care quality collaboratives (summarised from Øvretveit *et al.*[40]), showing comparable constructs from the diffusion of innovations literature.[3]

Topic chosen for improvement
- Focused and clearly demarcated area of interest (not, for example, 'to improve communication between primary and secondary care') – akin to *low complexity*.
- Robust evidence base with clear gaps between best and current practice – akin to *relative advantage*.
- Real examples of how improvements have been made in practice – akin to *observability*.
- Professionals feel that the proposed improvement is important – akin to *compatibility with individual norms and values*.
- Topic is strategically important to participating organisations – akin to *compatibility with institutional norms and practices*.
- Participants can exchange ideas and suggestions, which can be adapted and applied in different settings – akin to *trialability and reinvention*.

Participants
- Participants are motivated to attend (those who volunteer do better than those who are sent) – akin to the *persuasion, decision and action* stages in the adoption process.
- Participants are clear about their individual and corporate goals.
- Teams must work effectively together (teambuilding initiatives may be necessary as a precursor).
- There should be continuity of team leadership.
- Organisations must have a supportive culture and climate and be sophisticated in the use of process analysis and data collection tools.
- Organisations provide 'visible and real support' for the initiative; their goals align closely with those of the teams who attend the learning days.

Facilitators and expert advisers
- Facilitators must have time to plan and organise the work.
- Facilitators must resist didactic presentations and encourage horizontal networking between participants – akin to interpersonal influence based on *homophily*
- Experts must have credibility with participants – akin to criteria for *opinion leadership*.

The implementation process
- Organisers must provide a toolkit of basic change skills (e.g. how to gather data, set measurable goals, measure progress).
- Organisers must provide opportunities for discussion on the practicalities of implementation.
- Facilitators must provide adequate support outside the learning events for the teams attempting implementation of innovations in their organisations.

Maximising the spread of ideas
- Facilitators should encourage networking between teams in the action periods between learning days (e.g. via conference calls, emails and so on).
- Facilitators should encourage the spread of both specific ideas *and* process methods (e.g. change ideas, quality methods, data analysis methods) that can be used in the implementation of other innovations.

It is worth noting that many of the 'outcomes' of an effective knowledge manipulation initiative are not directly measurable. As well as transferring *particular* items of knowledge, individuals (and the teams and organisations they work in) develop a wider absorptive capacity (see Section 7.8, page 154). For example, they forge relationships and informal communication networks that can be used in the future; they gain confidence and skills in knowledge exchange; they develop an identity and social role as knowledge workers and so on. The tightly defined 'outcome measures' against which most of the projects listed in Table A.17 (page 278) evaluated themselves are not designed to measure these wider gains.

In summary, the relatively sparse literature on intentional spread strategies via multi-organisational improvement collaboratives suggests that such initiatives are popular but expensive and that the gains from them

(1) are difficult to measure;

(2) are contingent on the nature of the topic chosen and the participation of motivated teams with sophisticated change skills from supportive and receptive organisations; and

(3) can be explained from a theoretical perspective in terms of the knowledge creation cycle set out in Section 3.13 (page 70).

'Transfer of best practice' schemes: NHS Beacons

A comparable model of transfer of potentially better practice (also introduced into UK health care via the NHS Modernisation Agency) is the Beacon model. Beacons are specially selected organisations (hospital trusts, general practices and other NHS-funded centres) that have achieved a high standard of service delivery and are regarded as centres of best practice. The programme was launched in 1999. Beacons participate in the initiative for 2 years, and receive funding for the dissemination activities in one of the following theme areas: cancer, coronary heart disease, health improvement, human resources, mental health, outpatient services, palliative care, personality disorder (jointly sponsored by UK Home Office), primary health care, stroke and waiting lists and times. The idea of paying 'flagship' organisations to disseminate their ideas is not new. Rogers[3] (page 219), for example, notes that 'many change agencies award incentives or subsidies to clients to speed up the rate of adoption of innovation'.

The selection of new NHS Beacons has now come to an end, but the Beacon section of the Modernisation Agency website (www.modern.nhs.uk) has a database describing each of the Beacon services and advice on how to spread good practice. The Beacon Support Team at the Modernisation Agency continues to offer existing Beacons help and advice in promoting their Beacon status, identifying key audiences and contacts, identifying and linking to strategic networks and developing dissemination activities.

An independent evaluation of the NHS Beacon programme, commissioned by the Modernisation Agency suggested that Beacons had shown themselves able to

- encourage, recognise and reward best practice in the provision of health and social care services;
- motivate people to do the best they can, and be inspired to make improvements;
- facilitate sharing and learning (by passing on good ideas to raise standards overall and facilitate helping people to benefit from other's experience of implementing change but tailored to the local context);
- provide replicable models (providing blueprints for change to speed the process along and ease its conception and passage).

Benefits to the NHS were said to include supporting modernisation by creating a favourable climate for change, identifying and celebrating achievement, identifying what works and what does not and establishing a culture of sharing and learning.

The above evaluation was only published as an internal report and we do not have sufficient data to assess its methodological quality (for the full report see http://www.modernnhs.nhs.uk/nhsbeacons/1330/NHS%20Beacons%20Evaluation.doc). To our knowledge, no peer-reviewed evaluation of the NHS Beacon scheme has been published. However, a high-quality research-focused evaluation of the Beacon Council Scheme,[72] an integral part of the modernisation of local government (including social services) in the UK, was available and is reviewed below.

The Beacon Council Scheme, like the NHS Beacon Scheme, is based on principles and processes of interorganisational collaboration, learning and learning partnerships. Rashman and Hartley[72] undertook a qualitative study (focus groups and telephone interviews) of 59 participants from UK local councils who had attended Beacon events aiming to introduce potentially better practices in
(1) specific topic areas;
(2) overall service delivery;
(3) community involvement; and
(4) local political leadership.

The researchers hypothesised that councils would learn from Beacons, that this learning would lead to changes and that these changes would in turn lead to improved services.

Unlike the evaluations of the Collaboratives published in peer-reviewed journals and described in the previous section, Rashman and Hartley's study drew explicitly on knowledge creation theory to explain the *process* of organisational and interorganisational learning and knowledge transfer. The authors demonstrated that the transfer of knowledge is contingent on a number of conditions that facilitate or impede interorganisational learning.

Effective dissemination strategies were those that had selected appropriate learning methods that were matched to the different types of knowledge and the different learning needs of individuals in different roles. Explicit knowledge, which was more easily articulated and codified, was sought predominantly by individuals looking for specific performance statistics or guidance. Tacit knowledge, such as mental models, operational skills and know-how, was sought and acquired by means of shared practical experience through collaboration with colleagues and the creation of networks. This collaborative knowledge creation was found to depend critically on *enabling conditions for knowledge transfer* in the both the originating organisation (the system with Beacon status) and the recipient organisation (the system seeking to learn from the Beacon organisation). The originating organisation required a *developed framework for knowledge management* and learning and the *skills in converting tacit knowledge to explicit knowledge*.

The recipient organisation was only able to learn effectively from the Beacon organisation if it possessed *the capacity to learn as an organisation.** Critical dimensions of this capacity included effective methods for identifying problems and seeking new knowledge to address those problems, and the motivation and competence to assimilate and apply new knowledge (see page 532).[72] In addition, the successful recipient organisation was characterised by
(1) a facilitative rather than didactic leadership style;
(2) capacity for, and receptivity to, new knowledge;[†]
(3) mutual trust and common perspectives;
(4) problem setting;
(5) distributed decision-making; and
(6) strong internal networks.

The authors also found that homophily of organisational characteristics helped to support shared experience but that the complexity and uniqueness of local authorities presented particular challenges to effective knowledge transfer. They also identified some additional important barriers to knowledge transfer in these public sector organisations:
(1) initiative fatigue, usually associated with conflicting priorities;
(2) financial constraints and deficiencies; and
(3) limited guidance on the application of knowledge during the formal learning and training events.

The authors found that there were a number of tensions inherent to the Beacon model:
(1) the competitive award of Beacon status and subsequent collaborative exchange of knowledge;
(2) central control and local innovation; and
(3) an emphasis on performance management versus the need to promote innovation and capacity for change.

*See the summary section on the learning organisation in Section 3.13 (page 70).

†See the discussion on receptive context in Section 7.7 (page 150).

These three tensions also run through some of the literature on quality collaboratives (see above), and they may be common to any formal, organised initiative to promote horizontal spread of innovation in a targeted way.

Rashman and Hartley concluded that Beacon visits and Beacon learning events would benefit from being structured so as to promote knowledge acquisition and learning, and in particular to develop the skills of the recipients to transfer knowledge into their own context (a finding that aligned with that of Øvretveit *et al.* that the most valued parts of the event was the opportunity to exchange stories with other teams like them, and even to discuss these issues *within* their own team). Using Weick's conceptual framework of sense-making, all the research into interorganisational learning emphasises the need to create the conditions that enable the exchange and reframing of knowledge and the embedding of new understandings, practices and ways of working into the receiving organisation.

8.3 Empirical studies of environmental impact on organisational innovativeness

There is a vast body of literature relating to the wider environment in which organisations make decisions. It was beyond the scope of this study to examine this in detail, but we have included studies that addressed environmental impact as part of a research question focused primarily on diffusion, assimilation or routinisation of innovations. The prevailing external social and technical environments are thought to affect

(1) the nature of the innovations that are diffused between organisations;
(2) the attitudes of actors in organisations towards these innovations; and
(3) the type of organisations in which innovation and diffusion occur.

Van de Ven[123] suggests (page 601) that :

> The extra-organisational context includes the broad cultural and resource endowments that society provides, including laws, government regulations, distributions of knowledge and resources, and the structure of the industry in which the innovation is located.

We found eight studies – one was part of a meta-analysis[16] and seven were primary studies[36,38,59,63,64,73,76] – that examined a range of factors associated with the wider environmental context within which organisations function and which have been suggested as having an impact on the adoption of innovations. These are listed in Table A.18 (page 280) in Appendix 4.

Baldridge and Burnham[63] (whose work is also covered in Section 7.4, page 141, in relation to organisational determinants of assimilation) considered two dimensions of the wider environment – heterogeneity (in socio-economic status, ethnicity and so on) and changing environment in relation to innovation in schools. They hypothesised that both would increase innovativeness as organisations would be subject to varied pressure from outside. Whilst a small positive association was indeed found for environmental heterogeneity, environmental changes did not significantly influence the adoption of innovations by the school districts. Overall, they concluded, environment was an important variable to consider but its influence was relatively low compared with the structural characteristics of organisations.

Kimberly and Evanisko began their landmark 1970s study of innovation in US hospitals by suggesting that the importance of the organisation's environmental context for innovation had previously been acknowledged conceptually, but rarely examined empirically. They suggested three important 'environmental' variables: competition, size of city and age of hospital. Whilst we would not categorise 'age of hospital' as an environmental factor – preferring to classify it in terms of the characteristic of an organisation (our 'inner' context) – this was one of five factors that just reached significance in explaining variation in adoption behaviour for innovations in medical technology (but not for administrative innovations). Competition and size of city did not have a significant impact on the adoption of either technological or administrative innovations.

Meyer and Goes conducted comparative case studies (over 300 interviews, and observation and surveys) of 12 organisation-level medical innovations introduced into US community hospitals in late 1970s over a 6-year period (see Section 5.3, page 106, for more details of this study). Amongst a range of other variables, they explored whether the assimilation of innovations by organisations was influenced by the environmental variables of urbanisation, affluence and federal health insurance. The findings suggested that these environmental variables had little demonstrable impact.

As indicated in Section 8.1 (page 157), Fennell and Warnecke[36] sought to determine how the organisational environment in seven US head and neck cancer networks influenced the formation of diffusion channels for innovations in multi-disciplinary care and shared decision-making. 'Environment' in this study was taken to include changes in the environment (such as a declining population base, changing demographic character of the service area, decreasing revenues or increased competition from other hospitals) and the organisational make-up of a locality or region (the characteristics of those organisations competing for resources, patterns of resource development, allocation, and utilisation and the patterns of interaction among various organisations and key individuals). Through descriptive historical case studies of each network and a comparative analysis, the researchers found that, in general, network form (whether diffusion is through interpersonal or interorganisational networks) is dependent upon:

- The regional resource base (resource-'rich' led to interorganisational networks as opposed to interpersonal networks).
- The compatibility of the organisations participating in the programmes affects the ease with which the innovative program can be diffused (very diverse networks did not develop organisational diffusion channels whilst the most homogenous – or homophilous – did).
- The pre-existing relationships among the organisations in the environment (particularly the density, stability and 'domain consensus' – the recognition and acceptance of an organisation's. boundaries and appropriate tasks).

The significance of these findings is that where these factors were present, it was more likely that the innovations would spread via interorganisational networks: these were much more successful in bringing about sustained change in working practices than localities where diffusion was reliant on interpersonal networks.

In their study of the introduction of sessional fee remuneration for GPs in long-term hospitals in Canada over a 15-month period (covered in more detail in Section 5.3, page 106, in relation to the adoption process), Champagne *et al.*[64] included 'urbanisation' (the distance of the organisation from a large urban centre) as one of their independent variables. They found that the level of implementation of the innovation was positively associated with the level of urbanisation, but that the strength of association was again small compared with internal organisational variables.

In Castle's study of early adoption in 13 162 US nursing homes (discussed in Section 7.4, page 141, in relation to organisational size), the effects of seven environmental (referred to by the authors as 'market') characteristics on adoption of two groups of innovations – special care units and subacute units – were studied in addition to the organisational factors already discussed. Two of the characteristics increased the likelihood of early adoption: higher average income of residents ($p < 0.05$) and higher numbers of hospital beds per 100 000 population ($p < 0.01$). Two of the characteristics decreased the likelihood of early adoption: prospective reimbursement ($p < 0.01$) and less competition ($p < 0.01$). The final three characteristics (state legislative policies with regard to building of new facilities, the availability of hospital-based services and the age of the population) showed no significant association with the early adoption of the innovations studied.

Nystrom *et al.*,[76] whose study of the adoption of medical imaging technologies in US hospitals was discussed in Section 7.4 (page 141) in relation to organisational determinants of innovation, found that having an 'external orientation' (defined as those with boundary-spanning roles focusing particularly on the nature of communication links between the organisation and its patients/ community) interacted significantly ($p < 0.10$) with the dimension of organisational age to influence the adoption of medical imaging diagnostic technologies in US hospitals.

The authors proposed that older organisations can become complacent and isolated, so a climate that encourages a greater external orientation would lead to more innovativeness. External orientation also interacted significantly but negatively with size ($p < 0.05$) to determine innovativeness. This somewhat surprising negative association between external orientation and size and their combined effect on innovativeness was explained by the authors in terms of larger hospitals using a more functionally differentiated or decentralised structure.

In summary, Damanpour's 1996 meta-analysis of studies (mainly from the manufacturing sector) showed a positive but – in quantitative terms – unimpressive impact of environmental uncertainty on organisational innovativeness. The empirical studies reviewed in this section largely confirmed that finding specifically in the service sector.

8.4 Empirical studies of impact of politics and policymaking on organisational innovativeness

We found four empirical studies that considered the political and policymaking environment.[32,87,88,215] They are summarised in Table A.19 (page 283) in Appendix 4. Three are discussed in this section and the fourth[215] is discussed in Section 9.7 (page 195) in relation to whole-systems approaches to implementation and sustainability.

Hughes *et al.*[87] undertook in-depth case studies to evaluate five separate 'evidence into action' initiatives in the context of primary care in inner London in 1998–2000. The different initiatives were placed very differently on national (and local) policy agendas, ranging from one project to implement primary-care-led antenatal screening for haemoglobinopathies across a health district (driven by an enthusiastic local haematologist but with no corresponding national policy directive) to an initiative in a single general practice to improve proactive management of cardiovascular risk factors (which was closely aligned with a recent national policy directive).

The former initiative was never implemented and was associated with considerable resentment and frustration with the local GPs and community midwives; the latter was largely successful and went on to attract a stream of funding from the service sector once the research phase was complete. Hughes[87] *et al.* commented:

> [The cardiovascular project] clearly benefited from focusing on a topic that was high on national and local health policy agendas; promoting action that was congruent with current ideas; and working with participants whose awareness and enthusiasm had been stimulated by their involvement in a developmental initiative. A feeling of swimming with the tide and even of being ahead of the game in relation to other practices enhanced the project's attractiveness to participants and their commitment to seeing it through to completion.

Overall, a national policy 'push' was seen as an important facilitator for projects in the early implementation stages, but only if the local context was also favourable. Another prominent theme in all five case studies was the wider context of major structural changes that were occurring in UK primary care in the late 1990s, as well as a rapid stream of new policy documents from national government (representing the early stages of the modernisation agenda discussed in Section 1.2, page 22). Political pressures for change were not always unwelcome, and indeed often aligned with the goals of project teams, but the changes generally required frequent and flexible adaptation of the project's goals, milestones, methods and staffing structures. As Hughes *et al.*[87] concluded:

> [Political and policymaking] change is a normal part of the environment in which implementation projects take place. It is frequently disruptive and may be threatening to projects, although this is not necessarily the case. In some circumstances change may offer opportunities for increasing a project's impact. However, this depends on the project team being alert to such opportunities and able to adapt to take advantage of them. Rigidities of timescale, methods, objectives or resources

may prevent projects from responding constructively to contextual change.

Fitzgerald *et al.*,[32] whose work is discussed in more detail in Section 7.8 (page 154) in relation to sense-making within organisations, drew particular attention to the interplay of features of the 'inner' and 'outer' context in the UK NHS, where national policy priorities make strategic decisions in support of the diffusion of innovations that relate to priority targets more likely.* Their study focused on the influence of differing contexts as an integral component in the diffusion process. In their study of technological and organisational innovations they distinguished between the influence of context at two levels (macro and micro), which broadly relate to what we have termed the 'outer' and 'inner' context (Box 8.3).

Drawing on their eight case studies Fitzgerald *et al.*[32] suggest that their data 'demonstrate the critical and variable influence of context on the diffusion process' (page 1446). They also point out the crucial influence of limited funding on the diffusion process.

Another in-depth case study that explored the impact of politics and policymaking was undertaken by Exworthy *et al.*[88] in relation to local health care policymaking. They sought to study the adoption of policies to address health inequalities, and used three English health authorities as in-depth case studies, drawing for their theoretical framework on Kingdon's model of policy streams (Box 8.4). Exworthy and his team used a wide range of archival material as well as in-depth interviews, and as a result were able to search purposively for dissonance between their sources (e.g. between the public profile offered by official documents and the private accounts of individuals).

They found that although national policymakers viewed policies to reduce health inequalities as an innovation developed and supported centrally (and intended to be disseminated vertically to the local level), and although there was strong alignment in the *values* underpinning both central and local policymaking on inequalities, there was in reality little or no direct vertical cascading of this policy. In reality, what central government saw as uptake of the 'innovation' (policies to reduce inequalities) was actually rebranding of existing initiatives to fit the new category (and new budget) assigned to 'inequalities initiatives'.

Furthermore, competing imperatives imposed by national government (colloquially known as

Box 8.3 Contextual factors at macro- and micro-levels (from Fitzgerald *et al.*[32]).

Macro-level (primary and acute care contexts):
- Pattern of intra- and interorganisational relationships among doctors and their professional bodies
- Structures of organisations (and particularly the influence of the intermediate tier of the Health Authority in the primary care sector)
- Resourcing

Micro-level (within organisation):
- History, culture and quality of relationships
- Characteristics of the patient group
- Nature, type and strength of external networks
- Resourcing

Box 8.4 Kingdon's model of policy streams.[88]

Policy 'windows' open (or close) by the coupling (or decoupling) of three streams: problems, politics and policies.
- Problems come to light either as key events or crises or in response to systematic collection of data (often, because feedback is sought on existing policies).
- Politics comprises both national and local forces such as interest group lobbying, power bases, organisational interests, elections and so on.
- Policies (potential solutions to problems) float in a 'primeval soup' of potential actions, waiting to be selected and implemented. To gain selection, they must meet two key criteria: they must be technically feasible and congruent with prevailing values.

*Similar to Rogers'[3] concept of a 'mandate for adoption': a mechanism through which the system exerts pressure on individuals (or in this case organisations) to recognise the relative advantage of an innovation.

the 'must-dos', such as reducing waiting lists) leeched resources and energy away from local inequalities initiatives, resulting in a de facto mismatch of values between the periphery and the centre, and much local resentment that teams on the ground were being asked to square an impossible circle. Even when there was no explicit directive to wire funds elsewhere, Exworthy *et al.* found evidence that local decisions were often deferred in anticipation of the next 'must-do' directive. They comment on the irony that despite the widely held commitment to 'joined-up government', policies at the national level appeared to be 'vertically drilled down' rather than joined up centrally. Finally, local health authorities were repeatedly stymied by the need to meet short-term, easily measurable process-level indicators of dubious validity that became perverse incentives, rather than being allowed to plan longer term and measure their success by softer (but more 'real') indicators of progress.

In the in-depth case study of Canadian heart health programmes by Riley *et al.*, discussed in detail in Section 9.7 (page 195), the qualitative findings highlighted several key themes about politics and policymaking:

(1) the importance of synchronous interaction between external (national and regional) incentives and mandates and internal (organisational) activity;

(2) the long lead time (around 15 years) for outcomes to appear in a complex programme such as this; and

(3) that this lead time is increased if *what* to disseminate and implement is not clear.[215]

These four in-depth case studies are examples of a stream of potentially relevant literature from social and political sciences that attempts to look at the rich picture of how health care organisations make the decision to adopt, and go about implementing, innovations that are to some extent politically driven. All three studies demonstrated the critical importance not merely of political and policymaking forces but of their *dynamic interaction* with other variables (the nature of the innovation, the timing of key decisions and the presence of competing demands on energies and resources*) – conclusions that chime with the 'outer context' components of what Pettigrew *et al.*[78] have called 'receptive context for organisational change' (listed in Box 7.2, page 151). The sensitivity of implementation teams to these external forces, and their ability to respond adaptively to them, seems critical to implementation success. Few definitive conclusions can be drawn from the work reviewed here, but the studies raise a number of hypotheses that might direct further secondary and primary research.

---

*The EUR-ASSESS Subgroup on Dissemination and Impact, whose systematic review of dissemination and implementation strategies is reviewed in Section 9.3 (page 180) drew a similar conclusion from a handful of additional studies whose methodological quality was said to be poor overall; we have not revisited those primary studies.

Chapter 9

Implementation and institutionalisation

Key points

1. This chapter considers the highly diverse literature on approaches to implementing and routinising innovations. In Section 9.1 (page 176), we discuss some conceptual and theoretical challenges around the concepts of implementation and institutionalisation, including two alternative models of implementation: the 'ordered stage' model and the 'process' model. The more complex the innovation, the more iterative, complex and multidirectional will be the implementation process.

2. In Section 9.2 (page 178), we consider the methodological difficulties of researching the implementation and institutionalisation of innovations. The wide variety of primary studies, each of which was couched in a different context, tested a different aspect of implementation and hypothecated a different critical success factor (or combination of factors) make definitive conclusions impossible to draw.

3. Section 9.3 (page 180) discusses three systematic reviews and one narrative overview on implementation and institutionalisation: the EUR-ASSESS review on disseminating and implementing HTA reports, the review by Meyers *et al.* of implementing industrial process innovations, the review by Grimshaw *et al.* of implementing clinical guidelines and the review by Gustafson *et al.* of implementing change in organisations. Together, these reviews indicated that the success of an implementation initiative depends on (a) the nature of the innovation (relative advantage, low complexity, scope for reinvention) and its fit with the organisation's existing skill mix, work practices and strategic goals; (b) motivation, capacity and competence of individual practitioners; (c) elements of organisational structure (e.g. devolved decision-making, internal networks) and capacity (e.g. change skills, evaluation skills); (d) resources and leadership; (e) early involvement and cooperation of staff at all levels; (f) personalised, targeted and high-quality training; (g) evaluation and feedback; (h) linkage with the resource system from development of the innovation through to implementation; (i) embeddedness in interorganisational networks and (j) conducive external pressures, e.g. synchrony with local priorities and policymaking streams.

4. Empirical evidence from health services research on interventions designed to strengthen the predisposition and capacity of the user system (Section 9.4, page 186) was sparse. The findings of the systematic reviews listed above were broadly confirmed: initiatives that probably help the implementation process include provision of dedicated resources, targeted staff training, allocation of (and continuity in) defined staff roles, and forging of links to external agencies for support. In addition, individual project teams appear to benefit from teambuilding to develop motivation and trust and establish shared meanings and values in relation to a proposed innovation.

5. Section 9.5 (page 190) addresses evidence for initiatives to strengthen the resource system and change agency. Again, the evidence from the health care field is sparse. Such agencies are likely to benefit from training in communicating effectively with the potential users of innovations and in developing flexible, targeted support strategies based on a detailed assessment of the needs and capacities of different user systems.

6. In Section 9.6 (page 191), we consider linkage activities between different systems (e.g. resource system, user system, change agency) to support implementation. We review the detailed case study of one historically important linkage initiative, the US Agricultural Extension Model described by Rogers, who identified several critical features, including: (a) a research subsystem oriented to the utilisation of innovations; (b) consensual development of innovations based on shared concepts, language and mission between user system and resource system; (c) a high degree of interpersonal contact; (d) a spanable social distance across each interface between components in the technology transfer system and (e) co-evolution of the two systems rather than one reacting to changes in the other. The sparse empirical literature on linkage activities in implementing health care innovations is consistent with, but does not independently validate, these critical factors.

7. In Section 9.7 (page 195), we consider the evidence for 'whole-systems' approaches to implementation and institutionalisation. Whilst the published empirical evidence on this topic is limited, the theoretical principles of complexity theory explain why different primary studies in different contexts identify different key determinants of implementation success. We conclude that there remains – and there always will remain – a need to retranslate research and theoretical evidence into strategies, processes and tactics that incorporate unique contextual elements, and to use rapid-cycle feedback techniques to capture and respond to emerging data.

9.1 Overview of the implementation literature

This chapter considers the processes of implementation (assimilating an innovation within a system) and efforts to achieve institutionalisation or sustainability (when new ways of working become the norm). It asks: What are the features of effective strategies for implementing innovations in health service delivery and organisation and ensuring that they are sustained until they reach genuine obsolescence? Are there successful (or unsuccessful) models from which we might learn some general principles?

The literature on the implementation of innovations is particularly difficult to demarcate from the general literature on
(1) change management;
(2) organisational development; and
(3) quality improvement.

Perhaps unsurprisingly, we found multiple overlapping theoretical models and methodological approaches. As Klein and Sorra[237] stated in 1996:

> . . . because each implementation [of an innovation] case study highlights a different subset of one or more implementation policies and practices, the determinants of implementation effectiveness may appear to be a blur, a hodgepodge lacking organisation and parsimony. If multiple authors, studying multiple organisations identify differing sources of implementation failure and success, what overarching conclusion is a reader to reach? The implementation literature offers, unfortunately, little guidance.

Downs and Mohr[293] have echoed this view (page 701):

> Although cross-organisational studies of the determinants of innovation adoption are abundant, cross-organisational studies of innovation implementation are extremely rare. Most common are single, qualitative studies of innovation implementation . . . largely missing, however, are integrative models that capture and clarify the multidetermined, multilevel phenomenon of innovation implementation.

Despite this pessimistic introduction, it is possible to draw some clear messages from the literature, with the caveat that of all the areas covered in this review, implementation is the least well demarcated. The material in this chapter overlaps considerably with that already discussed in Chapters 4–8, since the success of implementation (and the chances of sustainability) are critically dependent on attributes of the innovation, the behaviour of individual adopters, the nature of communication and influence, and various structural and sociological features of the organisation and its wider environment. This overlap is evident in the theoretical literature. Shediac-Rizkallah and Bone,[399] for example, on the basis of a narrative overview of the health promotion literature, propose a conceptual framework for considering factors affecting the sustainability of innovations: (1) intraorganisational factors (several dimensions akin to what we have termed the inner context, described in Chapter 7, page 134);

(2) environmental factors (akin to what we have called the outer context, described in Chapter 8, page 157);
(3) programme design and implementation – including development of consensus amongst designers and stakeholders, resources, adequate time to judge effectiveness, evidence of perceived effectiveness training and planned length (long-term prevention programmes were especially unlikely to be continued).

Whilst most studies addressing the implementation and institutionalisation of innovations draw explicitly or implicitly on Rogers' diffusion of innovations theory, such an approach has been robustly challenged by a minority of critics (summarised by Yetton *et al.*[39]). These critics have argued that the diffusion of innovations model set out in Section 1.1 (page 20) only holds when
(1) the innovation is discrete and relatively fixed;
(2) it does not vary across the population of potential adopters; and
(3) the adopters are relatively homogeneous.

As we argued in Section 5.3 (page 106), none of these premises holds for most organisational innovations. In that section, we introduced two alternative models for the implementation process – the 'staged' model developed by Zaltman[227] and tested empirically in the health care setting by Meyer and Goes;[38] which sees assimilation as a series of linked decisions and planned actions in which implementation follows awareness, evaluation and strategic planning; and the more dynamic, organic model proposed more recently by Van de Ven *et al.*,[18] which emphasises the importance of intraorganisational relationships, negotiation and the iterative, back-and-forth movement between different 'phases' in the adoption-implementation process. The Van de Ven model aligned better with the findings of most of the empirical studies we reviewed in Section 5.3.

Reflecting these different approaches, Marble[400] has distinguished 'positivist' (logical, staged, planned, sequential) models of implementation from 'interpretivist' models (couched more in terms of engagement, involvement, communication, commitment, and values). In Sections 3.13 (page 70) and 3.15 (page 79), we present arguments from knowledge utilisation and complexity theory, respectively, that innovation in general is primarily to do with social interaction, exchange of ideas, and mutual sense-making, and only secondarily to do with institutionalisation or process control. It follows that according to these models the success of implementation must be measured (at least to some extent) in terms of effective human interaction and the reframing of meanings so as to accommodate the innovation in 'business as usual'.

One popular model for conceptualising the implementation process is known as implementation process theory, developed by Zmud[401] and others. Its central premise is that end users of innovations in the organisational context resist adoption until prompted (and unless supported) by their managers. Hence, the success of implementation at the organisational level will depend not primarily on the attributes of the innovation or the characteristics of the individual adopter, but on the strength of management and technical support and the presence of institutional incentives and sanctions.[39,401,402] Yetton *et al.* have produced a more sophisticated model that combines both diffusion of innovations theory and implementation process theory. Specifically, they propose that in situations where the innovation impacts primarily on the individual, the former model dominates; whereas in situations where the innovation impacts primarily on the group, team or organisation, the latter model dominates.*

A number of empirical studies relevant to this chapter have already been discussed in Section 5.3 (page 106) in relation to adoption. These include several in-depth qualitative studies of the process of assimilation – or rejection – of innovations by organisations (particularly Champagne *et al.*,[64] Denis *et al.*,[33] Fitzgerald *et al.*[32] and Timmons[49]). These studies provided a picture of the *process* of implementation in the particular setting of health

*Paul Plsek, who reviewed an earlier draft of this book, was unimpressed with the prominence given to implementation process theory in relation to the work of health care professionals. He commented: 'It is simply not my experience in working with professionals that they are just sitting and waiting to be prompted and supported to change by their managers.'

care organisations. The main focus of this chapter is studies that have evaluated *interventions* directed variously at health care organisations, the producers and purveyors of innovations, change agencies or the relationship between these stakeholders, aimed at making this implementation process more efficient, effective and sustainable.

9.2 Measuring institutionalisation and related concepts

A great deal has been written about measuring the institutionalisation of programmes within organisations and wider systems – some of it highly speculative and most of it relating to the commercial sector. Ledford[403] identified several synonyms for the institutionalisation of programmes within organisations: 'frozen', 'stabilised', 'accepted', 'sustained', 'durable', 'persistent' and 'maintained'. Others (reviewed by Goodman *et al.*[404]) have used the terms 'routinised', 'incorporated', 'continued' and 'built in-ness'. A recurring theme in all definitions is that the innovation becomes part of business as usual (the 'common-sense' world of practice) and ceases to be considered new.*

Goodman and Steckler,[406] writing in relation to health promotion programmes, draw an important distinction between implementation (putting the innovation into practice) and institutionalisation (akin to routinisation or sustainability). They speak from bitter experience – having set up a health promotion programme that won a national award for *implementation*, the programme nevertheless terminated on the day that its grant funding ended.[406]

Kaluzny and Hernandez[407] distinguish several stages in the institutionalisation of an innovation – including development of the innovation, initial adoption by the organisation, implementation and maintenance. They warn that these stages are distinct and separate, and that success in one stage does not assure success in the next. Many others have proposed similar staged models. See, for example, Nutbeam's[408] four-stage model of problem definition, solution generation (akin to innovation selection and adaptation), solution testing (akin to implementation) and solution maintenance (akin to institutionalisation or sustainability); the sequence given by Ashford *et al.*[203] for 'behaviour change strategies' (identify problem, examine context, consider literature, plan strategy, implement strategy and feedback/evaluate); and the recommended sequence for transfer of best practice using the benchmarking framework (search, evaluate, validate, transfer, review, routinise).[127,409,410] For a worked-up example of a staged benchmarking approach to introducing an innovation in a health care organisation, see the descriptive case study of implementing a computerised system for long-term care given by Ossip-Klein *et al.*[411]

All these models and approaches have in common the notion that the implementation process occurs as a sequence of stages that can be planned and controlled, and that planning, controlling and evaluating against predefined success criteria is the key to implementation. This assumption accords well with Marble's[400] 'positivist' school of implementation research but less well with the 'interpretivist' school.

Goodman and Dean[412] measured institutionalisation as a composite of five factors: three representing precursors (knowledge, performance, preference) and two representing true institutionalisation (normative consensus and value consensus). Many writers have commented on the difficult distinction between current implementation and future 'durability'. Yin[413] suggested that the degree of institutionalisation of a programme might be calculated by summing 'passages' (defined as formal transitions such as when a funding stream moves from temporary to permanent) and 'cycles' (repeated organisational events such as the annual budget allocation).

*Note that there is a largely separate literature on measuring the 'implementation' (i.e. adoption) of single-user innovations in organisations, most commonly with the Leonard-Barton frequency-of-use instrument.[405] However, this instrument appears to be losing favour to the more sophisticated measures of true organisational implementation discussed in this section.

Goodman *et al.*[*] drew on the work of the above authors to develop and validate a 'Level of Institutionalisation (LoIn) Scale', which measured the extent to which a health promotion programme is implemented and sustained. Using a taxonomy that is widely accepted in the organisation and management literature, they divided the organisation into four subsystems (production, maintenance, support and managerial), and for each of these considered the depth of institutionalisation of the programme (passages, routines and niche saturation):

- *Passages*. This initial LoIn comprises a production component (when a plan is formalised and approved), a support component (when funding moves from soft to hard money) and a managerial (administrative) component (when the programme 'appears on the organisational chart').
- *Routines*. Second-level institutionalisation is achieved when these features become routine and recurrent and their approval is expected and achieved at annual or other cyclical reviews.
- *Niche saturation*. This deepest LoIn is achieved when the programme has expanded to its optimum limits within the organisation's subsystems. For example, implementation of the programme is not only routine, but the programme has optimum staffing and reaches the maximum number of clients that it can sustain; stable funding is not only renewed annually but is at optimum level for the programme's goals; the programme is not only 'on the organisational chart' but has moved from a peripheral to a central position.

Goodman *et al.* used this matrix to develop a survey instrument, which they piloted and refined, and then distributed to 453 administrators in 151 health care organisations[†] in the USA. Following factor analysis they produced a 15-item questionnaire, which had high internal validity ($\alpha = 0.80$) and confirmed eight separate constructs (routines and niche saturation in each of the four subsystems described above). Their LoIn Questionnaire could potentially be used (or perhaps adapted) as a quantitative index of implementation and sustainability of organisational innovations in health care.

However, whilst the LoIn instrument has high internal validity, it was only designed to measure the perceptions of those working within the programme – and hence its *external* validity is probably questionable. The authors themselves point out this inherent weakness: the most important success criterion of a health promotion programme is surely the impact on the community and not the institutionalisation of the programme per se – hence, the LoIn questionnaire can never be more than an indirect measure of the programme's success.[‡] Citation tracking of their 1993 paper suggests that this instrument has rarely been used in empirical research – a fact that was confirmed by one of the authors (A. Steckler, personal communication, June 2003).[¶]

---

[*]The namesakes mentioned in this paragraph and the previous ones are different individuals from different research traditions: Paul Goodman is a US organisational theorist while Robert Goodman is a Canadian public health physician who drew on the work of the former.

[†]Public health units, schools (in their health promotion role) and non-profit health agencies.

[‡]All this may reflect the rapid and exciting changes in the research tradition of health promotion that have occurred over the past 20 years – from a focus on 'health education' and 'behaviour change' (in which the problem is implicitly couched in terms of individual knowledge and health choices) to a much greater focus on community development (see Section 3.8, page 62, for more discussion on this). This dramatic shift probably explains why the LoIn instrument was abandoned by the health promotion community. But in terms of measuring institutionalisation of other innovations in service delivery and organisation, it deserves further exploration.

[¶]The same group of authors subsequently developed questionnaires to measure 'level of use', 'awareness concern' (from Hall and Hord's CBAM – see Section 5.2, page 103), Rogers' innovation attributes and 'level of success'. Again, these scales, although rigorously developed, have not been taken up by other researchers (although the 'level of use' questionnaire has been published in a recent book of scales in patient education), and the authors suggest that they are almost certainly 'too cumbersome for routine use' (A. Steckler, personal communication, June 2003).

Shediak-Rizkullah and Bone suggest three possible measures of the implementation-sustainability continuum: maintenance of health benefits achieved through an initial programme, LoIn of a program within an organisation (see Section 9.2, page 178) and measures of capacity building in the recipient community (see Section 9.6, page 191). Øvretveit[414] offers a comparable four-level measure in relation to quality improvement initiatives:

(1) Are the results/outcomes of the activity sustained?

(2) Is the project itself sustained?

(3) Are the quality methods learned in *this* project sustained outside the project?

(4) Has the organisation's capacity to improve quality been strengthened?

This framework moves the focus of attention away from conceptualising the innovation as a 'thing' to be implemented and instead suggests a more organic model of continual adaptation and emergence.

Another important issue in implementation research is how to measure the *process* of implementation. How do we measure what gets done, by whom, in what order, how easy or difficult it is, and what are the barriers and facilitators? How do we distinguish instrumental from incidental factors? How do we measure the transferability of the findings of such studies to other innovations, organisations, and contexts? There are no easy answers to these questions, which is why implementation research is inherently fraught. It is easy to dismiss such research as 'methodologically flawed' since studies are of course conducted in the messy real world where potential confounders can never be fully controlled for (or even, in some cases, identified in the first place).

The empirical studies reviewed in this chapter have taken either a descriptive, in-depth case study approach (in which the causal relationship between variables is essentially inferred from the 'story' of the implementation effort*) or a more experimental approach in which the impact of particular variables on predefined measures of implementation success is tested prospectively. There are inherent strengths and limitations associated with both these approaches, which are discussed in the sections that follow.

It is worth noting that Pawson and Tilley[120] have developed a different (and potentially very powerful) conceptual framework for evaluating implementation studies and considering their transferability across different contexts and settings – known as realistic evaluation and illustrated in Box A.7, (page 240) in Appendix 2. None of the studies discussed in this chapter used this approach so we have not been able to apply Pawson and Tilley's framework further in our own analysis.

*See Section 3.12 (page 70) for a theoretical discussion of narrative inference.

9.3 Implementation and institutionalisation: systematic reviews and other high-quality overviews

We found no high-quality overviews that directly covered our own research question, but four were on closely related topics whose findings are relevant. These are summarised in Table A.20 (page 285) in Appendix 4 and described in detail in the following pages.

The EUR-ASSESS systematic review of dissemination and implementation of research findings

In 1997, Granados *et al.* (EUR-ASSESS Subgroup on Dissemination and Impact) published a review of primary studies that aimed to promote dissemination and implementation of the results of research (especially but not exclusively HTA reports). Their focus was thus different in key respects from our own focus on innovations in service delivery and organisation. In particular, the EUR-ASSESS review placed much greater emphasis on individual behaviour change amongst clinicians than on new ways of working for teams and organisations. The study also focused predominantly (although not exclusively) on influencing the behaviour of doctors† and on methods

†Since most HTA reports whose dissemination has been addressed in empirical studies relate to drugs, doctors are the most widely studied individuals in relation to such reports.

for spreading research information to the general public (which is not part of our own remit and so is not discussed further in this review).

Overall, the EUR-ASSESS Subgroup on Dissemination and Impact covered 110 papers, about half of which were primary studies. In common with our own team, they found that the empirical literature was complex and diverse, and that it drew on a wide range of underpinning theoretical frameworks (and, most usually, on no explicit theory at all). The main findings were as follows:

- The reviewers judged the methodological quality of most studies to be poor; most intervention studies were restricted to doctors in North America so their generalisability is in doubt.
- There was almost no relevant empirical work, and no controlled trials, on influencing the media or policymakers.*
- There was almost no relevant research on cost-effectiveness.
- Barriers to behaviour change in relation to disseminating and implementing research findings can be divided into (a) environmental factors (e.g. political climate, lobbying by special interest groups, and financial disincentives); (b) personal characteristic barriers (e.g. perception of risk, clinical uncertainty, information overload) and (c) prevailing opinion barriers (e.g. difficulty dealing with uncertainty, standards of professional practice, opinion leaders, social standards).
- The timing of dissemination strategies is crucial in policymaking. As the authors state: 'A piece of potentially influential research that arrives too early or too late in the policy drafting process may be ignored'.†
- Low scientific literacy (of both patients and professionals) meant that the targeted research findings were not adequately understood (and therefore not implemented).

*Our own view is that research into influencing policymakers is unlikely to be suited to 'intervention trials', but this was nevertheless identified as a gap in the literature by these authors.

†See the discussion of Kingdon's model of policy streams and Exworthy's work on policy innovations described in Section 8.4 (page 172), which also confirm (and expand on) the issue of 'timing'.

The EUR-ASSESS authors used a hierarchical approach to evaluating evidence in which randomised trial evidence was explicitly weighted more highly than more qualitative methods. Whilst this potentially allowed the magnitude of effects of particular strategies to be documented accurately, it did not allow an exploration of the *process* of the dissemination or implementation programmes.‡ Nevertheless, even though much of the evidence assessed by these authors was ranked 'low quality' in terms of their own hierarchy, and their overall conceptual framework differed in crucial respects from our own, their final conclusions and recommendations align closely with those set out in Chapter 10 (page 199) and with those of other systematic reviews of similar topic areas (see below).[11,91]

One important bottom line message from this review was that changing policy and practice is a complex process, and that the provision of more information does not necessarily foster more rational decision-making.¶ Note that HTA reports are not generally about organisational innovations, and are, in general, more easily amenable to 'intervention' type research. Whilst the hierarchy used by these authors to evaluate evidence might – arguably – have been appropriate for their own research question, it is inappropriate for our research question about the processes of dissemination, implementation and institutionalisation of complex innovations.

The Meyers *et al.* review of industrial process implementation

We found one overview of implementation strategies in industrial process innovations (i.e. innovations in the equivalent of 'service delivery and organisation' for industry and manufacturing), by Meyers *et al.*[91] This was not presented as a formal systematic review but we judged it to be

‡See Section 3.9 (page 64) for further discussion on this methodological issue.

¶Given the lead time for systematic reviews, and the prevailing stage of the meta-narrative of EBM in the mid-1990s (see Section 3.9, page 64), this conclusion was a seminal one at the time, although it may seem self-evident with the wisdom of hindsight.

systematic (there is an explicit, albeit brief, methods section), comprehensive (134 references), scholarly (they draw on a number of published theoretical frameworks and their conclusions derive logically from the data presented) and original (they present a new theoretical model that explains their findings and aligns closely with our independent findings) and to have important messages for our own review.

The findings of this extensive review closely match our own impression that whereas innovation, adoption, social influence and dissemination have been widely studied, very few empirical studies have specifically addressed the implementation, institutionalisation and sustainability of innovations. We describe their main findings below with the caveat that they focused exclusively on the commercial sector and their findings are unlikely to be *directly* transferable to the service sector.

Meyers *et al.* defined implementation as 'the early usage activities that often follow the adoption decision', and suggest that this stage is complete when the innovation becomes part of routine practice. They cite empirical work from the industrial sector that demonstrates the crucial importance of this initial post-adoption phase for the long-term acceptability and sustainability of the innovation. A swift and seemingly smooth adoption process may spell initial success, but (they warn) poor implementation can lead to underutilisation of the innovation, unmet expectations and widespread dissatisfaction. Furthermore, the story of an organisational failure, with its frustrations and wasted efforts, will inevitably be propagated through various individual and organisational networks and can serve as a powerful 'anti-adoption' message for comparable organisations.[91]

Meyers *et al.* explicitly omit consideration of innovation attributes* because, they say, this aspect of diffusion of innovations has been well summarised by previous authors. They consider the other influences on implementation of service innovations under four broad headings: characteristics of the user system (what they call 'the buyer'); characteristics of the resource system ('the seller'); characteristics of the interface between these systems ('the buyer–seller interface') and the wider environment. The factors that have been shown unequivocally in empirical studies to influence the success of implementation programmes are listed under headings based on our own terminology in Box 9.1.

*Relative advantage and so on, covered in this review in Chapter 4.

Box 9.1 Factors found in a systematic overview to be associated with successful implementation of service innovations in industrial process (from Meyers *et al.*[91])

Characteristics of the user system

Human resources

Appropriate and sufficient education and training at all levels

Positive motivation, attitudes and commitment towards the innovation

Organisational structure

An adaptive and flexible organisational structure

Strong communication mechanisms and networks across structural boundaries within the user system

Decision processes

Broad and strategic, as opposed to narrowly operational or technical, organisational goals

Greater and earlier involvement of the operational workforce in the implementation process

Top management support and commitment throughout the implementation process as well as the presence of champions

Cooperation among units within the user organisation

Slow and gradual rather than rapid and radical incorporation of the innovation

Technology fit

Familiarity with any new technology and availability of relevant skills within the user system

The more strategically critical the innovation the higher will be the commitment to it, thereby enhancing implementation

Characteristics of the resource system

Competence and capability of the resource system

A high level of technical capability, to allow successful 'installation' of the innovation in a range of settings

Strong communication skills, so that information about the innovation can be transmitted rapidly and efficiently
Project management expertise (especially important for large, complex projects)

Characteristics of the resource system–user system interface
Quality and depth of the linkage between systems
Joint product development
Constructive collaboration at the implementation stage
Knowledge transfer

Environmental factors
The wider context beyond the user and resource systems
More intensive networking within and across industries leads to greater exposure to new innovations and faster, more efficient implementation
Extensive governmental regulation impedes implementation

Whilst the findings of this review must be treated with caution in the context of our own research question, their overall taxonomy has high face validity, and we have used a similar taxonomy to organise the empirical studies for our own review in Sections 9.4–9.6 (page 186 et seq.). We suggest one limitation of the Meyers review, which is the lack of consideration of 'whole-systems' approaches (perhaps less relevant in the commercial sector than in the service sector), which we cover in Section 9.7 (page 195).

The Grimshaw *et al.* review of dissemination and implementation of guidelines

As discussed in Section 3.9 (page 64), the EBM movement has over the past 15 years become increasingly concerned with the issue of implementation of evidence-based guidelines. Initially implementation was construed in terms of 'clinician behaviour change' and addressed with educational approaches and behavioural incentives, but it is now recognised that guideline implementation often includes an organisational component. Grimshaw *et al.*[11] (a group of authors with a long tradition of conducting both empirical work and systematic reviews on EBM and guideline implementation) undertook a very large systematic review on interventions to improve the dissemination and impact of clinical guidelines.

Prior to their review, certain 'facts' had already been established about the implementation of guidelines (i.e. there was evidence in the literature to support these beliefs, which had begun to be propagated as 'received wisdom'):

(1) 'Top-down' initiatives (e.g. sending out reminders) are relatively ineffective.
(2) 'Interactive' initiatives (e.g. educational outreach programmes) are much more effective.
(3) 'Tailoring' guidelines to local priorities and circumstances improves their chances of being successfully implemented.
(4) Single interventions are less effective than multifaceted ones.

These conclusions had been reached largely on the basis of reviews that rated empirical studies as either 'positive' (an effect had been demonstrated) or 'negative' (it had not). Furthermore, many of the studies that had contributed to previous received wisdom were of marginal relevance or used subjective rather than objective outcome measures.

Against this background, Grimshaw's team sought to conduct a comprehensive review with clear eligibility criteria as set out in Box 9.2. Their search yielded 285 reports of 235 studies, describing 309 separate comparisons. Overall, methodological quality was judged poor (e.g. unit of analysis errors* were common); and the description of interventions was poor (i.e. there was very little process information provided in most studies, making them impossible to replicate faithfully).

Only 27% of studies considered in this review were judged to have drawn on theories or psychological constructs, and fewer than ten studies were presented as explicitly theory-driven. Only 29% of comparisons reported any economic data, and

*That is, randomisation was by one unit (e.g. hospital or ward) while analysis of data was by another unit (e.g. individual).

Box 9.2 The Grimshaw *et al.*[11] systematic review of guideline dissemination and implementation strategies: eligibility criteria.

- *Scope:* primary studies testing guideline dissemination and implementation strategies
- *Study designs:* experimental or quasi-experimental study designs (RCTs, non-RCTs, controlled before and after studies, and interrupted time series studies)*
- *Participants:* medically qualified health care professionals
- *Interventions:* guideline dissemination and implementation strategies
- *Outcomes:* objective measures of provider behaviour and patient outcome

*The authors have discussed choice of design from a theoretical perspective in separate commentary articles.[415,416]

of these, a mere four studies provided sufficiently robust data for consideration. The comparisons addressed by the primary studies are shown in Box 9.3.

The findings of the Grimshaw review were surprising and in some respects counter-intuitive:

- Improvements were shown in the intended direction of the intervention in 86% of comparisons – but the effect was generally small in magnitude.
- Simple reminders were the intervention most consistently observed to be effective.
- Educational outreach programmes only led to modest effects on implementation success – and were very expensive compared with less intensive approaches.
- Dissemination of educational materials led to modest but potentially important effects (and of similar magnitude to more intensive interventions).
- Multifaceted interventions were not necessarily more effective than single interventions.
- Nothing could be concluded from most primary studies about the cost-effectiveness of the intervention.

This important review has thus set the stage for reframing the widespread perception that the best way to promote implementation of guidelines is through multiple or high-intensity (and often costly) interventions. As with many reviews of the health services research literature, the focus on trials (and hence on a small number of predefined outcomes) means that the contribution of this review to illuminating the process of dissemination, implementation and institutionalisation is small. The authors acknowledge this and call for a greater breadth of study designs in future research.

Box 9.3 The Grimshaw *et al.*[11] systematic review of guideline dissemination and implementation strategies: comparisons addressed in primary studies.

Single interventions:
84 comparisons evaluated a single intervention against no intervention control including:

- 38 studies of reminders
- 18 studies of educational materials
- 12 studies of audit and feedback
- 3 studies of educational meetings
- 3 of 'other professional interventions'
- 2 studies of organisational interventions
- 8 studies of patient-mediated interventions

Multifaceted interventions
138 comparisons against a 'no intervention' control group

- Evaluated 68 different combinations of interventions
- Maximum number of comparisons of same combination of interventions was 11

85 comparisons against an intervention control group

- Evaluated 58 different combinations of interventions

In summary, the Grimshaw *et al.* systematic review should inject a note of caution into the current wave of enthusiasm for 'outreach' and 'linkage activities' (discussed further in Section 9.6, page 191). Whilst such approaches have strong theoretical and ideological appeal, the few rigorous randomised trials that have been undertaken have demonstrated only modest benefit – at a cost that is likely to be substantial but that was mostly unmeasured. Nevertheless, this finding may also be attributable to the fact that the benefits of complex interventions may go beyond what the unenhanced randomised trial can measure – a suggestion which in increasingly recognised by mainstream clinical triallists.[11] Grol and Grimshaw[417] have, incidentally, recently published a short summary of this review and related research in the *Lancet*.

The Gustafson *et al.* narrative review of change management in organisations

As discussed above, much material relevant to this chapter is to be found in the general change management literature, which we were unable to review comprehensively. However, one recently published overview from that literature deserves mention.[79] Gustafson *et al.* invited a panel of experts in organisational theory to suggest critical factors to account for the successful (or unsuccessful) implementation of organisational change projects. They combined this with a narrative review of the organisational change literature to produce an 18-item survey instrument (Box 9.4), which measured the Bayesian probability of successful change. They then tested this instrument retro-

Box 9.4 Factors contributing to Bayesian model for predicting success of organisational change initiatives, developed by Gustafson *et al.*[79,*]

The innovation ('the solution')
(1) *Exploration of problem and customer needs.* Ideally, a detailed needs assessment has been done (e.g. by talking first-hand to users) and fed into the design of the solution.
(2) *Radicalness of design.* The new process is not seen as a radical deviation from the organisation's existing philosophy and operation.
(3) *Flexibility of design.* The new process can be modified to the particular setting without reducing its effectiveness.
(4) *Complexity of implementation.* The implementation plan is simple and all understand it.
(5) *Evidence of effectiveness.* There is concrete evidence that the new process worked well in an organisation like this one.

The adoption decision
(6) *Advantages to staff and customers.* The proposed change is clearly understood by all stakeholders and perceived to have more advantages than disadvantages.
(7) *Staff needs assessment, involvement and support.* The change team have assessed staff needs and can successfully present the change as meeting those needs.

External links
(8) *Source of ideas.* Ideally these come from outside the organisation and have been tailored to fit.

User system – organisational antecedents
(9) *Work environment.* The organisational structure, leadership roles, incentive system and staffing are already set up to support the change.

User system – organisational readiness
(10) *Tension for change.* Ideally, staff feel strongly that the current situation is intolerable and actively seek a change.
(11) *Leader goals, involvement and support.* The change ('solution') aligns with leaders' prior goals; leaders are involved with the change and frequently consulted.
(12) *Funding.* Top management commits money to both problem-solving and implementation.
(13) *Middle manager goals, involvement and support.* The change ('solution') aligns with middle managers' prior goals; they spent time and resources to support the change.
(14) *Supporters and opponents.* Supporters of the change stand to gain more than its opponents.
(15) *Staff changes required.* Job changes are few and clear; high-quality protocols and training materials are available; coaching is provided.
(16) *Monitoring and feedback.* Good systems and measures are in place to get valid performance data and honest feedback from service users and staff.

Change agent and agency
(17) *Mandate.* Project leaders endorse both the change and any assigned change agent.
(18) *Change agent.* Has prestige, commitment, power, and is oriented to the service user.

*For ease of comparison with our own model (Figure 10.1, page 201), we have grouped the 18 items from the Gustafson review under comparable sub-headings, which were not used in by the original authors.

spectively against published studies of change initiatives in health service delivery and organisation. They found that it had very high sensitivity and specificity (area under the Receiver Operator Characteristic curve > 0.84) for distinguishing projects that were successfully implemented from those that failed or had only marginal success.

The Gustafson model has many parallels with the Meyers model (Box 9.1, page 182). Both, for example, emphasise the need for the innovation to align with the organisation's overall strategy and mission; the need for broad-based support and advocacy (from both top and middle management); attention to human resources (training and support) and meticulous monitoring of the impact of the change. The main differences were

(1) Gustafson *et al.* emphasised several key attributes of the innovation (which Meyers *et al.* explicitly did not review simply because these had been well covered by previous reviewers).

(2) Gustafson *et al.* placed less emphasis on external change agencies, linkage activities and networks (probably because the focus of their review was specifically on internal organisational change).

The critical importance demonstrated by Gustafson *et al.* of problem definition, assessment of 'fit', monitoring, evaluation and feedback accords strongly with advice given in more pragmatic articles in the quality improvement literature, which was beyond our remit to review comprehensively. We recommend, for example, the overview by Plsek[307] of management tools and techniques for quality improvement, which includes a toolkit of methods for process design, collecting and analysing data, collaborative working, quality planning and so on.

In summary, the article by Gustafson *et al.* has two limitations from the perspective of this review:

(1) Their model was developed in relation to change management in general rather than the assimilation of innovations in particular (although we can think of no theoretical reason why the latter – which is a subset of the former – should have substantially different success factors).

(2) Although developed very rigorously, their model has yet to be tested prospectively.

9.4 Empirical studies of interventions aimed at strengthening predisposition and capacity of the user system

Background literature

An organisation's capacity to embrace and implement *any* innovation (a critical component of what we have called 'system antecedents', covered in Chapter 7, page 134) is widely believed to be critical to the implementation of a *particular* innovation, and 'capacity-building activities' are widely promoted. But 'capacity' is not easy to define or measure, and the notion of a simple 'capacity checklist' or 'formula for building capacity' must surely be rejected. Organisations are complex, and 'capacity' must be defined, measured and enhanced flexibly according to the innovation and the context. We discuss some approaches to this task, drawn from different research traditions.

Parcel *et al.*[419] combined Rogers' diffusion of innovations theory and Green's[418] predisposing, reinforcing and enabling causes in educational diagnosis and evaluation (PRECEDE) model of health education in the context of community-based health promotion programmes (in which innovations tend to be especially complex and there are multiple contextual elements and confounding variables). Their model, which is discussed and developed further in relation to organisational change by Elliott *et al.*[96] to form the Survey of Capacity, Activities and Needs ('Organisation SCAN'), includes three key factors:

- *Predisposition.* Predisposing factors comprise the attitudes, beliefs, knowledge, perceptions and values that motivate individuals and organisations to implement a particular innovation. For example, dissemination of a health promotion programme at an organisational level is influenced by the motivation of the staff whose job is to deliver particular elements of the programme and the finance directors who are asked to find the budgets.
- *Capacity.* Capacity is the sum of the resources available to the organisation or system for the management and delivery of the implementation process. It is measured in terms of financial resources, staffing, training and technical assistance.

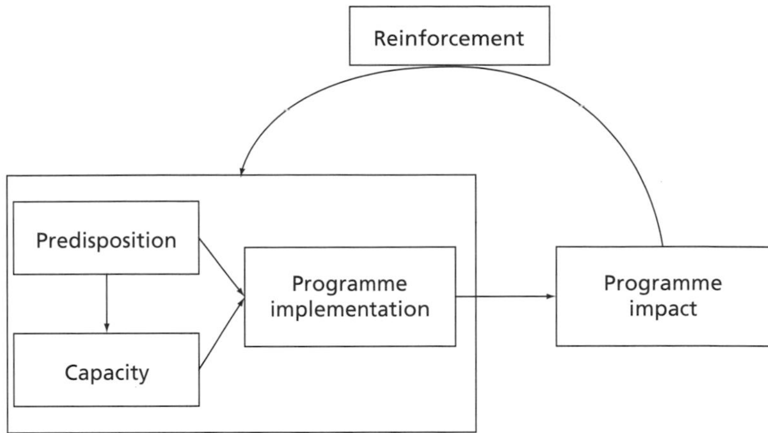

Fig. 9.1 Predisposition, capacity and reinforcement in programme implementation (based on Green *et al.*[418] and Elliott *et al.*[96]).

• *Reinforcement.* Sustainability of the programme depends partly on reinforcement by feedback about its impact on the target population (hence, implicitly, the systematic collection and feedback of such information will increase the sustainability of the programme providing a positive impact is demonstrated).

The relationship between these three dimensions is shown in Fig. 9.1.

Another conceptual framework worth noting in relation to the process of implementation, derived from evidence-based nursing, is the evidence–context–facilitation triad of Kitson, Rycroft-Malone *et al.*[93,420]:

• *Evidence.* The evidence for the innovation – divided into research evidence (clear, relevant, important), clinician experience (valued and systematically reflected upon) and patient experience (valued and systematically tapped).

• *Context.* The wider context in which the innovation is introduced – divided into organisational antecedents (clarity of organisational structure, power and authority processes, appropriate and transparent decision-making processes, information and feedback, receptiveness to change), organisational culture (explicit, values individual staff and clients, promotes 'learning organisation'*), leadership (role clarity, effective teamwork, democratic decision-making, transformational focus) and evaluation/feedback (occurs at individual, team and system levels; uses multiple sources and methods).

• *Facilitation.* People in role and processes in place to support the implementation across the organisation (systems for facilitation are in place, internal and external facilitators have been appointed, developmental and 'adult learning' principles are applied to staff training).

Whilst Kitson and colleagues have done considerable conceptual work to develop their framework, it is still at the hypothesis stage and they concede that its empirical support remains largely anecdotal.[421] 'Evidence' in this framework is akin to the attributes of innovations (most notably relative advantage and compatibility) discussed in Chapter 3. Different aspects of context and facilitation are broadly akin to elements of organisational capacity (with the addition of 'linkage activities' if the facilitation is provided or supported by an external change agency).

Predisposition and capacity of the user system: surveys

We found four surveys that looked specifically at the association between organisational capacity and implementation success *as perceived by the survey's respondents.*[90,96] These are summarised in Table A.21 (page 287) in Appendix 4. Two

*See Section 3.11 (page 68).

additional surveys, which included perceptions about user system capacity amongst other perceived determinants of implementation success, are covered in Section 9.7 (page 195) in relation to whole-systems approaches.

In a preliminary study aimed at exploring elements of organisational predisposition and capacity in the Canadian Heart Health Implementation Programme, Taylor *et al.* conducted semi-structured interviews on 56 key informants and questionnaire surveys on 262 staff from 42 separate organisations involved in health promotion innovations in Canada. They sought perceptions on organisational predisposition (i.e. its perceived readiness to become involved with new health promotion initiatives), and found five main motivators (collaboration with external agencies; high-level support, e.g. from the regional Board of Health; staff involvement and commitment; national directive from the Ministry of Health; and requests from the local community for change). Barriers to predisposition were broadly the converse of these.

Taylor *et al.* also identified five major elements that were perceived to facilitate actual implementation of the programmes: financial and material resources; staff experience, knowledge and skills; defined staff roles for the project; availability of good research evidence for the change; and links to external agencies. The five major perceived barriers to successful implementation were inadequate financial resources, inadequate staff, no (or too few) staff roles dedicated to the project, lack of coordination and lack of good research evidence for the change.[90]

The survey by Taylor *et al.*[90] suggests that, in terms of the *perceptions* of key actors, an organisation's predisposition (motivation, readiness) for implementing an innovation is determined substantially from external factors ('top-down' directives driven by national and regional policy, and external links both to other organisations and the local community), with the additional element of good research evidence; whereas the implementation process is largely determined by capacity variables within the organisation.

The Taylor study was an early publication relating to the wider Canadian Heart Health Initiative, Ontario Project (CHHIOP). In a subsequent publication, the authors report how they developed a survey instrument for health units – Organisation SCAN – that measured organisational predisposition (willingness to participate, measured on an 19-item scale that indicates 'the collective belief amongst staff of the importance of implementing the heart health activity') and capacity (a composite of per capita funding, whether the organisation has a 'line item' for heart health, whether there is a budget attached to this and whether the unit participates in coalitions) as independent variables, as well as an index of implementation (on a five-point scale from 'not aware of any organised activity' to 'high level of implementation') as the dependent variable. An additional, more detailed staff questionnaire (also mentioned in the Taylor paper) was also undertaken.[96]

The CHHIOP team demonstrated a strong correlation between predisposition (as assessed by respondents) and capacity (as assessed by respondents), and a moderate to strong correlation between capacity and implementation of health promotion innovations, but no direct relationship between predisposition and implementation. This suggests that predisposition is a necessary but not sufficient condition for successful implementation, and that it works via building capacity.[96] This finding makes sense, in that wanting to implement an initiative is a crucial prerequisite, but will not itself lead to effective action unless resources and skills are added.

As we noted previously (see Section 1.2, page 22), the validity and generalisablility of studies of perceptions is generally fairly weak, and at best these surveys raise some interesting hypotheses to bear in mind when considering empirical studies in which such influences have been formally tested.

Predisposition and capacity of the user system: intervention studies

We found no systematic reviews but did find three empirical studies (one randomised trial and two in-depth case studies) that measured interventions to improve predisposition (by improving motivation and commitment) and to improve capacity (by enhancing human resources, changing internal structures, improving decision-making processes or addressing technology fit) for the implementation of innovations in health service delivery and organisation. These studies are listed in Table A.22 (page 289) in Appendix 4.

It should be noted that 'capacity-building activities' (which in its broadest sense might include any staff training initiatives, allocation of resources to particular areas of activity, establishment of internal teams and so on) are widespread, and it was extremely difficult to delineate what did and did not count as a project whose main purpose was to build capacity specifically for the introduction of an innovation in service delivery and organisation. In particular, the distinction between 'quality improvement', 'change management' and 'implementation of an innovation' was often difficult to make. In order to exclude studies of marginal relevance (and hence improve the clarity if not the comprehensiveness of our findings), we used a stringent definition of innovation implementation (see Section 1.3, page 25), and also only selected studies in which capacity building was linked to the planned introduction of a particular innovation. The studies listed in Table A.22 should not therefore be considered an exhaustive list.*

One of the few RCTs in this literature was conducted by McCormick *et al.* They demonstrated (in the context of school-based health promotion programmes) that while intensive staff training did not enhance initial implementation of the innovation, it doubled the chances that the innovation would still be routine practice 4 years later (62% vs 30%). Furthermore, when individual staff were surveyed, awareness of the innovation and training, but not concerns about the innovation or personal interest in it, were significantly associated with successful implementation of the programme. This suggests that individual concerns and interests might be relatively less important when the innovation is adopted at an organisational level (i.e. when the adoption decision is authoritative). This finding aligns with the suggestion of Yetton *et al.* based on implementation process theory that if the impact of the innovation is mainly at the team or organisational level, innovation attributes and adopter factors will be relatively less important than internal organisational mandates, management support and training.[39] Incidentally, this study also showed a positive (but statistically non-significant) link between organisational size and climate and implementation success.

Green[92] undertook a detailed case study within a single US Health Maintenance Organisation of the implementation of ICPs. He used a highly systematic approach that involved major changes to the organisational structure, including the establishment of a cross-departmental multi-disciplinary collaborative to oversee the project and also interdepartmental multi-disciplinary implementation teams. Training was provided in a flexible, just-in-time manner tailored to the needs of different staff. Another striking feature of the project was the close attention to goals and milestones and to data collection, with systematic feedback to the implementation teams.

None of the hypothesised influences on implementation success was empirically tested against a control approach in this study, but in-depth qualitative methods supported the conclusion that eight key factors contributed to the project's success:

(1) 'just-in-time' training for team members and leaders;
(2) outcome-focused working;
(3) meticulous data collection and feeding this back tightly into the system;
(4) buy-in from both clinicians and top management;
(5) support and leadership;
(6) 'visual tools' to guide the process of the collaborative practice committees (e.g. plan–do–check–act);
(7) a culture of support, consistency and discipline; and
(8) attention to financial and operational issues.

*A peer reviewer of an earlier draft of this book pointed out that UNESCO has a wealth of know-how and 'grey literature' publications on strengthening the capacity of user systems and local change agencies in developing and transition countries in relation to community development, disaster relief, technology transfer, education and other initiatives. See www.unesco.org.

Overall, this study has some face validity, but given the single case approach and the lack of any consideration of negative influences or interaction between influences, it provides relatively weak support for the influences discussed.

The qualitative study by Edmondson *et al.*[95] of teams in 16 US hospitals implementing an innovative technology for cardiac surgery examined the collective learning process that takes place among interdependent users of a new technology during implementation. The fieldwork involved 165 interviews and observation over a 5-month period.

The study found that successful implementers underwent a qualitatively different team learning process than those who were unsuccessful. Successful implementers

(1) used enrolment to motivate the team;
(2) designed preparatory practice sessions and conducted early trials to create psychological safety and encourage new behaviours; and
(3) promoted shared meaning and process improvement through reflective practices.

The data did not tell a story of greater skill, superior organisational resources, top management support or more past experiences as drivers of innovation. Instead they suggested that face-to-face leadership and teamwork can allow organisations to adapt successfully when confronted with new technology that threatens existing routines.

This important study is one of the few that have explored the process of team learning. It may be that the reason why most studies to date have failed to find evidence for the importance of group-level inputs is that they did not look for such evidence, and further research is almost certainly needed at this level.

9.5 Empirical studies of interventions aimed at strengthening the resource system and change agency

The systematic review by Meyer *et al.* (Box 9.1, page 182) suggested that three features of 'the seller' (resource system) consistently influenced implementation by 'the buyer' (user system): a high level of technical capability (to allow successful 'installation' of the innovation in a range of settings), strong communication skills (so that information about the innovation can be transmitted rapidly and efficiently) and project management expertise (which was found to be especially important for large, complex projects). They recommend that 'sellers' should

(1) develop and share information about the innovation;
(2) develop the communication skills of their own staff; and
(3) develop and distribute tools and techniques for project management.

We should interpret these suggestions in the light of two important differences in the service sector: health care organisations do not see themselves in a buyer–seller relationship with the developers of innovations (the guideline 'industry', for example, is a case in point); and there is a growing industry of intermediaries (e.g. what Lomas[13] calls 'knowledge purveyors', and a range of change agencies of which the UK Modernisation Agency is perhaps a contemporary example) who increasingly ensure that the 'producers' of innovations and those who might adopt them is indirect rather than direct.

We found virtually no empirical studies focusing on approaches to enhance the input of the resource system in innovation implementation, and none at all from the health services literature. We found two relevant studies: one from the education sector and one from health care, both of which we rated as high quality, and which we feel raise interesting methodological issues.

In a highly original approach, but on a small scale, Dearing *et al.* conducted 27 interviews* of university academics (mostly engineers and industrial scientists) about the nature of their research findings (in this study, the innovation was the respondent's own research discoveries). The transcripts were independently coded and analysed, with 11 possible 'innovation attributes' (economic advantage, effectiveness, observability and so on) forming the basis for a formal content analysis.

*Nine academics were interviewed separately by three researchers for triangulation purposes

Of the 1600 codable sentences in the analysis by Dearing *et al.*, 93% could be coded in relation to the 11 attributes and 51% were classified as a 'positive' statement. But the majority of statements were simple description (77% contained no evaluative information), and overall, the innovators failed to convey the extent of their enthusiasm for their own innovation. An important recommendation is that innovators could and should help to 'create receptive capacity' for their innovations by learning to communicate more effectively (especially about the potential applications of the innovation) and by providing more evaluative information (e.g. stating why the innovation is 'better than X', rather than simply describing what it does).

Another critical finding in this study was the degree of *social construction of meaning* about the innovation between the interviewer and the respondent. The respondent did not simply *convey* information to the interviewer; rather, the meaning of the innovation developed during the course of the interview through questions, explanations, clarifications and negotiations. Dearing *et al.*[48] conclude that the dearth of research into knowledge transfer in this pre-adoption phase should be urgently redressed – a suggestion with which we concur.

Another study that is possibly relevant to this review in terms of raising ideas for how resource systems and change agencies might enhance their own capacity is the Nault *et al.*[422] work on fostering adoption of interorganisational information systems (two out of three were health service related – an IT system linking hospitals with suppliers of consumables and an ordering system for high street pharmacists). They used a mathematical modelling technique to demonstrate the value of a 'triage' approach to offering differential support packages to different organisations. Some organisations, they argue, adopt new innovations without support, whereas others will need considerable additional input – these can be identified using established measures of organisational innovativeness (see Chapter 7, page 134). Given that interorganisational information systems often require the cooperation of all stakeholders in a catchment area, the idea of proactively identifying the least innovative and targeting them for support from the outset deserves to be empirically tested.

A further gap in the literature was the complete absence of empirical studies addressing the role of the resource agency as a central resource of project management tools and techniques. Although many central agencies now offer such materials and support, we did not find any studies that explored whether and how they are being utilised. We were also disappointed not to find any studies comparing 'internal' change agents with 'external' agents provided by a resource agency. Again, this is a potentially fruitful area for targeted empirical research.

Overall, and in contrast to the findings from the commercial sector, there is almost no research aimed specifically at developing the role of the resource system or change agency. Perhaps this is partly because service delivery innovations are not a 'product' produced in a factory or laboratory, but it may also be because there is less commercial incentive for the resource systems to evaluate and enhance their own role.

9.6 Empirical studies of linkage activities to support implementation

Collaboration and knowledge transfer

Under this category, Meyers *et al.*[91] include 'joint product development', collaboration at implementation stage' and 'knowledge transfer'. They found in their systematic review of industrial process innovations (see page 181) that the greater the transfer of knowledge between resource system and user system, so that the former is involved in learning, diagnosing and shaping the usage patterns of the user system early in the use of the innovation, the more successful is the implementation.[91]

The notion of linkage between the developers (or purveyors) of an innovation and its intended adopters has been widely researched in the general sociological literature, and is well summarised by Rogers[3] (page 357 et seq.) in relation to the agricultural extension service. In his words:

> Change agent success in securing adoption of innovations by clients is positively related to increasing client ability to evaluate innovations.

> Unfortunately, change agents are often more concerned with such short-range goals as escalating the rate of adoption of innovations. Instead, in many cases, self reliance should be the goal of change agencies, leading to termination of client dependence on the change agent [for evaluating innovations].[3]

He suggests that linkage activities between the resource system and the user system should aim to achieve three things:

- A shared conception of the total system.
- Use of a common language by members of the system.
- A common sense of mission.

Towards this goal, the US agricultural research agencies joined forces with government and local agencies to develop a formal linkage (in their terms, 'extension') programme with farmers on the ground. Embryonic extension activities had begun as early as 1911, and by 1920 there were 3000 extension employees in the agricultural sector; in 1995 there were 17 000, funded by a composite stream including national (federal), state and local (county). Sixty-eight percent of the extension workers worked at a county level with individual farmers, taking a client-oriented perspective and gaining an understanding of their needs, priorities and concerns, and spending time teaching them how to evaluate new innovations. County extension workers linked in turn with state- and national-level extension workers, who were oriented towards the resource system (research institutions) and change agencies (government and other bodies pushing to 'roll out' innovations so as to achieve strategic goals). On the basis of over 80 years' experience with linkage in agricultural research, Rogers distils some principles (Box 9.5), which might be applied (with adaptation) to other areas.

The agricultural extension model is not without its critics, who have accused it of being centrally driven, bureaucratic and ideologically biased.* It is also, of course, only suited to those innovations that can be developed and driven in a reasonably formal manner by planned activity (many innovations, especially in service organisation, do not arise this way†). But to the extent that it was successful, this success is attributable to four factors:

(1) flexibility of the system, allowing it to respond adaptively to wider environmental change (e.g. to survive successive changes of central government);

(2) involvement of the users of innovations at all stages from identification of research priorities through design of innovations to their evaluation in practice;

(3) a financial reward system for researchers when their innovative ideas prove useful in the real world; and

(4) close spatial contact between extension workers and their clients (i.e. such individuals are paid not to sit in offices but to get on the road and 'press the flesh').

In contrast with the wealth of studies from marginally relevant traditions, and many opinion papers recommending linkage activities for promoting implementation of new health technologies, we found very few empirical studies on linkage activities for innovations in health service delivery and organisation. As with previous sections in this chapter, the greatest contribution was from Canadian public health, where heart health promotion initiatives have been extensively researched and evaluated over the past 15 years (and where champions for these ideas have worked hard to disseminate them). Again, the idea of linkage is widely discussed in a number of well-argued opinion papers (e.g. Orlandi[423] for a general overview and Stachenko[424] and Schabas[425] for a vision for delivering heart health promotion through formal linkage between research units who would provide the evidence, and local public health units who would be the main vehicle for delivering appropriate interventions).

*The agricultural extension model's pro-innovation bias, for example, led to the uncritical acceptance and widespread dissemination of the now-discredited intensive farming methods based on heavy use of chemical fertilisers.

†See Section 6.6 (page 131) for further discussion on innovations that arise more peripherally and spread more informally.

In their strategy papers, these Canadian authors closely reflect the principles of linkage as set out by Rogers (Box 9.5), and talk about 'creating engagement' at all levels (federal, local health unit and community), 'consensual development' of programmes (with input from all these players), 'sharing of resources and know-how' (both vertically and horizontally), 'building networks between user organisations', and providing demonstration projects from which others can learn. However, these papers were written before the project was properly underway, so they do little more than set out the early vision. Interim results from these long-term Canadian initiatives are just emerging and are discussed further in the next section.

Box 9.5 Principles of the largely successful US agricultural extension model that linked agricultural innovation research and their application in practice.[3]

(1) *A critical mass of innovations* – there must be a body of innovations of proven effectiveness with demonstrable advantages to the user system.
(2) *A research subsystem oriented to utilisation* – a major research programme must address the application of innovations in the real world, through (a) dedicated funding streams,
(b) rewards for researchers and
(c) appointment of researchers with an interest in applied science.
(3) *A high degree of user control over the technology transfer process* – potential users of the innovations must have explicit roles in developing and selecting innovations, a key say in research priorities and a formal channel for feeding back information to the resource system on whether (and to what extent) the innovations are working in practice.
(4) *Linkages among the extension system's components* – aiming for shared concepts, language and mission.
(5) *A high degree of client contact by the extension subsystem* – as discussed in Section 5.4, the change agent is effective only if he or she orients towards the client.
(6) *A spanable social distance across each interface between components in the technology transfer system* – 'social distance' in this context refers to heterophily in levels of professionalism, formal education, technical expertise, and specialisation.
(7) *Evolution as a complete system* – rather than having the extension system grafted onto an existing research system.
(8) *A high degree of control by the technology transfer system over its environment* – so that the system can actively shape the environment rather than passively react to change.

In another Canadian study, Potvin *et al.*[426] studied the specific issue of linkage with service users. In developing a school-based diabetes prevention ('healthy lifestyle') programme targeted at indigenous Indian groups, they worked in partnership with representatives from the local community from inception of the project to its evaluation. Their methodology used an action research framework specifically adapted for involvement of lay people from vulnerable groups.[427] Implementation of the project was deemed successful despite a funding hiatus midway, and was attributed to four interrelated factors:

(1) Integration of community people with researchers as equal partners at every phase.
(2) The structural and functional integration of the intervention and evaluation components.
(3) A flexible, responsive agenda.
(4) The creation of a project that represents learning opportunities for those involved.

Although these authors placed linkage with service users at the top of their list of critical success factors, it was not easy to achieve. The process of creating and sustaining shared meanings, goals and success criteria across multiple agencies and subcultures was demanding of time, energy and diplomacy, and required the setting up of a new infrastructure:

> ... a new organisational structure was created. A supervisory committee, with representatives from the local funding agencies, was given the mandate to oversee the project in order to ensure fiscal and administrative accountability of community funds. This phase required in-depth discussions in order to bridge the differences in expectations of the community agencies used to support service delivery in an institutional context and the

reality of supervising a multifaceted intervention and research project.[426]

Chen *et al.*[428] describe a small preliminary case study from Australia of an innovation comprising a new role for the community pharmacist and an associated change in the pharmacy services offered. A number of linkage initiatives between the community pharmacists and the local GPs were planned, including an initial 'scoping' meeting to promote social interaction and provide information, as well as a series of more formal review meetings by a joint committee. The method of a systematic evaluation is described in the published paper. The study showed positive outcomes against predefined criteria, but these results were only published as part of a PhD thesis.[429] The significance of the published paper by Chen *et al.* is the detailed theoretical model linking diffusion of innovations theory with a theory of implementation via explicit linkage initiatives.

The role of intermediary agents and agencies in linkage

The systematic review by Meyers *et al.* (page 181), whose findings generally seem very relevant to our own field of enquiry, did not discuss any studies that explored intermediary roles between the 'buyers' and 'sellers' of innovations. Yet such intermediaries are increasingly common in the health service. Several authors have described intermediary roles taken by a variety of agents and agencies in relation to implementing innovation in the service sector[13,430]:

- 'Knowledge purveyors' – media and public relations; conference organisers; publishers and distributors of books, journals and reports; guideline distributors, educational organisations, who package and present the results of research to the service sector.
- Professional change agencies, agents and aides (management consultancies, voluntary sector organisations) who mediate between one 'client' (the agency who seeks to spread innovation) and another (the potential user).
- Outsourced support and training services following the sale of a piece of technology (typically, an IT system).

In other words, in a modern health service, direct links between resource system and user system are increasingly rare, and formal linkage agents increasingly common. Despite enthusiasm for such roles (see, for example, Lomas's model of the cycle of evidence generation and use illustrated in Fig. 9.2, which rests heavily on linkage activities between the different groups of stakeholders), we found almost no studies that had systematically evaluated such roles in the health care sector.

The Canadian Heart Health Project reported by Riley *et al.*[431] (see Section 9.7, page 195) identified a small but statistically significant positive effect of a central 'resource centre' funded and coordinated by a central agency that provided (among other things) written materials and a responsive consultancy support service. We could find no other empirical studies that evaluated similar initiatives, but there are theoretical reasons why such a service might enhance the success of an implementation programme for complex technology-based innovations, and we recommend further research on this.

In a high-quality study from the wider literature, Attewell undertook a case study of the diffusion of IT computing systems in large US organisations. He drew on knowledge utilisation theory (see Section 3.13, page 70), which states that the diffusion of a high-technology system requires not merely 'know-what' knowledge (what the innovation is and what it does) but also 'know-how' knowledge (how do I make it work?). Whereas know-what knowledge diffuses readily through social systems, know-how knowledge does not travel well since it is generally grounded in practical skills and experience. This sets the stage for mediating firms (or indeed, subsidiaries) to establish themselves as suppliers of the 'know-how' associated with a particular technology, to be called upon for a range of packages including troubleshooting, after-sales service, bespoke training and so on. Attewell's case study mapped the growth of such 'computer bureaux' over the past generation.

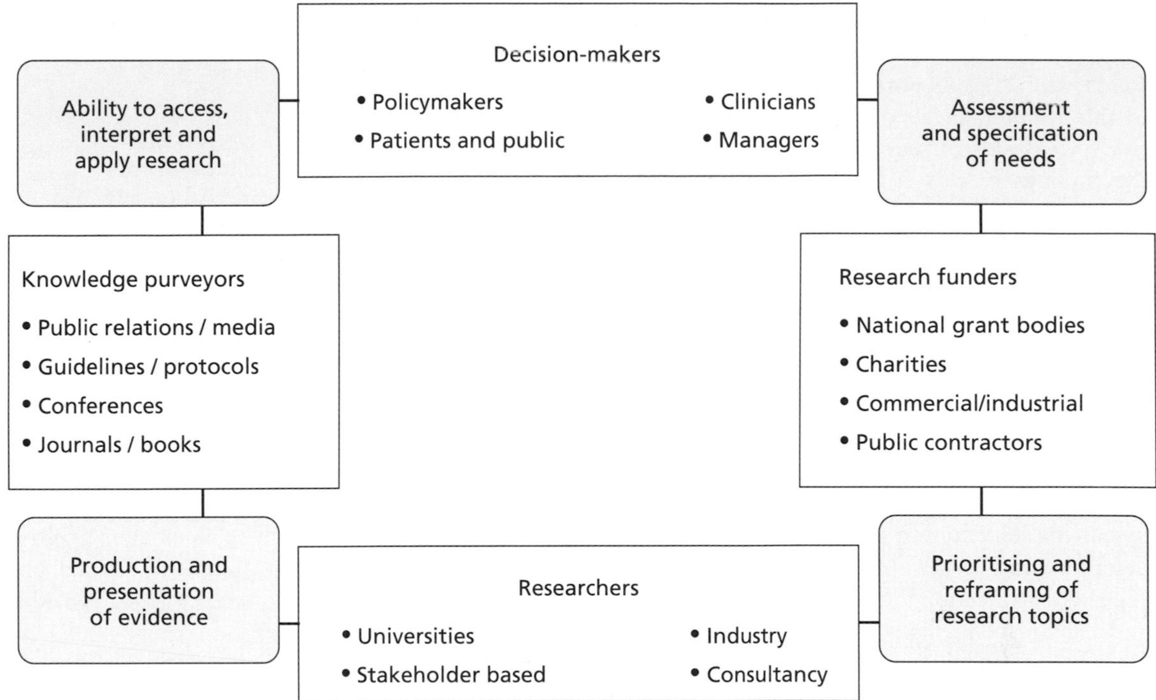

Fig. 9.2 The evidence generation and utilisation cycle, showing the critical need for linkage activities (shaded boxes) between different groups of stakeholders (adapted and reproduced with permission from Lomas[99]).

9.7 Empirical studies that have investigated 'whole-systems' approaches to implementation

As discussed in Section 3.15 (page 79), there is much to be said for addressing an implementation initiative from a whole-systems perspective – i.e. addressing the user system *and* the resource system *and* any intermediary activities *and* external links such as interorganisational networks in a coordinated programme. We found few such studies in the peer-reviewed literature, perhaps partly because 'whole-systems' approaches tend to be published in the 'grey literature'.

The Ontario Heart Health Promotion Project (comprising a total of 189 interventions on risk factor screening, courses for smoking cessation, healthy eating or physical activity, support groups to promote healthy lifestyles, environmental modification, dissemination of information) was the only recent large-scale programme identified in this review that was centrally designed around a 'whole-systems' approach. An in-depth case study of this initiative was published very recently,[215] and added to the results of a stakeholder survey published in 1998[349] and an organisational survey published in 2001.[431] These are listed in Table A.23 (page 291) in Appendix 4, and described briefly below.

In an attempt to capture a holistic picture of this programme, O'Loughlin *et al.*[349] conducted a survey to determine the perceived critical success factors in the sustainability of its different components. They interviewed key stakeholders in the programmes to ascertain which of these innovations were perceived as 'very permanent', 'somewhat permanent' and 'not permanent', and correlated these with a number of hypothesised independent variables. Independent correlates of perceived sustainability included 'intervention used no paid staff' (odds ratio 3.7), 'intervention was modified during implementation' (odds ratio 2.7), 'there was a good fit between the local provider and the intervention' (odds ratio 2.4) and 'there was the presence of a program champion' (odds ratio 2.3). As noted in the previous sections of this chapter, surveys of perceptions are a relatively weak design, but as with previous surveys, the findings of this study raise some interesting hypotheses.

Riley *et al.*[431] reported an extension of the 'Organisation SCAN' survey into the Ontario Health Health Project described above.[96] Organisation-level data were collected by surveying all 42 health departments in 1994, 1996 and 1997 with a view to explaining levels of implementation of heart health promotion activities in terms of both internal (organisational) and external factors. The data were analysed to examine relationships between implementation and four sets of possible determinants:

(1) the organisation's predisposition (motivation and commitment);
(2) its capacity (skills and resources);
(3) internal organisational (structural) factors; and
(4) external system factors (including interorganisational links and external facilitation).

The results are summarised in Box 9.6.

The same authors describe an in-depth case study of programme implementation, which used multiple methods (both qualitative and quantitative).[215] The aims of the case study were to describe and explain what they call 'the dissemination process' and what we have called implementation/institutionalisation (i.e. the development, delivery, mainstreaming and evaluation of the various heart health promotion activities provided by a total of 37 local coalitions). The factors hypothesised to influence implementation included innovation attributes (especially relative advantage over existing practice); user system capacity (what we would call 'system antecedents plus system readiness' – relevant skills and resources for systematic planning and delivery of the programmes, together with leadership and mandate) and external factors (interorganisational links, externally supported predisposing and capacity-building initiatives and contextual factors such as features of the local communities). In addition, of course, this high-profile initiative was

Box 9.6 Factors identified as critical to implementation success in the Ottawa Heart Health Promotion Project (from fieldwork by Riley *et al.*[215,431]).

Innovation development

- Synchrony of external political factors (strongly supportive of heart health) and internal mandate at a regional level for specific strategic developments in heart health.
- Change in organisational structure of regional resource agency – establishment of new section with brief to 'catalyse' innovation in this area.
- Establishment of demonstration projects and their systematic evaluation.
- Growing infrastructure for linking local public health units.

Strengthening predisposition and capacity of user systems

- Regional public health mandate.
- Responsive funding incentives for specific initiatives.
- Capacity-building funding at provincial level for increasing staffing levels, training (e.g. so staff could move from 'health education' focus to 'community development' focus), and promoting community partnerships.
- New organisational structures.
- Health promotion resource system comprising peer networks, funding incentives, training and consultation supports, and written resources.
- Major *barrier* identified at this stage was 'competing local priorities'.

Local implementation

- Five variables explained almost half the variance in implementation ($r^2 = 0.46$): organisational capacity ($\beta = 0.40$), priority given to heart health ($\beta = 0.36$), coordination of programmes ($\beta = 0.19$), use of resource centres ($\beta = 0.12$) and participation in interorganisational networks ($\beta = 0.09$). The other half of the variance remained unexplained by any factors.

Monitoring, evaluation and research

- Commitment of key political opinion leader (chief medical officer).
- External incentives (especially eligibility for research funding).
- Growing infrastructure to conduct public health research.

- Growing knowledge base and clinician interest in process evaluation.
- Early results of outcome evaluations positive (hence reinforcement of programme).

recognised as occurring within a highly positive political and fiscal climate (i.e. the 'outer context' was favourable).

The authors concluded that the findings confirmed their main hypotheses that 'dissemination' (i.e. implementation and institutionalisation in our terminology) is a lengthy, staged process that moves from defining problems to evaluating outcomes and that prior predisposing activities and concurrent capacity-building activities are essential. Riley *et al.* also highlighted:

(1) the importance of synchronous interaction between external (national and regional) incentives and mandates and internal (organisational) activity;

(2) the long lead time (around 15 years) for outcomes to appear in a complex programme such as this; and

(3) that this lead time is increased if *what* to disseminate and implement is not clear.

One critical factor linked with implementation failure in this and many other studies reviewed in this chapter was 'competing local priorities' – a finding that accords with common sense and emphasises the lack of transferability of the results of 'implementation research' that has failed to take account of local context and resources (see Box A.7, page 240, in Appendix 2). As Øvretveit[414] has commented in relation to the quality improvement literature:

> It is easier to get a promising project funded and started than it is later to make a project part of routine operations, no matter how cost-effective it is. Even if the project saves time and money in the long run, it is usually difficult to get finance to maintain it. Continuation usually requires that finance and personnel are moved from other activities to resource the project activities. Continuing activities is thus often linked to the difficulty of discontinuing activities elsewhere or switching funding.

In a non-health-care field (education), Ellsworth[432] has documented a whole-systems approach to the introduction of educational technologies in schools and universities. In a narrative overview (which we ranked as high quality) of the empirical literature from educational sociology and technology transfer, he describes a number of examples of whole-systems approaches including explicit linkage initiatives with potential users with a view to developing shared vision and shared meanings for the new technologies, strategies for gaining broad-based support across the organisation, approaches to changing organisational structure and approaches to staff development. A particular observation made by Ellsworth in his overview was the evident need to promote autonomy (the ability to make independent decisions) at every level in the organisation when implementing technology-based innovations.

The specific literature identified for this review on implementation and sustainability of health service innovations was fairly sparse and sometimes parochial, but we have alluded to a vast and disparate literature on related topic areas from which important lessons (and some new hypotheses) can be drawn. The key points from the literature reviewed in this chapter are summarised on page 175. These broad themes mask many important differences in the findings from different primary studies undertaken on different innovations in different contexts and settings with different teams. It is worth reflecting on the principles of complexity and general systems theory set out by Plsek[28] (see in particular Table 3.4, page 81), who cautions against assuming that health care organisations are largely similar and that results of an implementation study in one system will necessarily be transferable to the next, especially when presented as a list of (implicitly independent) 'factors' or 'determinants'. In reality, many of the determinants of implementation success (and of sustainability) are highly contextual and interact in a complex and often unpredictable way. The so-called 'receptive context' for successful implementation has no universal formula.

In conclusion, even when high-quality studies have demonstrated unequivocal success with a particular approach to implementation, we still cannot assume that a similar approach will work elsewhere. There remains – *and there always will remain* – a need to retranslate research and theoretical evidence into pragmatic strategies, processes and tactics that incorporate unique contextual elements of the organisation and the wider environment, and to use sensitive feedback techniques such as the rapid-cycle test-of-change approach[84,281] to capture and respond to emerging data.

Chapter 10
Case studies

Key points

1. This chapter draws together the findings from the studies presented in Chapters 4–9 into a single conceptual model, shown in Fig. 10.1 (page 201). We apply this model to four case studies on the diffusion of particular innovations in health service delivery and organisation.

2. Case studies were purposively selected to represent a range of key variables: strength of evidence for the innovation, technology dependence, source of innovation (central or peripheral), setting (primary or secondary care), sector (public or private), context (UK or international), timing (historical contemporary or under development) and main unit of implementation (individual, team or organisation).

3. In Sections 10.2–10.5 we explore four initiatives: integrated care pathways (ICPs) ('the steady success story', page 202), GP fundholding ('the clash', page 204), telemedicine ('the maverick initiative', page 206) and the electronic health record (EHR) in the UK ('the big roll-out', page 208).

4. In four summary tables, we analyse these cases in relation to characteristics of the innovation and the intended adopters (Table 10.2, page 211); aspects of communication and influence, and features of the organisations (Table 10.3, page 213); the wider environment and the implementation process (Table 10.4, page 215); and the role (if any) of external agencies (Table 10.5, page 217).

5. We conclude that the model provides a helpful framework for analysing the diffusion of organisation-level innovations in the three historical and contemporary case studies and for constructing hypotheses about the success of an ongoing initiative that is under development.

10.1 Developing and applying a unifying conceptual model

We have summarised the empirical findings relevant to this review in 'Summary Overview' (page 1). The model shown in Fig. 10.1 (page 201) attempts to depict our main findings diagrammatically and show how the different themes covered in Chapters 4–9 relate to one another. We developed the model on the basis of the many theoretical and empirical papers reviewed in earlier chapters.*

We are conscious that in presenting a one-page model of a complex reality, we risk encouraging a formulaic, 'checklist' approach in which arrows connecting different components are erroneously interpreted as simple causal relationships that can be controlled and manipulated in a predictable way. This, of course, is not the case. Nevertheless, in order to gain a theoretical understanding of innovation, spread and sustainability in organisations, we believe it is helpful to have some kind of conceptual model. We advise those who use or adapt the model to remain conscious of its inherent limitations, and we make no claims to its predictive value.

*We acknowledge one source as particularly influential in developing the notion of 'system antecedents', 'system readiness', and the influence of the innovation on moving between these.[433]

Selection of case studies

In order to test the validity of the model described previously, we sought to apply it to four case examples of the spread and sustainability of an innovation in UK service delivery and

organisation.* In the case studies that follow, we apply the model depicted in Fig. 10.1 on three levels: (1) We describe the individual components (the innovation, the adopters, the communication channels and processes through which the innovation is diffused or disseminated, the inner (organisational) context, the outer (environmental) context, the processes of implementing and institutionalising the innovation, and linkage activities with the external agencies).
(2) We highlight possible interactions between these different components.
(3) We consider the extent to which external agents and agencies can influence the structures, processes and outcomes depicted in the model.

We used a purposive sampling framework to select the four case studies (ICPs, GP fundholding, telemedicine and the EPR). The principles of purposive sampling for case studies are set out by Stake.[434] Briefly, because case studies require in-depth analysis of context and processes, there is a trade-off between representing sufficient numbers of cases and covering them in sufficient detail. As Stake comments, the transferability of case study findings to different settings is best judged via a detailed analysis of the 'rich picture' of the case itself rather than by seeking statistical inferences or conventional standards of generalisabilty. Ideally, a small number of studies should be chosen that together represent the full range of variables of interest to the researchers.

We drew up such a list and selected the cases so that each one illustrated a different combination of the following dimensions (Table 10.1, page 202):
• Evidence base for effectiveness and cost-effectiveness (strong, weak, or contested)
• Geographical (UK only vs international)
• Level of implementation (individual, team, organisational, interorganisational)
• Sector (private vs state)
• Setting (primary vs secondary care vs interface)
• Source of innovation (centralised, formal, policy driven vs decentralised, informal, locally driven)
• Technology dependence (high or low)
• Timing (historical vs contemporary vs 'under development')

Box 10.1 Key questions asked in case studies.

(1) What were the features of the innovation as perceived by the intended users (and also, separately, by top management and key decision-makers in the organisation)?
(2) What were the features of the individual adopters and the adoption/assimilation process?
(3) What was the nature of communication and influence that drove the diffusion/dissemination process?
(4) What was the nature of the inner (organisational) context and how conducive was this to the assimilation and implementation of innovations in general?
(5) What was the organisation's state of readiness for this innovation in particular?
(6) What was the nature of the outer (environmental) context and how did this impact on the assimilation process?
(7) Was the implementation and institutionalisation process (as opposed to the initial adoption process) adequately planned, resourced and managed?
(8) What were the nature, capacity and activities of any external agencies?
(9) What was the rate and extent of adoption/assimilation of the innovation, and to what extent was it sustained and developed? If these are considered as the dependent variables, to what extent do the answers to questions 1–8 explain them?

Applying the model

When constructing the case studies, we first researched the story of what happened in each of the cases from the published literature, and then asked nine questions (Box 10.1) based on our model, in order to fill out Tables 10.2–10.5:

*This case study exercise was not intended to be a piece of primary research, but a simple mapping of the different elements of the model against what was known about the different cases. Whilst its validity as 'research' is highly questionable, we believe this approach is defensible for the purposes of pilot testing the model as an interpretive schema.

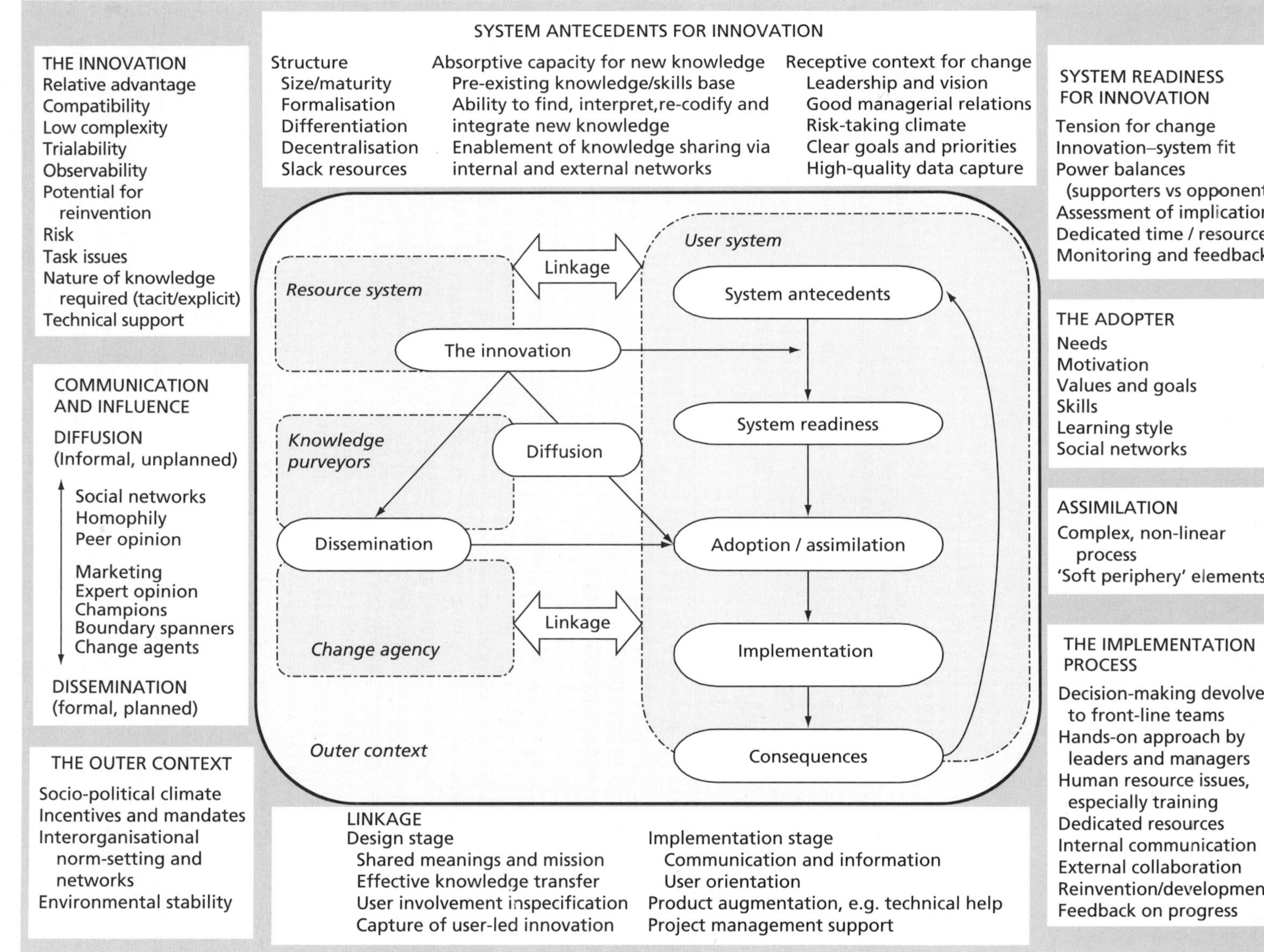

Fig. 10.1 A conceptual model for the spread and sustainability of innovations in service delivery and organisation.

Table 10.1 Criteria used to select a mix of case studies for testing the findings of this report.

Characteristic	*Integrated care pathways*	*GP fundholding*	*Telemedicine*	*Electronic patient record*
Evidence base for effectiveness and cost efficiency[a]	Potentially strong depending on the individual pathway	Contested	Moderate	Weak and contested
Geographical	International	UK	International	International
Level of implementation	Team	Organisation	Individual	Interorganisational
Sector	Private and public	Public	Mostly private	Private and public
Setting	Primary care, secondary care and primary–secondary interface	Primary care	Primary–secondary interface	Primary care, secondary care and primary–secondary interface
Source of the innovation	Decentralised	Centralised	Decentralised	Either/both
Technology dependence	Variable	Moderate to high	High	Very high
Timing	Contemporary	Historical	Contemporary (with major implications for future)	Under development

[a]This dimension maps broadly to 'relative advantage'.

10.2 Case study 1: integrated care pathways ('the steady success story')

ICPs (also known as anticipated recovery paths, case profiles, critical care paths, case maps, patient pathways, care tracks or care protocols) are predefined plans of patient care relating to a specific diagnosis or intervention, with the aim of making the management more structured, consistent and efficient.[435–437] The pathway typically incorporates standards and guidelines developed either as part of the pathway itself or (more usually) externally; it contains recommendations for particular investigations, drugs or therapies; and it includes checklists (with named roles assigned to particular tasks) and time frames. The ICP is intended to be used by staff across all professional and administrative groups to record information about care, investigation, treatment and outcome. Thus, in theory at least, important elements of care are less likely to be missed and information less likely to be mislaid.

The ICP can be useful clinically (and especially when things are suspected of 'going wrong') to gain a quick overview of the patient's history and the process of care, review progress and identify where any problems begin to occur. ICPs often have enormous potential to reduce inefficiency (e.g. double handling, unnecessary paperwork, unnecessary investigations, avoidable time delays, precipitous discharges with subsequent readmission and so on).[435] The structure of the ICP, especially if in electronic format, allows data to be collected in a standardised way (perhaps using standard codes), facilitating the production of aggregated data (e.g. for audit).

An ICP is generally developed collaboratively in a hospital trust (or occasionally, across the hospital–primary care interface) by doctors, nurses, other health professionals, administrators, technical staff and sometimes service users. Every patient is different, so it should be recognised that pathways are not prescriptive and that clinical (and administrative) judgement must also be used at every stage. However, in reality, controversy still surrounds this issue.[436,437] Some ICPs are kept 'at the end of the bed' or held by patients and the information presented in a user-friendly format, enhancing (perceived) involvement of users and carers.

It is probably self-evident that ICPs work best for patients when care and treatment is likely to follow a defined path (e.g. elective surgery in the acute setting[438,439]), and less well when there is likely to be a high degree of individualisation or variation in the course of the episode.[438–446] However, ICPs that allow for documentation (and justification) of a deviation from the pathway to suit the individual patient or a change in situation can be created. For patients with multiple pathologies, needs or uncertain diagnosis, ICPs can still (theoretically) be useful as tools or prompts that map broad processes and goals rather than outline the detail of treatment.

More sophisticated ICPs can serve as maps or algorithms to integrate and coordinate the input of different professionals and agencies to the care of service users with multiple and complex needs (e.g. children with special needs, mental health users with dual diagnosis).[435] Detailed discussion of inter-agency ICPs is again beyond the scope of this book, and little evaluative work has been published on such complex pathways, so we have not included these complex ICPs in the Tables 10.2–10.5.

Currie and Harvey[447] outline the original rationale for the introduction of pathways in different countries. In the USA, pathways were an explicit and planned response to the escalating cost of health care. In general, US insurance-based hospitals receive a negotiated fee for each patient depending solely on diagnosis, regardless of the services used or the length of stay. ICPs were introduced as a means of trying to ensure that patients would receive a standard, high-quality, but no-frills, package of care for a given diagnosis and that their length of stay would be predefined.

Oakley and Greaves[448] argue that the introduction of managed care and pathways in the UK occurred as a direct result of the restructuring of the NHS and the move towards patient-focused hospitals, clinical effectiveness and evidence-based practice. With the split between purchasers and providers that was prevalent at the time, pathways could be seen as a tool for purchasers to identify packages of care with defined outcomes. Despite the introduction of the internal market, foundation hospitals, and other 'market' style incentives, the culture of UK health care remains fundamentally different from that in the US. The *explicit* rationale for the introduction of ICPs in the UK, although connected with cost per case, has always had a strong quality/effectiveness emphasis, and there has been a strong professional call to distinguish 'rationalisation' of health care processes from 'rationing provision'.[448]

In theory, the ability of ICPs to combine process, practice and audit makes them potentially invaluable as tools to assist both clinicians and administrators (and both commissioners and providers) in meeting both quality and business objectives through cost-effective, integrated care. In practice, ICPs do not take the politics out of change management. They explicitly raise – but do not themselves answer – the difficult question of how to work effectively across professional boundaries to implement an innovation and how to reconcile (or at least, reach a compromise between) different value systems (e.g. evidence-based practice vs cost efficiency).

The effectiveness of particular ICPs (and the fascinating question of whether 'standardised' care benefits patients by making their care more evidence-based or penalises them with a 'one size fits all' approach) was beyond the scope of this review. But even without answering these important questions, we can consider ICPs as an innovation that was considered by enthusiasts to be a 'good thing' and that met relatively little resistance (although a vocal minority of opponents have described the concept as bureaucratic, unimaginative and a threat to clinical freedom).

As Tables 10.2–10.5 show, the ICP arose peripherally and spread informally via the professional networks of clinician enthusiasts. The relative advantage of well-constructed ICPs was generally apparent and uncontested. They aligned will with both professional and administrative values, and also chimed with prevailing political rhetoric about reducing variation in performance and improving efficiency and throughput. Usually, no new technology was required, and the ICPs generally fitted well with existing organisational routines. Because they were readily trialable and their impact observable, benefits were soon reaped and concerns about patients receiving 'rationed' rather than 'rationalised' care were rarely substantiated. Assimilation into hospitals was thus relatively unproblematic, helped by the fact that the innovation was resource-neutral to set up and probably resource-saving overall.

We were unable to find data on the types of organisational structure, or the prevailing cultures or climates that have supported the successful introduction of ICPs, but anecdotal evidence suggests that hospitals with a strong culture of interprofessional team working have the best track record.

ICPs are an example of an innovation that has shown steady – but not overwhelming – success. One important observation is that ICPs have not reached niche saturation, i.e. whilst there are many excellent examples of such pathways there are many more examples where they could be being used but are not. Furthermore, many poor quality ICPs are in circulation, and organisations may 'reinvent the wheel' because they are unaware of existing models that could be adapted. All this highlights the relative absence of interprofessional collaboration on ICPs, and suggests that were such collaborations to be developed and strengthened, further diffusion and greater sustainability might be achieved.

10.3 Case study 2: GP fundholding ('the clash')

We chose to look at GP fundholding because it is an innovation that came and went remarkably quickly, that was steeped in controversy from conception to demise, that had strong political overtones and that aroused (indeed, continues to arouse) strong emotions in stakeholders.*

GP fundholding can be seen historically as part of the 1991 reforms in UK health care, in which the then Conservative government introduced elements of a market allocation system into the NHS.† This internal market divided the health service – controversially – into 'providers' and 'purchasers' of health care. The purchasers, who included GP fundholders and Family Health Services Authorities (which subsequently evolved into Health Authorities and thence to Primary Care Trusts), 'bought' health care services for their patients from the providers who were the hospitals, GPs, pharmacists, dentists, opticians, community nurses and so on.[449–452]

The central idea of fundholding was that, although patients could not be given unlimited money to purchase their own health care, GPs could act as informed purchasers while keeping an eye on priorities. In this way patients and their advocates could be involved in shaping local services. GP practices who opted to become fundholders were allocated money on the basis of their historic expenditure, and in the first waves of fundholding, some regions ensured that the budgets were generous so as to 'pump prime' the new system. The fundholding budget paid for practice staff, certain hospital referrals, drug costs, community nursing services and management costs.

Fundholding GPs were both purchasers (of secondary care) and providers (of general practice care). Their provider role was not new. What was new – and again, highly controversial – was that some GPs were given budgets to purchase non-emergency health care services for their patients. The other purchasers were the Family Health Services Authorities, who purchased non-emergency secondary care for patients whose GPs were not fundholders and emergency health care for everybody. Family Health Services Authorities also purchased all primary health care. This involved contracting with GPs, dentists, pharmacists and opticians to provide, between them, the full range of primary care services.

The two stated aims of introducing fundholding in the UK (which historically came somewhat earlier than the more clinically oriented drives for EBM

*It must again be emphasised that we are not evaluating GP fundholding as such but using the case study to test a model for analysing the diffusion, assimilation and sustainability of organisation-level innovations in health services.

†When the concept of the market in the NHS was being developed, GP fundholding was not initially considered by policymakers, but it certainly aligned with this general strategy.

and clinical governance) were to promote better value for money and to improve consumer choice. Fundholders were free to choose the type, volume and location of care to be purchased, although they were obliged to indicate in their purchasing plans how they would address national policies such as the goals in the key policy documents of the day (such as the 'Health of the Nation' white paper[453] and 'The Patient's Charter'[454]). They were monitored by Family Health Services Authorities and Regional Health Authorities, whose main focus was on the financial management of the fund rather than on the actual purchasing decisions made.

It has been argued that the GP fundholding scheme was an afterthought in 1989 when the whole system of the internal market was being developed and that only subsequently did it become the forefront of the NHS reforms. In 1991 there were 720 GPs in 306 practices involved in fundholding.[455] In this initial phase, GP fundholding was limited to larger practices with over 11 000 patients, and their budgets averaged £1.3 million per practice. The minimum number of patients for a fundholding practice was later reduced first to 7000 and then to 5000. By 1994, 6% of the total NHS budget, equivalent to £1.8 billion, was being spent by fundholders. Importantly, substantial variation existed in the proportion of the local population covered by fundholders: 80% of the population was covered in well-heeled Derbyshire and Bury, but only 4% in the inner London borough of Camden and Islington.

In 1994, government ministers began to introduce a range of schemes to extend fundholding and encourage its assimilation by what might be called 'late adopting' and 'laggard' practices.[451] Individual or groups of practices with a registered population of over 5000 could opt to hold a budget to pay for specific hospital care; drugs; staffing in the practice; and community services – so-called standard fundholding. Practices with more than 3000 patients could hold a budget for community services and outpatient care only (so-called community fundholding). Practices could also opt for total purchasing, in which practices could buy any type of NHS care. Any type of fundholding practice could pool management resources with others to form a multi-fund. By April 1997, half of the population of England was covered by some system of GP fundholding. However, the change of government from Conservative to Labour in 1997 led to abandonment of the internal market and (as part of that) a rapid dismantling of the fundholding system, which ceased in 1998.

Rivett[456] has argued that the spread of GP fundholding was driven mainly by the GP initiative (i.e. GPs seeking, for honourable reasons, to improve services for their patients) and that – for the innovators in particular – it required courage, hard work and professional unpopularity with non-fundholding colleagues (who, implicitly, were less courageous and less hardworking, so had few genuine grounds for protest). According to him, it took hospital consultants a year to recognise the extent to which fundholding moved power to family doctors; then they added their voice to the opposition of other GPs. But the alternative argument was that fundholding was an innovation that played to the interests of well-resourced, well-organised suburban group practices with stable, compliant populations and relatively simple health needs (as opposed to mixed health and social needs).[457–459] Practices in inner cities, so the argument went, were often single-handed GPs working from poor premises and serving highly mobile populations with complex health and social needs. Their slow assimilation of fundholding was not because of lack of courage or laziness but because the innovation did not fit the needs of the practices or the populations they served (for whom broad-based community development, social capital and so on was presented as the way forward). Thus, somewhat unusually, both 'sides' laid claim to the moral high ground.

One of the most hotly contested issues was the amount of money that changed hands, and how it was spent. By the end of the second year of fundholding, fundholders had underspent by £31.7 million (3.6% of the budget allocated), of which £2.8 million was voluntarily returned to Regional Health Authorities by fundholders and the rest used in various schemes to 'improve services'. Against this, non-fundholders had overspent by £9.8 million in the same year. By 1995 the total underspend on fundholding budgets was estimated to be £120 million. Whether fundholders used their savings efficiently and appropriately is a controversy that is unlikely to be ever resolved. In a recent survey by the National Audit Office, fundholders reported using savings to buy equipment for their practices and the local hospital, to improve practice premises and information systems and to employ extra staff to provide services in house. Whilst many of these initiatives had clear benefits for patients, the controversy is whether they represented better value for money than what Health Authorities might otherwise have used the funds for, and whether it was appropriate for public funds to be spent on improving practice premises owned by the GPs themselves, who would benefit personally when the premises were sold.

Fundholding is an excellent example of an innovation whose relative advantage was perceived very differently by different players, which proved incompatible with certain value systems, for which some potential adopters had a good existing knowledge and skill base (e.g. in accounting) while others did not, where 'innovation–system fit' was highly variable across potential adopter organisations, and whose knock-on consequences were difficult to isolate or measure. It is also a good example of a centrally driven innovation that rose and fell with the prevailing political climate. Early adopters – who were probably highly homophilous with the change agents (and often shared their political persuasion) – were publicly groomed, supported and rewarded, but the strategy for dealing with later adopters and non-adopters was less well thought-out. The (alleged) wave-on-wave reduction in per capita fundholding budgets, for example, was widely publicised and interpreted as 'moving the goalposts', and the scheme began to lose credibility. As discussed above, fundholding was a unique innovation in that both adopters and non-adopters justified their arguments in moral terms, locking horns publicly over underpinning values. The lack of a formal pilot phase or rigorous evaluation programme means that this historical example will always remain controversial.[449,459]

10.4 Case study 3: telemedicine ('the maverick initiative')

We chose to look at telemedicine as one of our case studies because – almost uniquely for a complex health service innovation – it has been formally addressed from the classical 'diffusion of innovations' perspective in a number of empirical studies and theoretical papers,[460–465] because it tends to be introduced by individual enthusiasts rather than organisation-wide, and because it raises particular issues around sustainability.

Telemedicine is 'the use of telecommunications technology to provide medical information and services'.[461,465] Use of telecommunications technology to facilitate health care delivery has evolved over nearly four decades, beginning with pioneer programmes such as telepsychiatry consultations and teleradiology in the late 1950s. Telemedicine, with varying degrees of success, has subsequently been applied to a wide array of medical specialty areas including radiology, pathology, psychiatry, cardiology, neurology and neurosurgery.

Telemedicine is conventionally considered on three levels, dependent on the technology and infrastructure available as described in Box 10.2.

The benefits claimed to the patient from telemedicine include[460,461,463–467,*]:

- The patient enjoys rapid access to secondary and tertiary health care services and can gain the benefits of 'expert' care while maintaining continuity of care from the GP or local specialist.
- The patient is able to remain close to home, where family, friends and primary care team can provide support.

Box 10.2 Levels of telemedicine.

Level 1	Use of the telephone and fax technology for patient consultation and referrals
Level 2	File transfers for interactive still images, store and forward images or videoconferencing over low band width connections
Level 3	Full-motion video images that permit a full range of interactive diagnostic services

*As with previous case studies, it is beyond the scope this review to evaluate the validity of these claims; we are merely setting out the perspectives of the purveyors and enthusiasts for the innovation.

- Costly and traumatic patient transfers between hospitals are generally avoided (and when transfer is unavoidable, the receiving hospital can coordinate the preparation and transfer of the patient).
- Remote, underserved and possibly low-income areas can access specialty services – hence the 'inequality gap' is narrowed.
- Patient-borne costs (e.g. travel) are reduced.

The benefits claimed to practitioners include:

- Non-specialists have access to real-time consultations with experts.
- The transfer of knowledge between participants (notably GP and specialist) is mutually educational and richer than the equivalent exchange through outpatient letter or discharge summary (and occurs without taking time away from practice).
- Builds professional networks and allows collegial support.
- Potentially shifts power base of decision-making, allowing (for example) GPs to directly manage the care of their patients with support from specialists, rather than vice versa.

Historically, access concerns have driven much of the work to develop clinical telemedicine. Early applications often focused on remote populations scattered across mountainous areas, islands, open plains and Arctic regions where medical specialists and some times primary care practitioners were not easily reached. Dispiritingly, most telemedicine projects from the 1960s through the early 1980s failed to survive beyond the end of grant funding or trial financing. Telecommunications costs tended to be high, and the technologies were awkward to use and technically unreliable – especially in the early years. Few projects appeared to be guided by a business plan or an appreciation of the project features and results necessary for a sustainable program.[465]

More recently, telemedicine has been undergoing a resurgence driven by several factors. These include economic pressures to contain the rapid growth of health care expenditures, the increasing emphasis on fair resource allocation, the socio-political desire for decentralised and locally adjusted access to health care, rising demand and expectation for 'quality' health care (and hence for an expert opinion) and the availability of major research funding streams for e-health (including national and global information infrastructures and e-health collaborative activities).[461,462,468]

Another important reason for telemedicine's resurgence despite initial failures is that significant advances and development have been accomplished in both medical technology and IT. The pictorial archiving communication systems and advanced medical imaging systems such as computer tomography and magnetic resonance imaging are examples of exciting breakthroughs that were simply not available in the early years of telemedicine.[461,468,469] Teleconferencing and high-performance communication networks represent additional critical advances in the field.[469] These advances, along with the steady fall in price/performance ratio[308] have contributed crucially to the improved relative advantage of the innovation.

Enthusiasts say that the goal of telemedicine is to 'marry medicine with technology', capitalising on the advantages of technology to produce a robust system that 'reaches the parts other services do not reach', thereby delivering an enhanced service at an affordable price. Sceptics argue that face-to-face contact is fundamental to health care and that telemedicine can never be as good as the 'real thing', and that expansion of services is often driven more by doctors who are technology enthusiasts than by those genuinely seeking to expand services and redress inequalities.

Like all technology-based innovations, telemedicine should be thought of not as a piece of hardware but as a complex process between human actors that is supported by technology. This process has become much more feasible in the past few years as a result of technological advances and continuing cost reductions. It is also increasingly trialable, and clinicians who would not describe themselves as 'technical' are beginning to try it out. The evidence base for the overall effectiveness and cost-effectiveness of telemedicine remains contested,[464,469,470] but well worked up examples of particular initiatives that have shown clear benefit are now available in the literature.

The widespread adoption and assimilation of telemedicine could potentially have significant impacts on health care delivery systems as well as on intra- and interorganisational structures of health care organisations. In other words, if telemedicine were to 'take off' and reach anything approaching niche saturation, health care would look very different, since it threatens much of the structures and cultures underpinning and surrounding medical specialisation (e.g. the notion that a medical or surgical specialty develops in a particular area because there exists a sufficient regional population base to supply the service with clients).

Despite telemedicine's recent surge in growth, obstacles to its widespread use persist. For example, although many groups are working to develop hardware and software standards, it remains frustrating and difficult to put together systems in which the components operate predictably and smoothly, work in different settings without extensive adaptation and accommodate replacement components. Technical systems often remain poorly adapted to the human infrastructure of health care, i.e. the work environment, needs, and preferences of clinicians, patients, and other decision-makers. Moreover, sustainable telemedicine programmes require attention to organisational business objectives and strategic plans that is not always evident in current applications.

We have called telemedicine 'the maverick initiative' because the typical scenario is of a small team of enthusiasts setting up the service, often dedicating considerable time and personal resources to it, driven mainly by their own interest in the technology (and sometimes in the clinical relationships that it supports). But as Tables 10.2–10.5 show, a number of factors combine to conspire against its wider diffusion. As mentioned above, the technology is often fiddly and unreliable, and in most specialties there is remarkable little evidence for any clinical advantage of telemedicine over old-fashioned referrals (and almost no evidence of cost advantages). Furthermore, the innovator who introduces a telemedicine project (often on a research grant or short-term project funding) generally lacks the skills or interest to 'mainstream' the initiative within his or her organisation. The story of telemedicine at the organisational level has generally been one of 'boom and bust' as champions and short-term funding streams come and go (and, of course, whereas the 'boom' stories are often written up, the 'bust' stories rarely reach publication).

Times are changing, however. As Tables 10.2–10.5 show, several factors have recently come together to swing the risk–benefit equation much more in telemedicine's favour – most notably the development of more user-friendly technology, the fall in its price/performance ratio, and the increasing recognition by IT companies of the need for dialogue with the client both during initial development of the software and during implementation, allowing both a customised and an augmented product better tailored to the needs and skills base of the user.[461,468] Telemedicine is thus entering an interesting phase, and it is possible that its fortunes thus far (relatively poor spread and low sustainability) may at some stage be reversed.

10.5 Case study 4: the electronic health record ('the big roll-out')

In a health care system where sectors are highly differentiated and referral between them is a central feature, no single institution can hope to encompass a patient's entire health history. As we all know, patients' health care records are currently fragmented across multiple sites and sectors, posing obstacles to clinical care, administration, research and public health initiatives. EHRs and the Internet provide a technical infrastructure on which to build integrated, longitudinal medical records that can follow the patient to different locations, encounters and sectors.[471] The UK NHS Information Strategy offers the concept of levels of computerised record as well as two different varieties[472]:

• The EPR (electronic patient record) describes the record of the periodic care provided mainly by one institution (generally an acute hospital). Separate EPRs may also be held by other health care providers, for example, specialist units or mental health trusts.

• The EHR describes the concept of a longitudinal record of patient's health and health care – from 'cradle to grave' and across geographical, organisational and sectoral boundaries. It includes both information on primary health care contacts as well as subsets of information associated with the outcomes of periodic care held in the EPRs.

Although an integrated, electronic, 'cradle to grave' record is an appealing and (in some ways) conceptually simple notion, its implementation-in-use is highly complex and contentious, requiring new routines for individuals (most obviously, the systematic and consistent coding of information that was previously entered as free text) and a host of new systems for interpersonal, interdepartmental and interorganisational interaction. Weir *et al.* undertook a survey-based study of the impediments and facilitators to implementing the EHR. They identified multiple and diverse perceived impediments and critical success factors, which operated at every level from individual to interorganisational. They concluded that the application of the EHR 'involves multi-level changes in the whole system of care, from physicians' attitudes to interdepartmental relations'.[473]

Sicotte *et al.*[324,325] undertook an in-depth case study of a large initiative to implement an EHR system across four Canadian hospitals in the late 1980s in collaboration with two computer companies. The project aimed to 'make a paperless hospital a reality' by automating processes previously dependent on human labour, make record-keeping more structured and standardised, achieve 'spacelessness', avoid duplication of tasks, inform planning and aid later aggregation of data for audit purposes. But the entire system had to be withdrawn when both medical and nursing personnel boycotted its use. The main problems identified in this qualitative study were an increase (rather than the anticipated decrease) in routine clerical work, information overload, rigidity of work organisation and the negation of expert autonomy. The authors also observed that the mission to 'go paperless' became an end in itself rather than a means to improving communication and efficiency, and that staff focused on the output of putting data on the computer rather than what happened to the data once they were entered.

Another key observation made by Sicotte *et al.* was that the implementation of this complex technology was conspicuously removed from real-life medical and nursing practice. They comment:

> The project team attempted to identify the nature of the information from an idealized point of view rather than work closely with the delivery process. In this manner, the computerised patient record information architecture was inspired from the perspective of how nursing is taught and promoted in academic institutions and professional corporations rather than from the work site where nursing is truly practiced. A more comprehensive and integrated approach is needed to better understand the potential and limits of the IT, the constraints of nursing work, and how closely related these two aspects must be.[325]

This and other case studies in the literature suggest that widespread introduction of EHRs can turn out to be an expensive disaster. In the private sector, sharing data with 'competitor' institutions may be seen as commercially unviable.[474,475] Furthermore, concerns about confidentially and data protection have yet to be resolved (these are chiefly to do with the logistics of gaining consent rather than the fact that such consent is likely to be withheld[476–478]). Decisions about the structure and ownership of electronic records will have a profound impact on the health care system, as well as on the accessibility and privacy of patient information. Many of the technical challenges mentioned above in relation to telemedicine (as well as many of the potential advantages) also apply to the EHR.[474,475,479]

Despite all these unresolved issues, the palpable anxiety around electronic records amongst NHS staff, and major differences between potential users in level of appropriate knowledge and skills,[475,479] the NHS Executive has mapped out a detailed, three-phase programme for implementation with what some have described as a punishing schedule of milestones. Box 10.3 shows the milestones set out in 'Implementation for Health' for the EPR and EHR. The strong external mandate for the roll-out of the EHR will probably create predisposition in user organisations but will not in itself increase their capacity to deliver (see Section 9.4, page 186, for further discussion of this point).

As Tables 10.2–10.4 show, the 'big roll-out' of the EHR has considerable promise, and certain aspects of the programme so far are commendable (e.g. extensive consultation with pilot users of the record; major capacity-building initiatives focusing particularly on parts of the system with low absorptive capacity such as single-handed GPs; and material and financial incentives (such as free or cut-price computers). However, many major concerns remain – such as the functionality of the record (where will the 'soft' information go?), the pace at which the dissemination programme is being driven, the relative lack of piloting amongst users who are likely to have the most problems, the lack of detail on the level of outreach training and the 'after-sales service' to be provided and so on.

Overall, because of the extremely high complexity, questionable relative advantage and low ease of use of this innovation, its critical dependence on simultaneous adoption by multiple users, and the low absorptive capacity of so many parts of the system despite recent capacity-building input, we are not optimistic that it will spread and be sustained without major problems.

Box 10.3 Milestones for EPR and EHR implementation in England and Wales.[472]

1998–2000 (Phase 1)	Connecting all computerised GP practices to NHSnet Completing the national NHS email project Establishing local Health Informatics Services Completion of cancer information strategy
2000–02 (Phase 2)	35% of all acute hospitals to have implemented a Level 3 EPR Substantial progress in implementing integrated primary care and community EPRs in 25% of Health Authorities Use of NHSnet for appointment booking, referrals, radiology and laboratory requests/results in all parts of the country. A National Electronic Library for Health accessible through local litranets in all NHS organisations. Beacon EHR sites have an initial first generation EHR in operation.
By 2005 (Phase 3)	Full implementation at primary care level of first-generation person-based EHRs. All acute hospitals with Level 3 EPRs 24-h emergency care access to patient records

10.6 Conclusion

Overall, we were pleased with the ability of this preliminary model to prompt questions and reflections about the four innovations described in Section 10.1. We believe that it allows us to explain the different fortunes of these very different innovations.* We have also tentatively used the model to predict what might happen to the innovations in the future:

- ICPs will continue to spread slowly but may not reach niche saturation without more explicit interorganisational collaboration.
- An initiative comparable to GP fundholding should pay less attention to homophilous early adopters and more to developing shared meanings and value systems with heterophilous sceptics.
- Telemedicine (which has had a relatively disappointing history in terms of diffusion and sustainability so far) may have increased success now that the technology is more feasible, trialable, and easy to use.
- The national UK initiative to establish an EHR has done impressive groundwork but may prove a uniquely difficult challenge because of the extreme complexity (especially implementation complexity) of the innovation, the low receptive context of many intended adopters and the authoritative nature of the adoption decision.

*A recently published review on diffusion of innovations aimed at changing individual clinician behaviour, not available when we were developing our model, is highly consistent with our own findings, model and recommendations.[481]

Table 10.2 Innovation attributes and adoption in the four case studies.

	Integrated care pathways	*GP fundholding*	*Telemedicine*	*Electronic health record*
The innovation				
Key attributes of the innovation as perceived by intended user:				
(a) relative advantage;	(a) Relative advantage is potentially high.	(a) Relative advantage contested (see text).	(a) Relative advantage high in certain contexts, e.g. remote areas.	(a) Relative advantage potentially high but only if technical and practical barriers can be overcome (i.e. if it can be made to work well).
(b) Compatibility;	(b) Compatible with many professional values (e.g. evidence-based practice) *and* administrative ones (efficiency).	(b) Compatible with the values of some (innovative, business-driven) but not with traditional 'family doctor' ethos.	(b) Incompatible with traditional clinical values.	(b) Compatible with values of most but not all clinicians.
(c) complexity;	(c) Complex to develop because of multi-disciplinary input, but relatively simple thereafter.	(c) Complex.	(c and d) Initially complex and not easily trialable, but increasingly simple to use and trialable on a limited basis.	(c) Extremely complex.
(d) trialability;	(d and e) Highly trialable and observable.	(d) Not easily trialable.		(d) Not easily trialable.
(e) observability;		(e) Observable but many confounding influences.	(e) Impact highly observable.	(e) Impact readily observable.
(f) reinvention.	(f) High reinvention potential.	(f) Low reinvention potential.	(f) Moderate potential for reinvention.	(f) Moderate potential for reinvention.
Key operational attributes:				
(a) relevance to task;	(a–c) A good ICP will have high task relevance and usefulness, and will be feasible.	(a–b) Relevance and usefulness was contested ('improving services' vs 'paperwork').	(a–c) Task relevance, usefulness and feasibility vary depending on context, hence has 'taken off' in some fields more than in others.	(a–b) Potentially high task relevance and usefulness, but concerns about how to capture all health issues in computer codes.
(b) usefulness for task;				
(c) feasibility;		(c) Variable feasibility.		(c) Questionable feasibility.
(d) implementation complexity;	(d) May be very complex to implement initially.	(d) Very high implementation complexity.	(d) Implementation complexity high but getting lower.	(d) High implementation complexity.

Continued

Table 10.2 continued: Innovation attributes and adoption in the four case studies.

	Integrated care pathways	*GP fundholding*	*Telemedicine*	*Electronic health record*
(e) divisibility into components;	(e) Possibly divisible.	(e) Not initially divisible (but see text).	(e) Increasingly divisible.	(e) Possibly divisible.
(f) nature of knowledge needed.	(f) Knowledge generally highly codifiable and therefore transferable.	(f) Knowledge mostly highly codifiable and transferable.	(f) Knowledge moderately codifiable.	(f) High degree of tacit knowledge.
Adoption and assimilation				
Who are the potential adopters and what are their characteristics and needs?	Broad range of clinicians and administrators with widely differing needs and expectations.	Adopters – generally well-resourced, suburban group practices. Non-adopters – inner city, single-handed.	Adopters – technology enthusiasts plus remote practitioners. These two groups have very different needs.	Requires simultaneous adoption by several groups (clinicians, patients, administrators) across all sectors.
What is the meaning of the innovation to intended adopters?	For most, a way of improving and systematising patient care. For a minority, 'paperwork', 'interference'.	*Either* 'opportunity to improve services' *or* 'shifting administration' *or* 'two-tier system'.	Generally, seen as a means of improving efficiency and choice. Some see it as a superfluous gadget.	To some, a tool for efficiency and consistency of record-keeping. To a few, an imposition by 'Big Brother'.
What is the nature of the adoption decision (see page 105)?	Usually collective, although may be authoritative.	Collective within each practice (contingent on practice size).	Usually optional but contingent on service being available.	Currently, collective and contingent. Potentially authoritative.
What are the concerns of adopters at				
(a) pre-adoption stage;	(a) Will the pathway be evidence based? Will it make work (or save work) for me? Will it powerful interest groups impose their views?	(a) What is fundholding? What are the costs and benefits, especially personal workload and income? Do we have the capacity and skills?	(a) Can I make the technology work? Will the consultation lose richness at a distance? Will patients accept it? What will it cost?	(a) What does the EHR look like and how do I fill my bits in? Will I be able to acquire the necessary technical skills? Will patients accept it?
(b) early use stage;	(b) How can I overcome logistical barriers?	(b) How can we operationalise the purchasing process?	(b) Technology and logistical issues.	(b) Technology and logistical issues.
(c) experienced user stage, and to what extent are they met?	(c) How can we improve this ICP? Can we share with others?	(c) Can we set up a multi-fund?	(c) Can we extend the service to other specialties? Business spin-offs?	(c) Can we improve the EHR? What research can we do on the data?
Typical pattern of the assimilation process in organisations.	Usually relatively straightforward, perhaps because no 'budget line' or new equipment needed.	'Staged' model often followed with evaluation, planning, implementation, etc.	Typically, beset by shocks	Assumed 'staged' model driven by

Table 10.3 Communication and influence, and the inner context, in the four case studies.

	Integrated care pathways	*GP fundholding*	*Telemedicine*	*Electronic health record*
Diffusion and dissemination				
What is the nature of the networks through which influence about the innovation is likely to diffuse?	Innovations generally arise spontaneously at the local level and spread via informal, horizontal networks of professionals.	Fundholding spread partly by geographical proximity and also across homophilous groups, e.g. via National Association of Fundholders.	Two main mechanisms for spread: professional networks (technical special interest groups) and (once established) local spread via interpersonal influence.	A centrally driven, research-based innovation that is being spread mainly via vertical networks.
Who are the main agents of social influence and what are they doing?	Expert opinion leaders – mainly academics and quality improvement experts. Range of local champions.	Peer opinion leaders (practices with high social status).	Potentially, expert and peer opinion leaders, although sometimes no such individuals can be identified.	Peer opinion leaders, although many such 'early adopters' are not seen as typical and do not lead opinion.
The inner context				
What are the key structural features of the organisation? (a) size/maturity; (b) complexity/differentiation; (c) decentralisation; (d) slack resources.	ICPs have generally been adopted in hospital trusts with established 'multi-disciplinary team' structures. No data on slack resources.	Large size was a prerequisite for fundholding status. Slack resources were provided to early waves of fundholders but not to later waves, leading to resentment.	In the past, successful telemedicine projects have tended to occur in very large trusts involving groups of hospitals. As the capital cost of setting up telemedicine falls, size and slack may become less critical.	Not yet clear how size or other structural features will influence assimilation of EHR. The size of the NHS as a whole (and hence the massive scope of the project) has been mooted as a major barrier.
What is the organisation's absorptive capacity for this type of knowledge? (a) skill mix; (b) knowledge base; (c) transferable know-how; (d) ability to evaluate the innovation.	In general, a reasonably well run district general hospital would have the capacity to assimilate and adapt an ICP (i.e. the level of specialist knowledge, skills and know-how is relatively low).	Fundholding required a high level of business skills and also high clinical knowledge for purchasing. (when Primary Care Trusts were introduced, fundholders' knowledge base proved highly transferable).	Until recently, telemedicine required special hardware and internal technical knowledge). More recently, telemedicine consultations have become possible using largely 'ordinary' desktop equipment.	Absorptive capacity likely to be a major barrier for many organisations. NHS has recognised this and is funding an extensive capacity-building programme.

Continued

Table 10.3 continued: Communication and influence, and the inner context, in the four case studies.

	Integrated care pathways	*GP fundholding*	*Telemedicine*	*Electronic health record*
What is the organisation's receptive context for this type of change? (a) leadership and vision; (b) values and goals; (c) Risk-taking climate; (d) Internal and external networks?	No formal data but anecdotal reports suggest that it was the innovative, risk-taking hospitals who first tired out ICPs, and that these initiatives were led by pioneer clinicians who were widely networked externally.	No formal data. Fundholding practices tended to have an entrepreneurial and very businesslike culture. Some non-fundholders had a good receptive context but were unmotivated to adopt fundholding.	Data from several US case studies suggests a strong link between change-oriented culture and climate and successful telemedicine initiatives.[461,465,480]	Not yet clear. The prediction based on our model is that organisations with strong leadership, clear strategic goals, good managerial relations and a risk-taking climate will implement readily.
What is the organisation's readiness for this specific innovation? (a) organisational fit; (b) assessment of implications; (c) dedicated time/resources; (d) broad-based support.	In general, ICPs have been embraced enthusiastically and given appropriate support from top management (perhaps because relative advantage is clear to most players and cost is fairly low).	Readiness was formally developed and assessed during a shadow year. Dedicated resources were supplied. A minority of practices lacked consensus on readiness and many were unanimously opposed.	Several detailed case studies in the literature suggest that organisations that were enthusiastic but lacked specific readiness were able to adopt, but not sustain, telemedicine projects.[462,465]	Few NHS organisations would currently describe themselves as 'ready' for the EHR. Main barriers probably lack of organisational fit and low assessment of implications, although few hard data exist

Table 10.4 The outer context, and the implementation process, in the four case studies.

	Integrated care pathways	*GP fundholding*	*Telemedicine*	*Electronic health record*
The outer context				
What is the nature and influence of the socio-political climate?	Positive climate towards multi-disciplinary working, reducing variation in care, reducing waiting times, and increasing accountability, effectiveness and efficiency	Strongly in favour at inception; changed to strongly opposed with 1997 change of government	Until recently, not especially favourable but e-health now seen as a research priority and a means of improving accessibility and reducing inequalities	Currently, strongly positive in favour of EHR but there is also a strong civil liberties lobby opposing compulsory use of EHR
Are there any external Incentives and mandates?	No	There were many incentives at the outset ('first wave' fundholders) but these controversially diminished in successive waves	Not currently	Yes – see Box 10.3.
What are the prevailing norms from other comparable ('opinion leader') organisations?	ICPs increasingly seen as a 'good idea' but pressure from peer organisations not especially strong	Two opposing and powerful 'bandwagons' that became increasingly politicised – National Association of Fundholders, and various formal and informal networks who were ideologically opposed to fundholding	Interorganisational norms not especially strong, perhaps because telemedicine still generally arises in a somewhat ad hoc way and is driven through by individual champions rather than via organisation-wide policy	There is a growing interest in systems that have been shown to work (e.g. examples from other countries); whilst the interorganisational pressure to adopt the EHR is not yet strongly positive, this may well change in the near future
Implementation and institutionalisation				
What are the features of the implementation process in terms of (a) human resources; (b) involvement of key staff; (c) project management	In general, implementation of ICPs (a) requires no new roles or staffing; (b) requires and presupposes widespread staff involvement; (c) is inherently a project management initiative	Fundholding practices were generally characterised by (a) good human resources and HR practices and (b) A minority of practice staff felt the innovation was imposed on them (c) good project management skills.	This innovation can (and often is) implemented by individuals or groups of interested clinicians and only subsequently extended throughout the organisation; some never go beyond the 'maverick' stage.	Not yet established in most organisations; HR and project management issues are considered by some to be a major potential barrier to the success of this initiative in some organisations

Continued

Table 10.4 continued: The outer context, and the implementation process, in the four case studies.

	Integrated care pathways	*GP fundholding*	*Telemedicine*	*Electronic health record*
What measures are in place to capture and respond to the consequences of the innovation (e.g. audit and feedback)?	In general, the collection and analysis of audit data (or at least the facility to do so) are built into the ICP	Tight financial accounting and audit was a requirement of the system. Alleged knock-on consequences for patients of non-fundholders were not systematically measured	Variable approaches to audit and feedback; some projects at least lack a systematic approach to this, but others collect good data and use it systematically to improve services.	Not yet established.
What measures enable organisations to develop, adapt and reinvent the innovation (e.g. interorganisational networks and collaboratives)?	A weakness of ICP spread is that there are few well-developed networks, so development occurs slowly and in an ad hoc way	Strong collaborative support and knowledge sharing occurred (a) geographical localities and (b) through national associations	No formal collaboratives. Interested professionals can join a variety of networks (e.g. academic mailing lists and conferences)	Not yet established, but various pilot projects underway led by the NHS Information Authority

Table 10.5 The role of external agencies in the four case studies.

	Integrated care pathways	*GP fundholding*	*Telemedicine*	*Electronic patient record*
The role of external agencies				
Are the developers linked with potential users of the innovation at the development stage, and do they share value systems, language and meanings?	Not usually developed centrally	The extent to which potential users of fundholding were involved in its design is contested	Often good linkage between IT companies and telemedicine innovators, allowing modification of systems as they are developed	Some 'sentinel' sites work with developers but these may not be representative of all future users
What is the capacity and role of the external change agency (if any) to help organisations with operational aspects of assimilation?	No central change agency officially devoted to this innovation but National Electronic Library for Health is building a resource bank of downloadable ICPs	High-quality, flexible and responsive 'outreach' support was provided by local family health services authorities for practices in early stages of fundholding	No central change agency	Yet to be fully defined but it is already recognised that an 'outreach' support role will be needed
Who are the main external change agents and do they show (a) homophily; (b) positive relationships and client centeredness; (c) shared language and meaning	No external change agents; spread is by the professional networks of internal champions	External agents tended to have a formal political role. (a-c) High level of homophily, positive relationships and shared meaning with early adopters of fundholding but none of these with non-adopters.	No external change agents; spread is by the professional networks and interest groups of individual adopters	Yet to be fully defined but there is a danger that those selected for this role will be IT enthusiasts and lack sufficient homophily and credibility with the rank and file

Continued

Table 10.5 continued: The role of external agencies in the four case studies.

	Integrated care pathways	*GP fundholding*	*Telemedicine*	*Electronic patient record*
Does the dissemination programme follow social marketing principles (a) audience segmentation; (b) assessment of target group needs and perspective; (c) appropriate message and marketing channels; (d) good programme management; (e) process evaluation	No formal dissemination programme	The 'marketing' of fundholding was highly controversial and widely believed to have been inappropriately politicised	No formal dissemination programme	Yet to be fully defined, but because this is a centrally driven, compulsory initiative the main vehicle for spread will be formal, vertical channels (e.g. executive letters, NHS Information Strategy)
What is the nature and quality of any linkage relationship between the change agency and the intended adopter organisations?	NA	Main change agencies were local family health services authorities who enjoyed strong pre-existing links and high degree of shared language and meaning with fundholders	NA	'Performance management' approach rather than informal linkage, relationship building and sense-making activities; this may create resentment and resistance

Chapter 11
Discussion

Key points

1. This chapter considers the key findings from the systematic review, and discusses the different elements of the model introduced in Chapter 10 (see page 199). In Section 11.1, we discuss the complex and multifaceted nature of diffusion and implementation in relation to innovations in health service delivery and organisation and warn against an oversimplistic, deterministic interpretation of the available evidence.

2. In Section 11.2 (page 220), we provide some advice for applying the model in a service context. We note that because of the highly contextual and contingent nature of the diffusion process, it is not possible to make formulaic, universally applicable recommendations for practice and policy. Rather, we recommend a structured, two-stage process to guide reflection and action. In the first stage, the components of the model (attributes of the innovation, characteristics of intended adopters, potential agents of social influence, characteristics of the organisation, characteristics of the environment, nature of dissemination programme, nature of implementation programme) should be considered against the empirical evidence base presented in this book. In the second stage, we recommend a more pragmatic approach in which the complex interaction between these variables is considered in relation to a specific local context and setting.

3. In Section 11.3 (page 225), we suggest some potentially fruitful avenues for future research, which we divide into research that focuses on the separate components of the model and research that takes a 'whole-systems' approach and the dynamic interaction between components. We recommend further secondary research into areas that were beyond the scope of this review, notably into the largely untapped literature from cognitive psychology. In terms of whole-systems approaches, we recommend more studies that are explicitly applied in nature, which draw on multi-disciplinary research expertise and seek to develop and extend theoretical approaches to evaluative implementation research.

4. Throughout this chapter, we flag up a number of areas where further research is *not* needed, either because existing studies have already answered key questions or because the questions themselves have become obsolete.

11.1 Overview and commentary on main findings

This review has attempted to combine a large and diverse literature into a unifying model of diffusion of innovations in health care organisations. Our methods, described in Chapter 2 (page 32), were systematic and independently verifiable. However, the literature was vast and complex; our approach was emergent and somewhat unconventional; and many subjective judgements and serendipitous discoveries were involved. A different group of researchers setting out to answer the same research question would inevitably have identified a different set of primary sources and made different judgements about their quality and relevance. Their synthesis might have produced a different unifying model. This is, arguably, an inherent characteristic of any systematic review that addresses complex interventions and seeks to unpack the nuances of their implementation in different social, organisational or environmental contexts. In this respect, meta-narrative review can be thought of as a particular application of realist review, in which the interpretive judgements of the reviewer are integral to the synthesis process and can never be fully rationalised or standardised.[149,173] The findings presented here, and especially the model in Fig. 10.1, should therefore be seen as 'illuminating the problem and raising areas to consider' rather than 'providing definitive answers'.

Our review has affirmed many well-described themes in the literature – such as the useful list of innovation attributes that predict (but do not guarantee) successful adoption; the critical importance of social influence and the networks through which it operates; the complex and contingent nature of the adoption process; the characteristics (both 'hard' and 'soft') of organisations that encourage and inhibit innovation; and the messy, stop-start, and difficult-to-research process of assimilation and institutionalisation. We have also exposed some demons in this literature – such as the lack of empirical evidence for the widely cited 'adopter traits'; the focus on innovations that arise centrally and are disseminated through official channels at the expense of those that arise peripherally and spread informally; the limited generalisability of the empirical work on product-based innovation in companies to process innovation in service organisations; and the virtual absence of studies that focused primarily on the sustainability of complex service innovations.

The components of this model do not, of course, represent a comprehensive list of the determinants of organisational innovativeness and successful assimilation. They are simply the areas in which research has been undertaken and positive findings published. Conspicuously absent from most empirical work in the service sector, for example, is the important issue of internal politics (e.g. doctor–manager power balances), which was identified as one of several critical influences in a single qualitative study.[64] Our own team, in a previous evaluation of five projects to implement complex service innovations in primary health care, found that power relations (especially between a project steering group and the main project worker) were critical to successful implementation, but that they were extremely difficult to explore systematically and raised ethical issues for the research team.[87]

A striking finding of this extensive review was the tiny proportion of empirical studies that acknowledged, let alone explicitly set out to study, the complexities involved in spreading and sustaining innovation in service organisations. Most studies focused on a limited number of the components depicted in our model, and failed to take due account of their different interactions and contextual and contingent features. This, of course, is an inherent limitation of any experimental or quasi-experimental research – the shifting baseline of context and the multiplicity of confounding variables must be stripped away ('controlled for') to make the research objective.[173]

But herein lies a paradox. Context and 'confounders' lie at the very heart of diffusion, dissemination and implementation of complex innovations. They are not extraneous to the object of study – they are an integral part of it. The multiple (and often unpredictable) interactions that arise in particular contexts and settings are precisely what determine the success or failure of a dissemination initiative. Champions, for example, emerged in our review as a key determinant of organisational innovation – but no amount of empirical research will provide a simple recipe for how champions should behave that is independent of the nature of the innovation, the organisational setting, the socio-political context and so on. We make no apology for repeating the 'health warning' that we gave in Section 9.7 in relation to the fruitless quest for a simple formula for implementation: There will always remain a need to retranslate research and theoretical evidence into pragmatic strategies, processes and tactics that incorporate unique contextual elements of the organisation and the wider environment.

11.2 A framework for applying the model in a service context

Whilst the complex nature of this field of study precludes technical fixes and formulaic recommendations, we believe that it is still possible to apply a structured, evidence-based approach to diffusion and implementation of organisational innovations in a real-world context. We present below a two-stage framework that is based on the model depicted in Fig. 10.1 (page 201). The first stage is to consider the individual components of the model in turn: the attributes of the innovation; the characteristics and behaviour of individuals; the structural and cultural determinants of organisational innovativeness and so on. The second stage is to consider the interaction between these components with particular reference to local context, setting and timing. Whereas the first stage is largely a question of applying a literature-derived checklist and many questions can be addressed almost as a paper exercise, the second stage requires a high degree of practical wisdom, local knowledge and consultation.

Stage 1: considering the individual components of the model

The individual components of the model can be considered as a series of questions:

(1) What are the attributes of the innovation as perceived and evaluated by the intended users?

(a) In terms of the innovation itself, what is its perceived relative advantage, complexity, compatibility, trialability, observability and potential for reinvention in the eyes of key stakeholders?*

(b) In terms of its operational use, and for particular groups of staff, what is the relevance and usefulness of the innovation to particular tasks, and what is its feasibility, implementation complexity and divisibility into smaller 'chunks'? To what extent is the knowledge required to use the innovation codifiable and transferable (or could it be codified and made transferable)?

(c) How is the innovation perceived in terms of these attributes at the organisational level (e.g. by top management)?

(d) How might the perceptions of intended users and other key stakeholders be positively influenced – e.g. through creation of 'trialability space', production of rapid-cycle feedback data, demonstrations by opinion leaders or champions, visits to other departments or organisations and so on?

(e) How might the innovation be adapted ('reinvented') to change its key attributes as perceived by this group of intended adopters?

(2) What are the characteristics of the intended adopters and the adoption process?

(a) Who are the intended adopters and what are the relevant psychological antecedents (personality, learning style, pre-existing skills, values and goals) of different adopter groups?

(b) What are the perceived needs of the intended adopters that are relevant to the adoption decision?

(c) What meaning does the innovation have for the intended adopters, especially in relation to their work and professional identity?

(d) What are the key concerns that potential adopters have (i) in the pre-adoption phase (about what the innovation is, what it does, and the likely personal costs and benefits to them); (ii) in the early phase of use (about how to use the innovation in a specific task context); and (iii) as an established user (about the consequences of the innovation and the potential for adaptation and reinvention)?

(e) How might all the above influence the adoption decision? To what extent can they be influenced by planned interventions such as targeted training, familiarisation activities, provision of informal networking opportunities, adaptation of the innovation and so on?

(f) Is the adoption decision optional, authoritative, majority or contingent.[†] Can this be changed, e.g. by providing individual intended users with more (or less) autonomy?

(3) What is the nature of communication and influence about the innovation?

(a) What messages are conveyed about the innovation in official materials (e.g. policy documents), mass media and other communication sources? How do the content, style and medium of these messages align with the principles of effective marketing as set out in Sections 3.5 and 5.1?

*See Section 4.1 (page 83) for definitions of the terms used in this section.

[†]See Section 5.2 (page 103) for definitions.

(**b**) What are the main interpersonal (social) networks through which influence occurs in relation to this type of intervention? Where does the process of spread lie on the continuum from informal and unplanned ('diffusion') to formal and planned ('dissemination')?

(**c**) Who are the main agents of social influence (expert and peer opinion leaders, champions and so on) and by what processes and channels do key influences occur?

(**d**) How (if at all) might opinion leaders, champions, boundary spanners and so on be productively engaged in a planned programme of social influence?

(**4**) What is the nature of the organisational context and how conducive is this to the assimilation of innovations in general?

(**a**) Are there positive structural antecedents for innovation (large size, maturity, formalisation, functional differentiation, decentralisation and slack resources)? If such antecedents (especially differentiation, decentralisation and slack resources) are not present, can they be provided?

(**b**) To what extent does the organisation have the capacity to absorb new knowledge ('learning organisation' values and goals, pre-existing knowledge and skills base, pre-existing technologies, leadership and enablement of knowledge sharing through facilitated internal networking and external networking via organisational boundary spanners)? Can these features be enhanced and if so, how (e.g. knowledge-sharing events, appointment of knowledge workers)?

(**c**) To what extent does the organisation have a receptive context for change (strong leadership, clear strategic vision, good managerial relations, risk-taking climate, effective monitoring and feedback systems and so on)? Can this be enhanced and if so, how?

(**5**) What is the organisation's level of readiness for this innovation in particular?

(**a**) To what extent does the innovation fit with the existing strategies, goals, values and ways of working of the organisation? To what extent is it appropriate to consider a change in any of these to accommodate the innovation – and if so, how might it be achieved?

(**b**) Is there specific tension for change (ideally, do staff feel that the present situation is intolerable and that change in the direction of the proposed innovation is needed)? How might such tension be promoted or enhanced?

(**c**) To what extent is the innovation supported and advocated by (i) top management; (ii) middle (operational) management; (iii) technical staff; (iv) administrative staff? Do the perspectives of these groups align and if not, what can be done about this?

(**d**) Have the implications of the innovation for the organisation (in terms of the 'soft periphery' of structures, systems, specific training needs, and supporting technologies) been fully and positively assessed? In particular, are job changes full and clear, has training been adequately resourced and appropriately targeted and has relevant augmentation been provided (e.g. manuals, helpdesk, hotline)?

(**e**) Have adequate dedicated time and resources been allocated to the implementation and maintenance of the innovation? If necessary, how might time and resources be redeployed from other projects?

(**f**) To what extent is the organisation capable of evaluating and monitoring the innovation? In particular, does it have the capacity and capability to collect and analyse high-quality data about the impact of the innovation in a timely manner? If not, how might this capacity be enhanced?

(**6**) What is the nature of the outer (environmental) context and how will this impact on the assimilation process?

(**a**) What are the current social norms and expectations from other comparable organisations (e.g. as communicated via interorganisational networks)? If necessary, how might these be influenced?

(**b**) What is the current availability of (and what is the future scope for) intentional spread strategies to promote interorganisational networking? For example, is there scope for collaborative quality improvement initiatives or 'Beacon' schemes? Might new technologies be used more effectively in this context?

(c) To what extent is the external environment providing pressure for change? What are the prevailing political, economic, sociological and technological influences? To what extent can these be manipulated (e.g. by providing incentives or mandates)?

(d) What specific national and local policy initiatives are ongoing or planned? What is their specific timing and how might the innovation be aligned with them?

(7) Is the implementation and maintenance process (as opposed to the adoption by individuals) adequately planned, resourced and managed?

(a) Are the resources, skill mix and level of staffing appropriate? How might these be enhanced?

(b) Are all key staff involved from an early stage?

(c) Can the relevant individuals and teams make and implement decisions autonomously? Can changes be made to improve decision-making autonomy?

(d) What type and structure of employee incentives and rewards will promote assimilation and implementation of innovations? Can these be introduced and if so, how and at what cost?

(e) Are plans for project management adequate (e.g. goals and milestones, operational management)? How might these be improved?

(f) What measures and procedures are in place to capture and respond to the consequences of the innovation (e.g. method and type of data collection for audit and feedback)? How might these be improved?

(g) What measures and procedures are in place to enable individuals and teams to make sense of the innovation and if necessary reframe it in terms of relevant meaning systems, values and goals (particularly through intraorganisational networking and sensemaking initiatives)? How might such initiatives be introduced?

(h) What measures and procedures are in place to enable organisations to develop, adapt and reinvent the innovation (particularly through interorganisational networks and collaboratives)? If such networks are not already in place, how might they be introduced?

(8) What (if any) is the nature, capacity and activities of external agencies? In particular

(a) If the innovation is formally developed (e.g. in a research centre), to what extent are the developers linked with potential users of the innovation *at the development stage*, and do they share value systems, language and meanings? How might this linkage be enhanced?

(b) If a formal change agency exists, does it have the capacity, commitment, technical capability, communication skills and project management skills to help organisations with operational aspects of assimilation? How might these features be proactively enhanced so that the innovation can routinely be disseminated as an augmented product (e.g. with tools and resources, technical help and so on)?

(c) Who are the main external change agents and to what extent do they meet the criteria of (i) homophily with intended adopters; (ii) positive interpersonal relationships and client centeredness; (iii) shared language and meanings with the intended adopter about the innovation? What might be done to optimise these critical conditions?

(d) If a formal dissemination programme is used, to what extent does it follow the established principles of social marketing (audience segmentation, assessment of target group needs and perspective, appropriate message and marketing channels, good programme management, rigorous and timely process evaluation)? What changes are needed to the programme to improve its alignment with these principles?

(e) What is the nature and quality of any linkage relationship between the change agency and organisations attempting to assimilate an innovation (e.g. are human relations positive and supportive; do the two systems share common language, meanings and value systems; is there sharing of tools and resources in both directions; does the change agency enable and facilitate external networking and collaboration between organisations; is there joint evaluation of the consequences of innovations and so on)? How might this linkage be enhanced?

Stage 2: considering the interaction between components

As the example in the last paragraph of Section 11.1 (page 219) illustrated, the studies reviewed in Chapters 4–9 caution against thinking of the individual components of our model as 'cogs in a machine'. The whole is more than the sum of the parts. Although the model suggests a long list of possible determinants and moderators of spread and sustainability, none of these can be thought of as simple variables whose influence can be predicted or manipulated either in experimental research or in practice and policymaking. For example:

- Innovation attributes are not fully predictable because different people have different perceptions of the same innovation – and indeed, attributes such as relative advantage are to a large extent socially constructed within particular contexts and systems.
- The adoption process is not fully predictable because different adopters have different perceived needs even in similar situations, and certainly when operating in different ones.
- Social influence is not fully predictable because different individuals identify different others as 'influential' and different types of influence are perceived as credible for different innovations.
- Organisational structure is not fully predictable because the impact of structural determinants is contingent on time (e.g. whilst more structurally complex organisations may *adopt* innovations relatively early, less structurally complex organisations may be able to *spread* innovations internally more effectively, and the balance between these different processes varies).
- The organisational context is not fully predictable because (among other things) the same individual behaves differently in different contexts and at different times, and because multiple confounding (unmeasured) variables from within and outside the organisation are often present.
- External incentives and mandates are not fully predictable because a crucial moderating influence on the impact of such factors is timing – an incentive or mandate that appears at the wrong time in relation to other confounding influences will have a far weaker impact.
- The environmental context is not fully predictable because an environment that facilitates the spread and sustainability of a particular innovation in one organisation will inhibit its spread and sustainability in a different organisation.
- The implementation process is not fully predictable because much depends on human motivation, capability and behaviour, and because of the impact of multiple competing priorities and forces.

Interactions like these are necessarily highly contingent. It is not possible, *nor will it ever be possible*, to provide prescriptive and transferable recommendations on how different parts of the model will interact with one another in a particular situation. Rather, such interactions might best be explored in relation to particular initiatives using an open-ended question format. For example:

Interaction between the adopter and the innovation: How does this particular adopter perceive the attributes of this particular innovation (and can he/she be supported to change these perceptions)?

Interaction between opinion leadership and the nature of the innovation: What is the overall perceived potential of this particular innovation by the more influential members of this particular social group, and what impact is this likely to have on the behaviour and choices of the 'rank and file'?*

Interaction between the task (innovation-in-use) and the boundary role: What impact does the nature of the task(s) associated with the innovation have

*In Section 5.2 (page 103), for example, we described a study by Becker in which an innovation perceived as 'high potential' was adopted earlier by individuals of high social status within the network and spread rapidly, whereas an innovation perceived as 'low potential' was adopted earlier by individuals of lower social status and spread much more slowly.

on the preferred boundary-spanning role (linking the organisation with the external world)?

Interaction between organisational structure and stage of assimilation: For this particular innovation, what is the balance between high structural complexity (hence promoting innovativeness and hence adoption) and low structural complexity (hence facilitating diffusion of the innovation within the organisation)?*

Clearly, the number of possible interactions is extremely high, and practitioners must use situational judgement to prioritise the key questions in a particular initiative. One structured approach for applying situational judgement, realistic evaluation, is considered in Section 11.3 (page 227) in relation to the research agenda on 'whole-systems' approaches.

11.3 Recommendations for further research

When undertaking this review, we were struck by the duplication of empirical studies, and also by the number of studies that had been undertaken without a comprehensive review of relevant research already undertaken, many of which had asked what appeared to be obsolete questions. We highlight below some specific areas where we believe further empirical research is – and equally importantly, where we believe it is not – needed.

(1) **Innovations.** Further research into the attributes of innovations that promote their adoption is probably not needed. Instead, research in this area should be directed at these questions:

(a) How do innovations in health service organisations arise, and in what circumstances? What particular mix of factors tends to produce 'adoptable' innovations (e.g. ones that have clear advantages beyond their source organisation, low implementation complexity, and are readily adaptable to new contexts)?

(b) How can innovations in health service organisations be adapted so that they are perceived as more advantageous, more compatible with prevailing norms and values, less complex, more trialable, with more observable results, and with greater scope for local reinvention? Is there a role of a central agency, resource centre or officially sanctioned demonstration programs in this?

(c) How do innovations arising as 'good ideas' in local health care systems become reinvented as they are transmitted through individual and organisational networks, and how can this process be supported or enhanced?

(d) How might we identify 'bad ideas' that are likely to spread so that we can intervene proactively to prevent this?

(2) **Adopters and adoption.** We do not recommend further descriptive studies on patterns of adoption by individuals. We believe the main unanswered questions are:

(a) Why and how do people (and organisations) reject an innovation after adopting it? (In over 200 empirical research studies covered in our review, only one explicitly and prospectively studied discontinuance[283]).

(b) What are the transferable lessons from cognitive and social psychology about the ability and tendency of individuals to adopt particular innovations in particular circumstances? For example, what can we glean from the mainstream literature about how individuals process information, make decisions, apply heuristics and so on? A particularly fruitful area is likely to be the psychological literature on human-computer interaction as it applies to the adoption and assimilation of information and communications technology (ICT) innovations in the service sector.

(3) **Dissemination and social influence.** We do not recommend further 'intervention' trials of the use of opinion leaders in efforts to change the behaviour of potential adopters. We already know from published research that opinion leadership is a complex and delicate process, and research that fails to capture these process elements is unlikely to add to what we already know. We recommend that research into dissemination addresses the following questions:

*See Section 6.3 (page 126).

(a) What is the nature of interpersonal influence and opinion leadership in the range of different professional and managerial groups in the health service, especially in relation to organisational innovations? In particular, how are key players identified and influenced?

(b) What is the nature and extent of the social networks of different players in the health service (both clinical and non-clinical)?* How do these networks serve as channels for social influence and the reinvention and embedding of complex service innovations?

(c) Who are the individuals who act as champions for organisational innovations in health services? What is the nature of their role and how might it be enabled and enhanced?

(d) Who are the individuals who act as boundary spanners between health service organisations, especially in relation to complex service innovations? What is the nature of their role and how might it be enabled and enhanced?

(4) **The organisational context.** We do not recommend further survey-based research to identify structural determinants of innovativeness in health care organisations, since the small but significant effect of key structural determinants is well established. We suggest the following questions as possible directions for further research†:

(a) To what extent do 'restructuring' initiatives (popular in health service organisations) improve their ability to adopt, implement and sustain innovations? In particular, will a planned move from a traditional hierarchical structure to one based on semi-autonomous teams with independent decision-making power improve innovativeness?

(b) How can we improve the absorptive capacity of service organisations for new knowledge? In particular, what is the detailed process by which ideas are captured from outside, circulated internally, adapted, reframed, implemented and routinised in a service organisation, and how might this process be systematically enhanced?

(c) How can leaders of service organisations set about achieving a receptive context for change – i.e. the kind of culture and climate that supports and enables change in general? A systematic review centring on the mainstream change management literature (which we explicitly excluded from this review) is probably the most appropriate first step for this question.

(d) What is the nature of the process that leads to *long-term* routinisation (with appropriate adaptation and development) of innovations in health service delivery and organisation?

(5) **System readiness for innovation.** There is relatively little systematic research into the development of system readiness (i.e. the steps that organisations can make to assess, prepare for and anticipate the impact of an innovation). The following questions should be addressed:

(a) What steps must be taken by service organisations when moving towards a state of 'readiness' (i.e. with all players on board and with protected time and funding), and how might this overall process be supported and enhanced? In particular, (i) how can tension for change be engendered?; (ii) how can innovation–system fit best be assessed?; (iii) how can the implications of the innovation be assessed and fed into the decision-making process?; (iv) what measures enhance the success of efforts to secure funding for the innovation in the resource allocation cycle?; and (v) how can the organisation's capacity to evaluate the impact of the innovation be enhanced?

(b) What are the characteristics of organisations that successfully avoid taking up 'bad ideas'? Are they just lucky – or do they have better mechanisms for evaluating the ideas and anticipating the knock-on effects?

(6) **The outer context.** Aside from questions in the fields of political science and macroeconomics, the

*In Section 9.1 (page 176), we note that the more complex the innovation, the more crucial are external networks in enabling the individual and the organisation to operationalise and adapt it. Hence, this is a particularly ripe area for future research.

†There may be existing literature on all these questions, hence secondary research may be more appropriate than empirical work.

main research questions on the environmental context are:

(a) What is the nature of informal interorganisational networking in different areas of activity, and how might this be enhanced through explicit knowledge management activities (such as the appointment and support of knowledge workers and boundary spanners)?

(b) What is (or could be) the role of professional organisations and informal interprofessional networks in spreading innovation between health care organisations?

(c) What is the cost-effectiveness of structured health care quality collaboratives and comparable models of quality improvement – and how might this be enhanced? To what sort of projects in what sort of contexts should resources for such interorganisational collaboratives be allocated?

(d) What are the harmful effects of an external 'push' (such as a policy directive or incentive) for a particular innovation when the system is not ready? What are the characteristics of external pushes that tend to be more successful in promoting the assimilation and implementation of innovations by health service organisations?

(7) **Implementation.** Overall, we found that empirical studies on implementing and maintaining innovations in service organisations: had been undertaken from a pragmatic rather than an academic perspective and been presented as 'grey literature' reports (which for practical reasons we did not include in this review); were difficult to disentangle from the literature on change management in general; and were impoverished by lack of process information. We recommend that further research focus on two questions:

(a) By what processes are particular innovations in health service delivery and organisation implemented and sustained (or not) in particular contexts and settings, and can this process be enhanced? This question, which was probably the most serious gap in the literature we uncovered for this review, would benefit from in-depth mixed-methodology studies aimed at building up a rich picture of process and impact.

(b) Are there any additional lessons from the mainstream change management literature (to add to the diffusion of innovations literature reviewed here) for implementing and sustaining innovations in health care organisations? This question would of course require in-depth qualitative methods aimed at building up a rich picture of the process being studied,[142] and is discussed further in the next subsection on whole-systems research.

Recommendations for 'whole-systems' research

As discussed in Section 11.1 (page 219), a consistent theme in high-quality overviews and commentaries on the diffusion and implementation of organisational innovations is that empirical research has generally been restricted to a single level of analysis (individual *or* team *or* organisation *or* interorganisational), has implicitly or explicitly assumed simple causal relationships between variables, has failed to address important interactions between different levels (e.g. how different organisational settings moderate individual behaviour and decision-making) and between both measured and unmeasured variables within these levels and has failed to take due account of contingent and contextual issues.

To some extent, these criticisms apply to organisational research in general, which has tended to consider either the 'micro' level (the behaviour of individuals within organisations) or the 'macro' level (the structural and cultural aspects of the organisation as a whole). House *et al.*[77] make a cogent case for developing a 'meso paradigm' in organisational behaviour that explicitly addresses the interaction between these macro and micro levels.

A 'meso' approach could potentially produce fruitful research on the impact of different organisational structures and cultures on the decisions of particular groups of individuals (e.g. whether nurses are more or less likely to adopt a technology-based innovation when working in a large hospital trust as opposed to a small general practice). But like much previous organisational research, this approach ultimately seeks a level of generalisability that is inherently unattainable for most questions relating to the dissemination and implementation process.

In an important theoretical article, Potvin argues that because of the highly complex and relentlessly contextual nature of dissemination programmes, they should be treated as a 'special case' in research:

> Dissemination programmes are at the far end of an applied research continuum. ... We can forget the experimental and quasi-experimental paradigms as one-size-fits-all methodological kits for dissemination research.[482]

In another reflective overview on the epistemological challenges in dissemination and implementation research, Professor Larry Green, veteran director of numerous community-based health promotion programmes, echoes this sentiment:

> A common misunderstanding about health promotion research is that it seeks or should seek a magic bullet, a package to put on a shelf in any community where professionals can pull it off and apply it. ... Yet, because generalizability or external validity is one of the criteria of good science, we are at risk of undermining confidence in health promotion if we make too much of a point that our research cannot be expected to produce highly generalizable findings. What needs to be clarified is that health promotion research can promise to produce a generalizable process for planning, not a generalizable plan. The products of health promotion research are ways of engaging the community, ... ways of assessing resources, ways of planning programmes, and ways of matching needs, resources and circumstances with appropriate interventions.[483]

Although Green is talking specifically about health promotion, his comments apply directly to any research into the dissemination and implementation of complex interventions in the service sector. 'Best practice', he stresses, should be thought of as a process or a general approach, and not as an 'intervention package'.

Where does this leave the research agenda for 'whole-systems' approaches to dissemination and implementation? Both Potvin *et al.* and Green have suggested some key requirements for applied health promotion research, which we drew upon to develop some general recommendations for research into the dissemination, implementation and routinisation of innovations (listed in Box 11.1).

Action research might be a particularly useful approach for the kind of applied research that would meet the criteria listed in Box 11.1, since it has the following key features:

(1) it focuses on change and improvement;
(2) it involves participants in the research process;
(3) it is educational for all involved;
(4) it looks at questions that arise from practice;
(5) it involves a cyclical process of collecting, feeding back, and reflecting on data; and
(6) it is a process that generates knowledge.[278,*]

We recommend that this approach be explored further in this context.

Another approach that we believe has important potential is the 'Would it work here?' framework developed by Gomm,[116] who in turn drew on Pawson and Tilley's[120] 'realistic evaluation', and which we adapted for considering the spread of organisational innovations in Box A.7 (page 240) in Appendix 3.

As mentioned briefly in Section 2.7 (page 42), the goal of realistic evaluation is to *critically examine the mechanisms of success or failure* in different efforts to implement an innovative practice throughout a sector, and hence, in general terms, address the question 'what works for whom under what circumstances?'[140] (Fig. 11.1). Pawson and Tilley developed this method specifically to consider and compare policy implementation programmes, and we initially thought that we would be able to apply this method to many of the primary studies in this review. In practice, we found that few if any published studies contained sufficient detail to allow us to apply the framework – confirming the

*For an example of how action research was used in organisational development in a hospital trust see Bate (2004).[97]

Box 11.1 Recommended characteristics of an applied, 'whole-systems' research agenda into dissemination and implementation (adapted form Potvin,[482] Rootman *et al.*[484] and Green[483]).

Applied research into the process of dissemination, implementation and routinisation should be

- *Theory-driven*: it should aim to explore an explicit hypothecated link between the determinants of a particular problem, the specific mechanism of the programme and the expected changes in the original situation.
- *Process- rather than 'package'-oriented*: it should explicitly avoid questions framed with a view to causal inferences, such as 'Does programme X work?' or 'Does strategy Y have this effect?'. Rather, research questions should be framed with a view to illuminating a process – e.g. 'What features account for the success of programme X in this context and the failure of a comparable programme in a different context?'
- *Participatory*: it should engage practitioners as partners in the research process. In experimental research, the researcher is 'in charge' of the study, frames the problem, makes any key manipulations and interprets the data. But in process evaluation it is the practitioners who frame the problem, make the manipulations and interpret the data while the researcher observes. Locally owned and driven programmes will produce more useful research questions and data that are more valid and reliable.
- *Collaborative and coordinated*: it should aim to prioritise and study key research questions across multiple programmes in a variety of contexts, rather than small isolated teams 'doing their own thing'. In this way, the impact of place, setting and context can be systematically studied.
- *Addressed using common definitions, measures and tools*: it should adopt standardised approaches to measuring key variables and confounders (e.g. quality of life, implementation success) to enable valid comparisons across studies.
- *Multi-disciplinary and multi-method*: it should recognise the inherent limitations of experimental approaches for researching open systems, and embrace a broad range of research methods with the emphasis on interpretive approaches.
- *Meticulously detailed*: it should document extensively the unique aspects of different programmes and their respective contexts and settings to allow for meaningful comparisons across programmes. Such detailed descriptions can be used by future research teams to interpret idiosyncratic findings and test rival hypotheses about mechanisms.
- *Ecological*: It should recognise the critical reciprocal interaction between the programme that is the explicit focus of research and the wider setting in which the programme takes place. The latter provides a dynamic, shifting baseline against which any programme-related activity will occur; each will influence the other. Programme-setting interactions form a key element of data and are a particularly rich source of new hypotheses about mechanisms of success or failure.

observations made independently by Potvin and Green that current reporting of intervention programmes is insufficiently systematic or detailed.

A realist approach to evaluating a service innovation from the diffusion/assimilation/implementation perspective would seek to provide a detailed description and interpretation of how the innovation fares in more than one organisation or setting. Pawson advocates an in-depth case study approach, focusing on both the context and the detailed mechanism of each separate implementation project. Using the headings illustrated in Fig. 11.1, the researcher should ask for each of them 'what are the differences and to what extent do these differences explain the outcome'?

The realist framework potentially allows a highly structured comparison across studies. The key questions for undertaking a realistic synthesis (i.e. a cross-programme comparison) are listed in the far right column of Box A.7 (page 240). In Pawson's[140] words:

> The reviewer's basic task is to sift through the mixed fortunes of the programme, attempting to discover those contexts that have produced solid and successful outcomes from those contexts that have induced failure.

Pawson suggests that we learn as much – perhaps more – from the study of programmes that 'failed' as from the study of those that succeeded. The

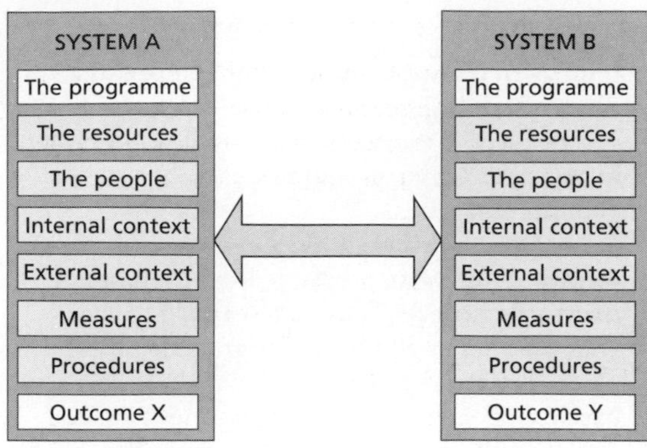

Fig. 11.1 Realistic synthesis framework for considering spread and sustainability initiatives across different organisations and projects.

realist synthesis framework can be used retrospectively to guide a summative evaluation of an initiative already undertaken, or more prospectively and formatively (and hence probably more usefully) for addressing the planned implementation of a possible innovation.

We strongly recommend that the realist approach be explored further and that future research and evaluation studies of the adoption and implementation of innovations by health service organisations should

(1) meet the criteria for applied dissemination research listed in Box 11.1 (page 229) and

(2) prospectively collect the kind of data recommended by Pawson and Tilley[120] and listed in Box A.7 (page 240).

A standard framework for describing and reporting implementation studies will allow more meaningful comparison of service initiatives (in particular, better lessons about what leads to success or failure), and will potentially also allow the subsequent synthesis of findings from process evaluations and 'grey literature' documents.

Were such information to become available in relation to the topic areas relevant to this review, the stages of realist synthesis might look something like this:

(1) Classify the primary research studies of dissemination and implementation according to the proposed mechanism through which the programme was assumed or intended to work.

(2) For each different mechanism, consider each primary study in detail, and ask three questions:

(a) What was the historical, social, political and ideological context of the programme(s) in the study?

(b) What were the outcomes (intended and unintended) of the programme(s)?

(c) Given the context of the programme, and using the sub-headings shown in Fig. 11.1 as a guide, what was the likely mechanism through which the programmes produced the outcomes?

(3) For each mechanism, synthesise these data across studies to produce a set of realist hypotheses about dissemination and implementation of innovations in service delivery and organisation such as 'programmes based on mechanism A are particularly useful in contexts such as B or C, but are less likely to succeed if factor D is present or if factor E is absent'.

In summary, most of the existing empirical research relating to the spread and sustainability of innovations has focused on a limited number of components in the model depicted in Fig. 10.1 (page 201), often based on experimental (and, some would argue, reductionist) designs. Such research has produced findings that may or may not be generalisable to the complex realities of real-world implementation in particular contexts. A relatively new research tradition is emerging in UK health services research, some based on the evaluation of initiatives led by the NHS Modernisation Agency, as described in Section 1.2 (page 22). This research is qualitative, interpretive and emergent rather than experimental, and is arguably better suited to drawing meaningful lessons from complex implementation projects.

We strongly support this direction of enquiry, but we urge the commissioners and coordinators of research programmes to note carefully the draft principles for ensuring the quality of such research (listed in Box 11.1, page 229). As a first step towards a coordinated programme of illuminative research, we recommend that this preliminary list be debated, refined and ratified by the research community. Once formal quality criteria are established, they should be meticulously and proactively adhered to, so as to maximise the rigour and transferability of this particularly challenging research agenda.

11.4 Conclusion

We believe that this extensive systematic review has produced three important outputs:
(1) a parsimonious and evidence-based model for considering the diffusion of innovations in health service organisations;
(2) clear knowledge gaps where further research on the diffusion of innovations in service organisations should be focused; and
(3) a robust and transferable methodology for undertaking systematic reviews of complex research evidence.

Research commissioners should note in particular our suggestions for where further research is unlikely to add substantially to the knowledge base. We encourage other research teams to test both our proposed model for the diffusion of service innovations and our proposed methodology for systematic review of diffuse bodies of literature.

Appendix 1
Data extraction form

AUTHOR/TITLE OF PAPER

NAME OF REVIEWER

A. Is the paper relevant to our research question and worthy of further consideration?

1. **Relevance.** Is the paper about the diffusion, spread or sustainability of innovation in service delivery or organisation?
2. **Worth.** Does the paper go beyond superficial description or commentary – i.e. is it a broadly competent attempt at research, enquiry, investigation or study?

[If the answer to one or both of these questions is 'no', do not consider the paper further]

B. How does the paper fit into our taxonomy?

Paradigm. What is the predominant theoretical 'lens' used? [if more than one, put double circle round the dominant one]	1. Complexity/general systems theory	2. Social network theory	3. Social influence theory (classical adoption)	4. Communication theory
	5. Marketing theory (including social marketing)	6. Political influence theories	7. Knowledge utilisation theory	8. Behaviour theories (e.g. concerns-based adoption model, TBP)
	9. [Adult] learning theory	10. Organisational theory	11. Classical management theory	12. Classical economic theory
	13. Others (specify)	14. None discernible	Notes	
1. **Type of paper.** What is the research design or review style [classify as the main pitch of the paper]	1. Theory or conceptual framework	2. Editorial review, commentary or opinion	3. Systematic review	4. RCT
	5. Non-RCT experimental or quasi-experimental study	6. Questionnaire survey	7. Qualitative interview study (including focus group)	8. Ethnographic study ('anthropological' case study)
	9. Mixed-methodology case study	10. Action research	11. Tool/checklist/ model	12. Guideline/protocol
	13. Comparative case study	14. Network analysis	15. Attribution study	
	16. Others (Specify)			

Continued

B. How does the paper fit into our taxonomy? *(continued)*						
2. **Unit of analysis** [encircle one or more] Notes	Individual	Group or team	Organisation	Interorganisational	Regional/national	Multi-level

C. Bottom line for this review (complete this after Section D)			
1. **Relevance**. Does the paper have an important message for our research question? [encircle one]	Essential to include	Relevant but not essential	Marginal relevance
2. **Methods**. Does the paper fulfil the established quality criteria for papers in its domain? [encircle one]	Outstanding	Some limitations	Many important limitations

D. Appraisal questions for primary studies

(e.g. Oakley 2000[500]: 'The distinguishing mark of good research is the awareness and acknowledgement of error and [hence] the necessity of establishing procedures which will minimise the effect such errors have on what counts as knowledge.')

1. **Question.** Did the paper address a clear research question and if so, what was it? In particular, were complex terms such as 'hospital at home', 'private finance' defined clearly and unambiguously?
2. **Design.** What was the study design and was this appropriate to the question?
3. **Funding.** Who funded the study?

1. National government	2. International (e.g. EU)	3. Research charity	4. No external funding
5. Private (e.g. pharma)	6. Service (e.g. NHS, HMO)	7. Profession (e.g. RCN)	8. Not stated

4. **Actor 1 ['resource system'].** In this study, from whom is the innovation said to come?
5. **Innovation.** What is the nature of the innovation?
6. **Context.** What was the context of the study? Was this sufficiently well described that the findings can be related to other settings? [*Note*: Transferability of case study findings to different settings is best judged via a detailed analysis of the 'rich picture' of the case]
7. **Actor 2 ['user system'].** Who is receiving the innovation (or to whom is it being sent or marketed)?
8. **Dissemination process.** What (if any) were the elements of the active dissemination process?
9. **Implementation process.** What (if any) were the elements of the active implementation process?
10. **Sampling.** Did the researchers include sufficient cases/settings/observations? [could conceptual rather than statistical generalisations be made?]
11. **Data collection.** Was the data collection process systematic, thorough and auditable?
12. **Data analysis.** Were the data analysed systematically and rigorously? Have sufficient data been presented to allow the reader to assess independently whether analytical criteria have been met? How were disconfirming observations dealt with?
13. **Results.** What are the main results and in what way are they surprising, interesting, or suspect? [Include any intended and unintended consequences]
14. **Conclusions.** Did the authors draw a clear link between data and explanation (theory)? If not, what are your reservations?
15. **Critical factors.** What factors does the paper identify as critical to the spread/sustainability of innovations?
    Hypothetical or assumed
    Actually demonstrated
16. **Reflexivity.** Are the authors' positions and roles clearly explained and biases considered?
17. **Any ethical reservations?**

Appendix 2

Critical appraisal checklists

Box A.1 Quality checklist for experimental (randomised and non-randomised controlled trial) designs.

1. Research question and design

- *Was there a clear research question, and was this important and sensible?
- *If the study was non-randomised, could a randomised design have been used?

2. Baseline comparability of groups

- [RCTs only]: Was allocation adequately concealed by a rigorous method (e.g. random numbers)?
- Were appropriate measures of baseline characteristics taken in all groups before the intervention, and were study groups shown to be comparable in all characteristics likely to influence outcome?
- Was there a baseline measure of performance and patient outcomes, and were study groups comparable in these at baseline?

3. Outcome measures

- *Was the primary outcome measure valid (i.e. do two independent raters agree that this was a sensible and reasonable measure of performance or outcome)?
- Was the primary outcome measure reliable (i.e. do two independent raters agree on the nature and extent of change)?

4. Protection against contamination

- Is it unlikely that the control unit of allocation (professional, practice, institution, community) received the intervention through contamination?

5. Protection against bias

- Were outcomes measured by 'blinded' observers or were they objectively verified (e.g. quantitative measures recorded prospectively and independently)?

6. Follow-up

- Was there complete follow-up of professionals (ideally >80%)?
- Was there complete follow-up of patient groups (ideally >80%)?
- *Was follow-up continued for long enough for the primary outcome measure to show an impact and for sustainability to be demonstrated?

Source: Modified from Cochrane EPOC checklist.[141] Asterisks mark the places where we have added to, or deviated from, the standard EPOC criteria for reasons explained in Section 2.5 (page 38).

Box A.2 Quality checklist for quasi-experimental (interrupted time series) designs.

1. Research question and design
- *Was there a clear research question, and was this important and sensible?
- *Could a randomised or non-randomised controlled design have been used?

2. Protection against secular changes
- Was the intervention independent of other changes over time?
- Were there sufficient data points to enable reliable statistical inference?[a]
- Was a formal statistical test for trend correctly undertaken?

3. Outcome measures
- Was the primary outcome measure valid (i.e. do two independent raters agree that this was a sensible and reasonable measure of performance or outcome)?
- Was the primary outcome measure reliable (i.e. do two independent raters agree on the nature and extent of change)?

4. Protection against detection bias
- Was the intervention unlikely to affect data collection (e.g. sources and methods of data collection were the same before and after the intervention)?
- Were outcomes measured by 'blinded' observers or were they objectively verified (e.g. quantitative measures recorded prospectively and independently)?

5. Completeness of data-set and follow-up
- Does the data-set cover all or most of the episodes of care (or other unit of analysis) covered in the study (ideally, >80%)?
- *Was follow-up continued for long enough for the primary outcome measure to show an impact and for sustainability to be demonstrated?

[a]See EPOC handbook for full list of criteria for the different statistical methods.
Source: Modified from Cochrane EPOC checklist.[141] Asterisks mark the places where we have added to, or deviated from, the standard EPOC criteria for reasons explained in Chapter 2 (page 38).

Box A.3 Quality checklist for attribution studies.

1. Predictive rather than descriptive design
- Did the study predict, rather than describe *post hoc*, the relationship between particular attributes and adoption (i.e. were the postulated attributes identified before rather than after adoption was measured)?

2. Going beyond the decision to adopt
- Did the study assess the fact of adoption rather than merely the decision to adopt? (In organisational studies this will require an assessment of whether and to what extent the innovation was implemented).

3. Methodological rigour
- Was the research undertaken according to a reliable and reproducible method?
- Was the study adequately powered?

4. Perspective
- Were the attributes of the innovation established from the perspective of the research participants (rather than assumed by the research team)?

5. Comparative rather than dichotomous approach
- Were more than one (and preferably several) attributes of the innovation studied in order to provide data on their relative importance?
- Were more than one (and preferably several) different innovations studied in order to improve the generalisability of conclusions about particular attributes?

6. Emphasis on organisational innovation
- Would the innovations studied be adopted by organisations rather than simply by individuals (i.e. does it fit the definition of an innovation in service delivery and organisation as given in page 28)?

Source: Modified from Tornatsky and Klein.[62]

Box A.4 Quality checklist for questionnaire surveys.[153]

1. Research question and design
- Was there a clear research question, and was this important and sensible?
- Was a questionnaire the most appropriate research design for this question?

2. Sampling
- What was the sampling frame and was it sufficiently large and representative?
- Did all participants in the sample understand what was required of them, and did they attribute the same meaning to the terms in the questionnaire?

3. Instrument
- What claims for reliability and validity have been made, and are these justified?
- Did the questions cover all relevant aspects of the problem in a non-threatening and non-directive way?
- Were open-ended (qualitative) and closed-ended (quantitative) questions used appropriately?
- Was a pilot version administered to participants representative of those in the sampling frame, and the instrument modified accordingly?

4. Response
- What was the response rate and have non-responders been accounted for?

5. Coding and analysis
- Was the analysis appropriate (e.g. statistical analysis for quantitative answers, qualitative analysis for open-ended questions) and were the correct techniques used?
- Were adequate measures in place to maintain accuracy of data?

6. Presentation of results
- Have all relevant results ('significant' and 'non-significant') been reported?
- Is there any evidence of 'data dredging' (i.e. analyses that were not 'hypothesis driven')?

Note: Attribution studies were assessed using criteria in Box A.3, page 236.
Source: Boynton and Greenhalgh.[153]

Box A.5 Quality checklist for qualitative studies.

1. **Question.** Did the paper address a clear research question and if so, what was it?
2. **Design.** What was the study design and was this appropriate to the research question? In particular, was a qualitative approach suitable and was the right design used?
3. **Context.** What was the context of the study? Was this sufficiently well described that the findings can be related to other settings?
4. **Sampling.** Did the researchers include sufficient cases/settings/observations so that conceptual rather than statistical generalisations could be made?
5. **Data collection.** Was the data collection process systematic, thorough and auditable? Were attempts made to identify and explore disconfirming examples?
6. **Data analysis.** Were data analysed systematically and rigorously? Did the analysis take account of all observations? Were sufficient data presented? How were disconfirming observations dealt with?
7. **Results.** What were the main results and in what way are they surprising, interesting, or suspect? Were there any unintended consequences and if so, what were they?
8. **Conclusions.** Did the authors draw a clear link between data and explanation (theory)? If not, what were the limitations of their theoretical analysis?
9. **Reflexivity.** Were the authors' positions and roles clearly explained and the resulting biases considered? Were the authors' preconceptions and ideology adequately set aside?
10. **Ethics.** Are there any ethical reservations about the study?
11. **Worth/relevance.** Was this piece of work worth doing at all, and has it contributed usefully to knowledge?

Note: This checklist was used for interview and focus group studies; in-depth case studies and other process-focused designs were assessed using criteria in Box A.6 (page 239).
Source: Adapted from Mays and Pope.[154]

Box A.6 Quality checklist for mixed-methodology case studies and other in-depth complex designs.

1. **Question.** Did the paper address a clear research question and if so, what was it? In particular, were complex terms such as 'hospital at home', 'private finance' defined clearly and unambiguously?
2. **Design.** What was the study design and was this appropriate to the research question?
3. **Funding.** Who funded the study and what was their perspective?
4. **Resource system.** In this study, from whom was the innovation said to come?
5. **Innovation.** What was the nature of the innovation?
6. **Context.** What was the context of the study? Was this sufficiently well described so that the findings could be related to other settings?
7. **User system.** Who was receiving the innovation (or to whom was it marketed)?
8. **Dissemination mechanism.** What (if any) were the elements of the active dissemination process and how did they interact?
9. **Implementation mechanism.** What (if any) were the elements of the active implementation process and how did they interact?
10. **Sampling.** Did the researchers include sufficient cases/settings/observations so that conceptual rather than statistical generalisations could be made?
11. **Data collection.** Was the data collection process systematic, thorough and auditable?
12. **Data analysis.** Were data analysed systematically and rigorously? Were sufficient data presented? How were disconfirming observations dealt with?
13. **Results.** What were the main results and in what way are they surprising, interesting, or suspect? Were there any unintended consequences and if so, what were they?
14. **Conclusions.** Did the authors draw a clear link between data and explanation (theory)? If not, what were the limitations of their theoretical analysis?
15. **Reflexivity.** Were the authors' positions and roles clearly explained and the resulting biases considered?

Ethics. Are there any ethical reservations about the study?

Source: Adapted from Mays *et al.*[118]

Box A.7 Quality checklist for comparison of 'real-world' implementation studies.

	System A	System B	Desirability or feasibility of changing practice, procedures and context of system B to match those of system A
The innovation	What are the salient features of the innovation currently being used in system A?	What are the salient features of the innovation intended to be used in system B?	Where there is a mismatch, could and should system B adopt the same innovation as is used by system A?
The resources	What resources were used in producing the outcomes (staff time, money, equipment, space, etc.) in system A?	What resources are available to system B?	Has system B got the resources to emulate the practice of system A? If not, would it be feasible or desirable for system B to enhance or redeploy resources?
The people	What are the salient characteristics of the key actors in system A in terms of expertise, experience, commitment and so on?	What are the salient characteristics of the key actors in system B?	Insofar as there is a mismatch, would it be desirable or feasible to recruit different staff, invest in training, go through teambuilding activities, etc.?
Institutional factors	How far were the outcomes dependent on organisational/ departmental structure, organisational culture, etc.?	How far does the organisational structure and culture of system B determine practice?	Insofar as there are differences, would it be feasible or desirable to change the institutional structures and cultures in system B?
Environmental factors	How far were the outcomes dependent on particular environmental factors (e.g. political, legislative, etc.)?	How far is the external environment of system B comparable?	Insofar as there is a difference, would it be feasible or desirable to change the external environment of system B?
Measures	What baseline, process, outcome and other measures were used to evaluate success?	Does system B (or could it) use the same measures?	Would it be desirable or feasible for system B to change the way it measures and records practice?

Continued

Procedures	What exactly was done in system A that led to the outcomes reported?	Does system B do exactly the same (or could it)?	Insofar as there are differences, would it be desirable or feasible for system B to change what it does?
Outcomes	What were the key outcomes, for whom, at what cost, and what are they attributable to? What was the cost per successful outcome?	What key outcomes are measured in system B? Are they achieved for the same actors as in system 1? What outcomes does system B achieve that system A does not? To what are these outcomes attributable? What is the cost per successful outcome in system B?	Insofar as the outcomes are different, to what are the differences attributable? Are there desirable outcomes that system B is not achieving? Could system B achieve the same outcomes at a lower cost? Would system B have to forgo some current outcomes in order to achieve the same outcomes as system A?

Source: Adapted from the 'Would it work here?' framework developed by Gomm[116] who draws on the work of Pawson and Tilley[120] on realistic evaluation.

Box A.8 Quality checklist for action research designs.

1. Is there a clear statement of the aims and objectives of each stage of the research, and was there an innovation?

- Did the authors clearly define the aims and objectives of the project?
- Were the aims and objectives appropriate?
- Was an innovation being considered at the outset, or did one arise during the course of the project?

2. Was the action research relevant to practitioners and users?

- Did it address local issues?
- Does it contribute something new to understanding of the issues?
- Was it relevant to the experience of those participating?
- Is further research suggested?
- Is it stated how the action research will influence policy and practice in general?

3. Were the phases of the project clearly outlined?

- Was a logical process in evidence, including problem identification, planning, action (change or intervention that was implemented), and evaluation?
- Did these influence the process and progress of the project?

4. Were the participants and stakeholders clearly described and justified?

- Did the project focus on health professionals, health care administrators, or health care teams?
- Is it stated who was selected and by whom for each phase of the project?
- Is it discussed how participants were selected for each phase of the project?

5. Was consideration given to the local context while implementing change?

- Is it clear which context was selected, and why, for each phase of the project?
- Is there a critical examination of values, beliefs and power relationships?
- Is there a discussion of who would be affected by the change and in what way?
- Was the context appropriate for this type of study?

6. Was the relationship between researchers and participants adequately considered?

- Is the level and extent of participation clearly defined for each stage?
- Are the types of relationships that evolved over the course of the project acknowledged?
- Did the researchers and participants critically examine their own roles, potential biases and influences, i.e. were they reflexive?

7. Was the project managed appropriately?

- Were key individuals approached and involved where appropriate?
- Did those involved appear to have the requisite skills for carrying out the various tasks required to implement change and research?
- Was there a feasible implementation plan that was consistent with the skills, resources and time available?
- Was this adjusted in response to local events and participants?
- Is there a clear discussion of the actions taken (the change or the intervention) and the methods used to evaluate them?

8. Were ethical issues encountered and how were they dealt with?

- Was consideration given to participants, researchers and those affected by the action research process?
- Was consideration given to underlying professional values? How were these explored and realised in practice?
- Were confidentiality and informed consent addressed?

Continued

9. Was the study adequately funded/supported?
- Were the assessments of cost and resources realistic?
- Were there any conflicts of interest?

10. Was the length and timetable of the project realistic?
- Is a timetable given for the project and, if appropriate, an indication of where the section being reported fits into the overall timetable?

11. Were data collected in a way that addressed the research issue?
- Were appropriate methods and techniques used to answer research questions?
- Is it clear how data were collected, and why, for each phase of the project?
- Were data collection and record-keeping systematic?
- If methods were modified during data collection, is an explanation provided?

12. Were steps taken to promote the rigour of the findings?
- Were differing perspectives on issues sought?
- Did the researchers undertake method and theoretical triangulation?
- Were the key findings of the project fed back to participants at key stages?
- How was their feedback used?
- Do the researchers offer a reflexive account?

13. Were data analyses sufficiently rigorous?
- Were procedures for analysis described?
- Were the analyses systematic? What steps were made to guard against selectivity?
- Do the researchers explain how the data presented were selected from the original sample?
- Are arguments, themes, concepts and categories derived from the data?
- Are points of tension, contrast or contradiction identified?
- Are competing arguments presented?

14. Was the study design flexible and responsive?
- Were findings used to generate plans and ideas for change?
- Was the approach adapted to circumstances and issues of real-life settings: i.e. are justifications offered for changes in plan?

15. Are there clear statements of the findings and outcomes of each phase of the study?
- Are the findings and outcomes presented logically for each phase of the study?
- Are they explicit and easy to understand?
- Are they presented systematically and critically – can the reader judge the range of evidence/research being used?
- Are there discussions of personal and practical developments?

16. Do the researchers link the data that are presented to their own commentary and interpretation?
- Are justifications for methods of reflection provided?
- Is there a discussion of how participants were engaged in reflection?
- Is there a clear distinction made between the data and their interpretation?
- Have researchers critically examined their own and others' roles in the interpretation of data?
- Is sufficient evidence presented to satisfy the reader about the evidence and the conclusions?

17. Is the connection with an existing body of knowledge made clear?
- Is there a range of sources of ideas, categories and interpretations?
- Are theoretical and ideological insights offered?

Continued

Box A.8 Quality checklist for action research designs (*continued*).

18. Is there discussion of the extent to which aims and objectives were achieved at each stage?
- Have action research objectives been met?
- Are the reasons for successes and failures analysed?

19. Are the findings of the study transferable?
- Could the findings be transferred to other settings?
- Is the context of the study clearly described?

20. Have the authors articulated the criteria upon which their own work is to be read/judged?
- Have the authors justified the perspective from which the proposal or report should be interpreted?

Source: Adapted slightly from Waterman *et al.*[278]

Appendix 3

Descriptive statistics on included studies

In total, we considered over 100 books or book chapters and 6000 titles or abstracts from electronic sources, of which 495 (excluding 13 duplicate publications) ultimately contributed to our final report. We added a further 10 references at proof stage to support statements queried by proofreaders, but these references were not considered in detail in our analysis. Our sources are summarised in Figure 2.1 (page 36) and in Tables A.1 and A.2.

Our early 'non-systematic' searching (e.g. browsing) provided much of the background to the study. This early fluid phase allowed us to conceptualise a structure for this book that was based on the research traditions set out in Chapter 3, though this was by no means a straightforward task. In addition to Rogers'[3] key work, 16 books provided particularly authoritative reviews of the primary literature.[27,46,78,98,137,227,240,241,260,308,485–490] We found that books often provided better descriptions of concepts and theoretical models (and were sometimes a better source of empirical studies) than journal articles. Books were generally better identified by asking experts than by formal search of bibliographic databases.

The yield from our hand search is shown in Table A.3 (page 249). The number of potentially relevant journals to hand search was very high; but with very few exceptions (e.g. *Administrative Sciences Quarterly*), the yield from any one journal turned out to be extremely low. For example, we searched a total of 8000 articles in the *Annals of Internal Medicine* and found a single article relevant to our search! Nevertheless, as shown in Table A.1 (page 247) some important sources were identified exclusively by this method. The yield from electronic searches is shown in Table A.4 (page 252). Again, because the literature was so widely dispersed and inconsistently indexed, we found that the signal-to-noise ratio was high and the electronic search proved laborious, time-consuming and often disheartening.

Scanning the references of papers that we had identified as high quality and relevant was a far more fruitful technique than 'cold' searching by hand or electronically. Electronic citation tracking of the 15 papers that we identified as likely to be 'seminal' (including all the systematic reviews and meta-analyses), of which 5 actually proved seminal, produced a further 36 valid and relevant hits, including over 20 recent high-quality empirical studies. Figures for citation tracking are shown in Table A.5 (page 254). The main reason why some potentially seminal papers had rarely been cited was probably their year of publication: we found that papers less than 5 years old had generally only been cited in editorials and non-systematic overviews, but had not yet shown a direct influence on empirical research. As mentioned above, we found that many seminal texts, especially in the management literature, were books rather than journals and not easily amenable to electronic citation tracking.

A surprisingly high proportion of valid and relevant papers came our way informally, when colleagues (and contacts of colleagues) who knew we were doing this review kindly sent material unsolicited. These included two high-quality systematic reviews[41,91] that were not initially uncovered by the more formal and systematic approaches. Finally, a small but important group of sources was discovered serendipitously, when we chanced across a relevant paper when looking for something else.

A number of previous research teams have attempted to summarise and synthesise the literature on diffusion of innovations and related topics. Their scope and emphasis is summarised in Table A.6 (page 255). Given the extent and complexity of the literature, the well-described limitations of meta-analysis of non-experimental data (see Chapter 2), and the low analytical power that was possible in the meta-analyses published in this field[14–16,62] (e.g. Section 4.2, page 87; Section 6.2, page 118; and Section 9.3, page 180), we believe that the 'expert narrative overview' followed by most reviewers listed in Table A.6 is a defensible methodological approach (indeed, arguably, it is the preferred approach[2]). Because of the constraints of this project and our own main focus on organisational innovations, we did not attempt to validate independently the primary studies presented by the authors of previous overviews, except where these studies fell directly within the scope of our own study.

The main meta-analyses of experimental data included were Grimshaw *et al.*[11] (235 primary studies reviewed), Grilli *et al.*[218] (17 primary studies), Zwarenstein *et al.*[221] (1042 primary studies), Freemantle[219] (11 primary studies), and O'Brien[54] (8 primary studies). We also referred to other meta-analyses that were of tangential relevance (e.g. our case studies of the electronic health record and telemedicine in Chapter 10).

The main meta-analyses of non-experimental data included in this review were Tornatsky and Klein[62] (75 primary studies), Granados[89] (about 100 primary studies, which included a small number of experimental studies), Damanpour[14] (23 primary studies), Damanpour[15] (20 primary studies), and Damanpour[16] (21 primary studies).

In total, we found 27 different primary research designs, which we grouped into 9 broader categories (Table A.2, page 248).

Table A.1 Main sources and yield of papers, books and book chapters.

	Empirical research studies	*Theoretical or 'overview' sources*	*Total*
Electronic database search [see Table A.2, page 248]	75 (35%)	51 (18%)	126 (26%)
Hand search	12 (6%)	12 (4%)	24 (5%)
Tracking references of references	87 (41%)	131 (44%)	218 (43%)
Citation tracking[a]	26 (12%)	8 (3%)	34 (7%)
Sources known to research team[b]	15 (7%)	70 (24%)	85 (17%)
Social networks of research team[c]	4 (2%)	25 (8%)	29 (5%)
Serendipitous[d]	2 (1%)	3 (1%)	5 (1%)
Raw total including double counting[e]	220 (104%)	300 (107%)	520 (105%)
Total papers in final report	213 (100%)	282 (100%)	495 (100%)

[a]Using electronic search methods to track forwards a particular paper to identify subsequent papers that cited it in the reference list.
[b]Books and journal articles of which the research team were aware before the study began.
[c]Passed on by a colleague in response to a personal or email request for relevant books or papers.
[d]Finding a relevant paper for this study when looking for something else.
[e]Numbers add up to more than 100% because some sources were located by more than one method. The proportion of sources 'double counted' is probably a substantial underestimate since (for example) we did not flag a paper identified in a reference track if we already had it on file.
Note: This book contains 10 additional references not included in this table. Nine of these were added at proof stage to back up statements that had been queried by proof readers of a previous draft. We also added a newly published systematic review that had been detected by an automated electronic search command but which appeared too late to be included in our main analysis.[481]

Table A.2 Breakdown of studies included in the book.

Research design	*Number of studies contributing to final report*
Experimental and quasi-experimental designs	
Randomised controlled trial	8
Other comparative trial	1
Quasi-experimental (e.g. interrupted time series)	2
Non-experimental designs	
Action research	6
Attribution study (i.e. assessing the attributes of innovations)	11
Case study (in-depth, mixed methodology, comparative)	56
Case study (in-depth, mixed methodology, single)	37
Mathematical model	13
Network analysis	26
Qualitative interview or focus group	2
Survey (including in-depth qualitative and questionnaire)	49
Unclassifiable	2
Total primary studies	**213**
Secondary research (excluding non-systematic reviews or editorials)	
Narrative systematic review	7
Meta-analysis that included experimental data	11
Meta-analysis of non-experimental data	4
Total secondary studies (covering a total of around 600 additional primary studies)	**22**

Note: Numbers add up to more than 100% as some studies included more than one design; the low number of randomised controlled trials was partly due to our decision not to review primary studies if they had already been included in published meta-analyses.

Table A.3 Yield from hand search of journals.

			Number of papers found		
Body of literature	*Journal*	*Years searched*	*Total found in initial search*	*Contributed to final report*	*Comment*
Biomedicine	*American Journal of Medical Quality*	1990–2002	4	0	Overall, the yield from hand searching, especially biomedical journals, was disappointing and the reasons for this are discussed in the text (page 245)
	Annals of Internal Medicine	1985–2002	10	1	
	British Medical Journal	1985–2002	20	17[a]	
	British Journal of General Practice	1990–2002	6	1	
	Health Service Journal	1990–2002	0	0	
	Health Services Research	1990–2002	4	0	
	Health Technology Assessment	1990–2002	0	0	
	International Journal of Quality in Healthcare	1990–2002	1	0	
	International Journal of Technology Assessment in Healthcare	1990–2002	2	1	

Continued

Table A.3 continued: Yield from hand search of journals.

			Number of papers found		
Body of literature	*Journal*	*Years searched*	*Total found in initial search*	*Contributed to final report*	*Comment*
	Journal of American Medical Association	1990–2002	10	7	
	Journal of Evaluation in Clinical Practice	1990–2002	1	1	
	Joint Commission on Quality Improvement	1990–2002	4	0	
	Journal of Management in Medicine	1990–2002	3	0	
	Journal of Quality in Clinical Practice	1990–2002	1	0	
	Lancet	1990–2002	2	1	
	Medical Care	1990–2002	5	2	
	New England Journal of Medicine	1990–2002	3	1	
	Qualitative Health Research	1990–2002	2	2	
	Quality [& Safety] in Healthcare	1990–2002	11	6	

	Social Science and Medicine	1985–2002	11	5	
Organisation and management	*Academy of Management Review*	1997–2002	12	6	Many additional articles from the management journals were of tangential relevance, but in view of the potentially vast scope of our review, we made a pragmatic decision to exclude studies that did not contribute centrally to our research question
	Administrative Sciences Quarterly	1997–2002	18	7	
	American Journal of Sociology	1997–2002	7	3	
	Californian Management Review	1997–2002	4	2	
	Human Relations	1997–2002	8	3	
	MIS Quarterly	1997–2002	1	0	
	Policy and Politics	1997–2002	0	0	
	Organisation Studies	1997–2002	11	7	
	Organisational Dynamics	1997–2002	6	2	
	Organisational Science	1997–2002	11	7	

[a] *British Medical Journal*, with which the hand searcher was particularly familiar, provided many background articles (e.g. on the nature of policymaking and the methodology of synthesis), but no empirical papers that contributed to the final report.

Table A.4 Yield from search of electronic databases.

Body of literature	Journal	Years accessed	Number of papers found		Comment
			Papers pulled	*Contributed to final report*	
Biomedical	Medline (general search as set out in Chapter 2)	1966–2002	70	49	The entire EPOC database (3200 references) was searched by hand since all were potentially relevant; several relevant primary studies listed on EPOC had been included in systematic reviews so were not pulled. Biomedical databases revealed a vast literature of potential relevance on the dissemination of evidence-based guidelines, which we did not review because a major systematic review was being undertaken by colleagues (now published[11]).
	Medline (search for named authors)	1966–2002	34	19	
	Medline (search for 'champion' and 'opinion leader')	1966–2002	12	6	
	EmBASE	1980–2002	18	14	
	CinAHL	1980–2002	19	12	
	Cochrane Database of Systematic Reviews	1995–2002	15	11	
	DARE			1	
	Effective Practice and Organisation of Care (EPOC) Database	1980–2002	25	6	
	CareData	1980–2002	2	2	
Social sciences and management	ZETOC	1980–2002	5	1	Electronic searching of social science and management databases proved less fruitful than hand searching and tracking references of references, largely because of inconsistency of index terms.
	ASSCI	1980–2002	13	6	

	Dissertation Abstracts International	1990–2002	12	3	
	Health Management Information Centre (incorporating DHdata and Kings Fund Database)	1980–2002	9	3	
Education	British Education Index	1986–2002	15	4	Educational databases provided some important sources that were not otherwise identified, especially in relation to models of adoption.
	ERIC	1985–2002	57	18	
Psychology	Psychinfo	1985–2002	33	10	Psychological databases indicated an important source of additional data from cognitive science on how individuals make decisions, which we did not review because of time and resource constraints.
	Psyclit	1985–2002	3	1	

[a]Using electronic search methods to track forwards a particular paper to identify subsequent papers that cited it in the reference list.
[b]There was a high degree of overlap between these closely linked meta-analyses (many papers cited all three); the results are therefore merged.
[c]Two paired editorials/reviews published in the same journal. Their results are presented as merged data.

Table A.5 Yield from electronic citation tracking[a].

		Number of references found			
Author/year	*Description of paper*	*Total citations of article*	Full text requested	*Valid and relevant*	*Comment*
Tornatsky and Klein (1982)[62]	Meta-analysis of attributes of innovations that determine their adoption in organisations	243	42	18	Very high yield of methodologically sound and relevant articles, with many new primary research studies. These two citation tracks produced an overlap of 8 papers – i.e. yield from both these sources was 29 papers.
Damanpour (1991),[14] (1992),[15] (1996)[16,b]	Three meta-analyses of characteristics of organisations that determine their innovativeness	170	57	19	
Green and Johnson (1996),[102] Johnson and Green (1996)[180,c]	Overview of past research and future priorities in dissemination of innovations in health promotion	18	9	4	These editorials summarised current thinking following a major 'blue skies' conference in Canada on dissemination of health promotion programmes; many papers that subsequently cited them were written by those who had attended the original conference.
Granados *et al.* (1997)[89]	Systematic review of approaches to disseminating health technology assessment reports	24	1	1	Surprisingly few citations of this major EU-funded review of the biomedical literature on dissemination, which assigned most weight to RCTs and dismissed qualitative studies of process evaluation.
Kraft *et al.* (2000)[491]	Overview and primary research study of health promotion programmes, which includes systematic review of diffusion of innovations literature from a technology transfer and knowledge utilisation perspective	7	2	1	Recent overview and conceptual piece, as yet only cited by other editorial/opinion papers.
Potvin *et al.* (2001)[10]	Overview of methodological challenges in evaluation of dissemination programmes	4	2	1	Recent overview and conceptual piece, as yet only cited by other editorial/opinion papers.

Note: Several additional 'seminal' reviews were published very recently[11,41,79,91,223,492] but in view of the diminishing yield from citation tracking on recently published papers we did not pursue these.

Appendix 4

Tables of included studies

Table A.6 Narrative overviews used as key sources in this review.

Author/year	*Field of study*	*Scope of the review*	*Method used*	*Comment*
Rogers 1995[3]	Sociology	Focuses primarily on the 'classical diffusion theory' – i.e. spread of ideas and practices between individuals via social networks, with an emphasis on the author's own field (rural sociology). Provides limited discussion of organisational research.	Narrative review. Falls short of formal systematic review (synthesis method 'based on past writing and research', page 208).	Undoubtedly an informed and scholarly summary by the acknowledged 'world authority' on classical diffusion
Wolfe 1994[174]	Organisation and management	A broad overview of innovation research in the organisation and management literature. Good sense of vast expansion in empirical work in this tradition in the 1980s and 1990s, e.g. identified 1299 journal articles and 351 dissertations addressing 'organisational innovation'.	Eclectic review of vast literature. No clear search strategy but highly systematic framework for analysis.	Useful source on key theoretical influences in organisational research
Strang and Soule 1998[124]	Sociology	An overview that begins on territory similar to that covered by Rogers – classical diffusion from a sociological perspective – but also includes a critical analysis of a wider body of literature relevant to diffusion of innovations in organisations.	Narrative review. Selection of primary studies seems eclectic and quality criteria are not given.	A sound and readable review whose strength is its scholarly and creative commentary
Meyers *et al.* 1999[91]	Organisation and management	Reviews a large, fragmented body of work on implementation in organisations, including process engineering, information technology, human resource management and marketing. Synthesises findings to develop a conceptual framework and derives propositions about effects of key factors on implementation.	Narrative review. Search strategy was not given and inclusion and quality criteria were implicit rather than explicit.	Well-written review with conceptually clear taxonomy, which is summarised in Section 9.3 (page 180)

Continued

Table A.6 continued: Narrative overviews used as key sources in this review.

Author/year	*Field of study*	*Scope of the review*	*Method used*	*Comment*
Gustafason 2003[89]	Change management	Review of primary studies from the change management literature relevant to implementation of innovations, linked to some empirical work (see Section 9.3, page 180). Synthesises primary and secondary research to develop a Bayesian model for predicting success of organisational change initiatives.	Search strategy not given in detail. Authoritative but not comprehensive overview of a vast and disparate literature.	An important complement to this book since we explicitly omitted 'mainstream' change management research from our own synthesis
Ellsworth 2003[432]	Education	Provides overview of the educational sociology literature, based on a wealth of primary studies, on a range of whole-systems approaches with different linked interventions at different levels.	Search strategy not given in detail. Appears comprehensive in relation to the educational literature but does not go beyond it.	In-depth overview; we have only included brief details in this book
Wejnert 2003[41]	Social and political sciences	Reviews the literature on diffusion of innovations in fields relatively distant from the focus of this review (political science, social movements, geography, environmental studies). Develops a conceptual framework that groups independent variables into 3 components: (a) characteristics of the innovation; (b) characteristics of the actors/adopters; (c) characteristics of the environmental context.	Narrative review. Search strategy was not given and inclusion and quality criteria were implicit rather than explicit.	An up-to-date, extensively referenced and theoretically robust narrative review

Note: One additional systematic review was identified as this book went to press. It focussed mainly on the diffusion of innovations in clinical behaviour.[481]

Table A.7 Empirical studies of attributes of health care innovations in the organisational setting (discussed in Section 4.3, page 90).

Author/year	*Field of study*	*Innovation*	*Target adopter*	*Type of study and number of participants*	*Attributes tested*	*Attributes found to predict adoption*	*Comment*
Marshall 1990[30]	Information services	Electronic database searching	Doctors and nurses	Survey of 150 clinicians	Relative advantage, compatibility, complexity, trialability, observability	Relative advantage and complexity were significant predictors of current use.	This study was undertaken before widespread Internet access to these databases.
Grilli and Lomas 1994[37]	Evidence-based practice	Clinical guidelines	Doctors	Survey of 23 studies involving 143 recommendations	Complexity, trialability, observability	Complexity, trialability and observability together accounted for 47% of variance in adoption.	Attributes evaluated by authors; perceptions of potential adopters were not measured directly.
Dirksen *et al.* 1996[29]	Surgery	6 surgical endoscopic procedures, e.g. appendicectomy, cholecystectomy	Surgeons in the Netherlands	Survey of 138 surgeons (82% response rate)	Perceptions of 3 attributes of the procedure, 6 of the system context, 3 social influence factors, plus perceived 'competition'	Different surgical procedures had very different adoption patterns, and different attributes had *different* impact depending on the procedure. 'Extra benefit' was a precondition for further evaluation by potential adopters.	This was a retrospective attribution study whose predictive power is therefore weak.

Continued

Table A.7 continued: Empirical studies of attributes of health care innovations in the organisational setting (discussed in Section 4.3, page 90).

Author/year	*Field of study*	*Innovation*	*Target adopter*	*Type of study and number of participants*	*Attributes tested*	*Attributes found to predict adoption*	*Comment*
Meyer *et al.* 1997[31]	American public health (cancer prevention)	3 cancer prevention projects undertaken in an interorganisational cancer information network	Mainly managers	Survey of 89 professionals (96% response rate)	Innovation attributes (relative advantage, compatibility, complexity, trialability, observability, adaptability [reinvention], riskiness, acceptance)	Relative advantage, complexity, reinvention, riskiness. Observability and trialability were not related to adoption. Compatibility proved impossible to measure accurately.	Authors suggest that impact of trialability and observability may have been overshadowed by strategic interorganisational decision to adopt these innovations.
Yetton *et al.* 1999[39]	Australian public health care system	IT system for human resource management	Managers	Survey of 133 potential users (67 usable replies)	Innovation attributes (task relevance, task usefulness) plus adopter characteristics and organisational variables	Only 3 factors were significant in the final model: task relevance, task usefulness, and physical access to the innovation.	Conclude that innovation attributes dominate for innovations whose impact is on the individual; but organisational variables dominate at team level.
Lia-Hoagberg *et al.* 1999[297]	Canadian public health	Practice guidelines	Nurses	Survey (51 replies) plus semi-structured interviews	Relative advantage, compatibility, complexity, trialability plus open questions	Complexity, competing agency demands, lack of time.	Small study of borderline methodological quality but shows creative use of free text questions.

Lee 2000[296]	Ambulatory care	Electronic medical record	Clinicians, managers, administrators	Survey of 115 individuals (83% response rate)	Compatibility, ease of use, image, relative advantage, result demonstrability, trialability, visibility, voluntariness	Different groups rated different attributes differently. Doctors perceived the EMR significantly less favourably than nurses and non-clinical respondents.	Actual adoption was not measured, but the finding that perceived attributes differ between professional groups is important and possibly generalisable.
Aubert and Hamel 2001[35]	Ambulatory care	'Smart card' medical record	Doctors, nurses, pharmacists, paramedics	287 (66% response rate)	Perceptions of 7 attributes of the innovation, 3 of the system context, plus 'satisfaction' and 'quality of support' (see text)	Ease of use, compatibility, perceived quality of support, voluntariness, and information were significant predictors of use of the record.	Possible Hawthorne effect – see page 93.
Dobbins *et al.* 2001[42]	Public health	Systematic reviews	Pubic health doctors	147 (96% response rate)	Relative advantage, ease of use, compatibility	Ease of use was the only attribute that proved significant in the final model.	Organisational attributes (size, differentiation, slack resources) did not influence use.
Foy *et al.* 2002[34]	Gynaecology	Clinical practice recommendations	Gynaecologists	Over 4000 clinical records; number of clinicians not stated	13 attributes (see page 91 for list)	Compatibility with values, no change needed to routines.	Incompatibility with values associated with greater *change* in behaviour after audit and feedback.

Table A.8 Empirical studies that focused on the *process* of adoption in health care organisations (discussed in Section 5.3, page 106).

Author/year	*Context*	*Innovation*	*Study design*	*Size and scope*	*Hypotheses tested*	*Main findings*	*Comment*
Meyer and Goes 1988[38] [see Tables A.12, A.14 and A.18]	US private (non-profit) community hospitals in 1980s	Health-related technologies (main focus was large pieces of equipment)	Comparative case study with over 300 interviews, and observation and surveys	12 innovations in 25 hospitals over 6 years; 300 potential adoption decisions	Assimilation of innovations by organisations is influenced by (a) environment, organisational context and leadership; (b) attributes of the innovation and (c) interaction between these	Assimilation of innovations was a lengthy and complex process. Hypotheses were broadly confirmed. Innovation attributes explained 37% of variance.	The notion of 'assimilation' as a 9-stage process rather than an all-or-none event is a potentially useful framework for studying organisational adoption
Gladwin and Wilson 2000[493]	A low-income African country	A health management information system	In-depth (ethnographic) case study	Innovation implemented nationally but extent of data collection not clear	Adoption of a high-technology health service innovation will be primarily determined by its degree of 'organisational fit'	Process of adoption was complex and barriers were identified at multiple levels. Many barriers were technological.	Compares diffusion of innovations theory and dynamic equilibrium organisational change theory as explanatory models
Champagne *et al.* 2001[64] [see Tables A.14 and A.18]	Canadian community hospitals	Sessional fees for GPs	Multiple case studies and correlational analysis	67 interviews in 27 long-term care hospitals over a 2-year period	Adoption of innovations is partly determined by the centrality of the innovation in relation to the actor's goals	Micropolitical factors (actors who controlled the power bases had greater influence on adoption than did structural factors)	One of the few studies that explicitly considered micropolitical factors

Timmons 2001[49]	3 UK hospitals	Computerised care planning system	Semi-structured interviews	Numbers not given	Explored perceived barriers to use of the new computer system by nurses	A wide range of tactics was employed by nurses, aimed at ensuring non-adoption	Explained in terms of internal power relations and meaning of the system for staff
Fitzgerald *et al.* 2002[32] [see Tables A.14, A.16 and A.19]	UK health care	8 'evidence into practice' initiatives	Comparative case study	8 case studies	How is complex evidence implemented at an organisational level?	The nature of diffusion is highly interactive. There is no single, all-or-none adoption decision	Authors comment on the ambiguous, contested and socially mediated nature of new scientific knowledge
Denis *et al.* 2002[33]	Canadian hospitals and primary care	4 innovations selected as a maximum-variety sample	Qualitative cross-case analysis	4 in-depth case studies	Adoption of complex innovations is determined by subtle and complex interactions between multiple variables	Hypothesis was confirmed	The methodology of cross-case analysis is potentially very powerful if in-depth qualitative methods are used

Note: See also Table A.22, page 289, especially Edmundson *et al.*[95]

Table A.9 Network analyses of interpersonal influence in health care organisations (discussed in Section 6.1, page 114).

Author/year	*Context*	*Innovation*	*Study design and size*	*Nature of social group(s)*	*Hypotheses tested*	*Main findings*	*Comment*
Fennell and Warnecke 1988[36] [see also Tables A.10, A.16 and A.18]	US cancer care	Cancer management strategies	Descriptive historical case study of each network and a comparative analysis	Clinicians	Homophily between clinicians will enhance communication of innovations	Homophily was an independent predictor of spread	See Table A.10, page 263, Table A.16, page 276, and Table A.18, page 280, for additional hypotheses from this study
West *et al.* 1999[51]	UK NHS hospital trusts	Findings of research – i.e. evidence-based policies and practices	Network analysis (via semi-structured interviews)	Clinical directors (doctors and nurses)	To what extent can (a) network density; (b) centrality; and (c) centralisation explain the diffusion of innovations amongst doctor and nurse clinical directors?	Professional socialisation and structural location are important determinants of social networks. Doctors and nurses are differently situated in their respective social networks – doctors have denser, more horizontal networks and are better at promoting adoption through informal influence, whereas nurses' networks are more vertical and hence better suited to dissemination through formal channels	See article for good discussion on implications of the findings for spread of ideas in contemporary health services

Note: Opinion leadership studies are covered separately in Table A.10.

Table A.10 Empirical studies of opinion leadership in health care organisations (discussed in Section 6.2, page 118).

Author/year	*Context*	*Innovation*	*Study design*	*Sample*	*Hypotheses tested or question explored*	*Main findings*	*Comment*
'Opinion leader' identified through sociometric analysis							
Coleman *et al.* 1966[5]	US ambulatory care in the 1960s	Tetracycline prescribing	Network analysis via semi-structured interviews	128 doctors	Interpersonal influence and mass media (journal advertisements) both have an impact on a doctor's decision to start prescribing a new drug	Mass media creates awareness but interpersonal influence vastly more important in changing behaviour	'Landmark' book that gave rise to the idea of opinion leadership in the medical literature and to drug company 'detailers'
Becker 1970[52,192]	US public health	(a) Measles immunisation ('low uncertainty'); (b) Diabetes screening ('high uncertainty')	Network analysis via questionnaire survey	95 directors of public health departments across 3 US states	The nature of the innovation (high or low uncertainty) *and* the influence of interpersonal communication will determine time to adoption	Measles immunisation was adopted quickly by public health departments; diabetes screening spread very slowly at first then took off	See page 120 for discussion of different dissemination patterns for these different innovations – which suggests a complex interaction between variables
Fennell and Wernecke[36] [see also Tables A.9, A.16 and A.18]	US cancer care	Cancer management strategies	Network analysis via questionnaire survey	Cancer clinicians in 88 hospitals (number not given)	Opinion leaders lie at critical points in the social network	Hypothesis confirmed. Opinion leaders also have linkages outside the group to sources of information regarded as important by its members	See Table A.9, page 262, Table A.16, page 276, and Table A.18, page 280 for additional hypotheses from this study

Continued

Table A.10 continued: Empirical studies of opinion leadership in health care organisations (discussed in Section 6.2, page 118).

Author/year	*Context*	*Innovation*	*Study design*	*Sample*	*Hypotheses tested or question explored*	*Main findings*	*Comment*
'Opinion leader' as an intervention in randomised trials (see Table A.11 for details of primary studies in this review and two additional trials left out of this table for clarity)							
O'Brien *et al.* 2003[54]	[Cochrane review]	'Evidence-based' clinician behaviour	Systematic review of controlled trials	8 trials involving a total of 293 health professionals	The presence of an opinion leader will improve the uptake of evidence-based recommendations	Opinion leaders had no significant impact on process or outcome of care in 6 of 8 studies	See separate summary of primary studies in Table A.11. See page 122 for discussion on limitations of RCT design
'Knowledge utilisation' approach to evidence-based medicine taken by social scientists							
Dopson *et al.* 1999[369] and Locock *et al.* 2001[53]	UK health care	A wide range of 'evidence into practice' initiatives	In-depth case studies (mainly qualitative)	22 case studies; hundreds of interviews	How is complex evidence implemented at the organisational level?	Opinion leadership is an important variable; 2 main types: peer and expert	In general, qualitative studies showed a much more powerful and diverse impact of opinion leaders on the adoption and assimilation of innovations than was shown in controlled trials (see text for discussion)
Fitzgerald *et al.* 2002[32,356]	UK health care	8 'evidence into practice' initiatives	Comparative case study	8 case studies	How is complex evidence implemented at the organisational level?	Opinion leadership is an important variable; three main types: peer, expert, and boundary spanner	

Table A.11 Controlled trials of opinion leaders as an intervention in health care organisations (discussed in Section 6.2, page 118).

Author/ year	*Context*	*Innovation*	*Intervention/ control*	*Sample size*	*How was opinion leadership measured?*	*Main outcome variables*	*Main findings*
Studies included in the Thomson O'Brien systematic review (last updated November 1998; accessed June 2003)							
Stross 1980[501]	US hospitals	Rheumatoid arthritis guideline	Opinion leader vs none	6 hospitals; 174 patients	Questionnaire (Hiss *et al.*[337])	Process of care in line with guideline	Small but non-significant impact in favour of intervention
Stross 1983[502]	US hospitals	Pulmonary disease guideline	Opinion leader vs none	16 hospitals; 510 patients	Questionnaire (Hiss *et al.*[337])	Process of care in line with guideline; mortality	Small but non-significant impact in favour of intervention
Stross 1985[503]	US hospitals	Osteoarthritis guideline	Opinion leader vs none	6 hospitals; 586 patients	Questionnaire (Hiss *et al.*[337])	Process of care in line with guideline	Small but non-significant impact in favour of intervention
Hong 1990[504]	Hong Kong hospitals	Correct catheter use	Opinion leader vs lecture vs both	220 nurses; 255 episodes of care	Knowledge and the ability to influence peers'	Process of care in line with guideline	Significant impact in favour of intervention
Lomas *et al.* 1997[338]	Canadian hospitals	Patient-centred obstetric care	Opinion leader vs audit/feedback vs none	16 hospitals; 76 physicians	Questionnaire (Hiss *et al.*[337])	Process (trial of labour offered) and outcome of care (vaginal delivery achieved)	Significant impact in favour of intervention
Hodnett 1996[505]	Canadian hospitals	Patient-centred obstetric care	Opinion leader vs none	20 hospitals	Questionnaire (Hiss *et al.*[337])	Outcome of care (interventional delivery)	No overall difference in outcome between groups
Elliott 1998[96]	US cancer care	Evidence-based pain management	Opinion leader + outreach vs none	6 hospitals	Questionnaire (Hiss *et al.*[337])	Physician knowledge and attitudes; patient pain score	No overall difference in outcome between groups

Continued

Table A.11 continued: Controlled trials of opinion leaders as an intervention in health care organisations (discussed in Section 6.2, page 181).

Author/ year	*Context*	*Innovation*	*Intervention/ control*	*Sample size*	*How was opinion leadership measured?*	*Main outcome variables*	*Main findings*
Soumerai *et al.* 1998[339]	US hospitals	Myocardial infarction management	Opinion leader + education vs audit and feedback	37 hospitals; 2938 patients	Questionnaire (Hiss *et al.*[337])	Process of care in line with guideline	Small but non-significant impact in favour of intervention
Additional studies identified in our search that met the criteria used in the above systematic review							
Searle *et al.* 2002[340]	Australian hospitals	Gynaecological surgery	Opinion leader + guideline vs no intervention	62 gynaecologists in 6 units	Questionnaire (Hiss *et al.*[337])	Reduction in unnecessary gynaecological procedures	Clinical behaviour changed in line with guidelines but no impact on procedure rates
Berner *et al.* 2003[341]	US hospitals	Quality improvement initiatives (5 target conditions)	3 arms: quality improvement with or without opinion leader vs no intervention	21 hospitals	Questionnaire (Hiss *et al.*[337])	Success of quality improvement initiative	Opinion leader arm did significantly better in only one of the five target conditions

Table A.12 Empirical studies of impact of champions in health care organisations and selected other examples (discussed in Section 6.3, page 126).

Author/year	*Context*	Innovation	*Study design and size*	*Type of champion*	*Hypothesised role of the champion*	*Main findings*	*Comment*
Meyer and Goes 1988[38] [see Tables A.8, A.12, A.14 and A.18]	US private (non-profit) community hospitals in 1980s	Health-related technologies (main focus was large pieces of equipment)	Comparative case study of 12 innovations in 25 hospitals over 6 years	Chief executive officer (CEO) advocacy	Innovations are more likely to be assimilated when CEOs are influential proponents	CEO advocacy added significantly to a multiple regression model for assimilation of innovations, but the absolute magnitude of effect was small	'Advocacy' of CEO measured as a composite of his or her (a) support for the innovation and (b) decision-making influence
O'Loughlin *et al.* 1998[349] [see Table A.21]	Community-based heart health promotion in Canada	212 separate innovations, e.g. risk factor screening, smoking cessation	Telephone survey of 189 key informants (93% response rate)	Programme champion (person who 'strongly advocated' for continuation of the programme)	Programme champion is a necessary criterion for the sustainability (institutionalisation) of a health promotion programme	Presence of programme champion was highly significantly associated with sustainability of the programme (odds ratio 2.3)	Programme champion was one of 40 variables tested in a closed questionnaire. Categorised dichotomously as 'present' or 'absent'
Backer and Rogers 1998[57]	US occupational health in mid-1990s	Work-site AIDS policies based on Business Response to AIDS (BRTA) model	4 in-depth case studies of companies considering BRTA	An individual who gains attention and resources for an issue	Variable role but hypothesised that without a champion the adoption decision is delayed considerably	The two 'early adopter' firms had a clearly identifiable champion; the other two firms did not	Small study with little methodological detail; hard to judge whether researchers were merely confirming their preconceptions

Continued

Table A.12 continued: Empirical studies of impact of champions in health care organisations and selected other examples (discussed in Section 6.3, page 126).

Author/year	*Context*	Innovation	*Study design and size*	*Type of champion*	*Hypothesised role of the champion*	*Main findings*	*Comment*
Valois *et al.* 2000[350]	School health programmes in southern USA	Coordinated school health program (CSHP) infrastructure	Detailed questionnaire survey completed by evaluation team	7 schools in 3 separate communities	'Project management/liaison/facilitation'; a designated staff member who engaged with the programme, desired additional responsibility, was well respected by peers, and embraced the championing role.	Of 8 hypothesised factors needed for successful implementation, 4 proved significant, including presence of identifiable champion	Used non-standard method for producing quantitative values, which did not allow the contribution of each factor to be assessed relative to others; hence results should be interpreted with caution
Riley 2003[215] [see Tables A.14, A.19 and A.23]	Community-based heart health promotion in Canada	Wide range of community-based heart health interventions	In-depth comparative case study	Internal champion with decision-making authority	No prior hypothesis as this was an in-depth case study	Champion with public health background and decision-making authority appeared critical to programme success	Authors comment that *interaction* between champion and external factors (e.g. nature and strength of evidence) was particularly noteworthy in some programmes

Table A.13 Meta-analyses that addressed the impact of the organisational context on adoption of innovations (discussed in Section 7.2, page 135).

Author/year	*Source of studies*	*Sample size*	Aim of meta-analysis	*Main findings*	*Comment*
Damanpour 1991[14]	Sociological abstracts (1960–1988), plus references from recent review articles and other sources[a]	23 (21 papers and 2 books)	To test the hypothesis that the rate of adoption of multiple innovations (organisational innovativeness) is determined by particular organisational factors ('determinants'). In all, 14 structural, process, resource and cultural variables were tested.	Statistically significant association between 10 of the 14 determinants and organisational innovativeness. The strongest and most significant determinants were specialisation, functional differentiation and external communication (see Table 7.1, page 136, for definitions).	Results suggest that relations between these determinants and innovation are stable across studies, casting doubt on previous assertions of their instability.
Damanpour 1992[15]	Sociological abstracts; psychological and economic abstracts (no date range supplied), plus other sources as above (see footnote)	20 (18 papers and 2 books)	To specify the strength of the association between organisational size and organisational innovativeness, and to delineate the role of various moderators of this association.	Organisational size is positively related to innovation. Moderators included the measure of size (e.g. relation between size and innovativeness increased if size was measured by turnover rather than number of staff), type of organisation (for-profit companies had a closer correlation between size and innovativeness), and stage in the innovation process (more closely related to implementation than initiation), but not to the nature of the innovation.	Size was probably a proxy for other variables, e.g. slack, complexity (see subsequent study in row below).

Continued

Table A.13 continued: Meta-analyses that addressed the impact of the organisational context on adoption of innovations (discussed in Section 7.2, page 135).

Author/year	*Source of studies*	*Sample size*	Aim of meta-analysis	*Main findings*	*Comment*
Damanpour 1996[16]	Sociological, psychological and economic abstracts (1991); empirical studies (published 1960–1990) in English language	21 studies including 27 separate correlations on complexity and 36 correlations on size	To explore further the relationship between organisational complexity (independent variable) and innovativeness (dependent variable). Two measures of complexity were used: (a) structural complexity and (b) organisational size. Also considered 14 'contingency factors' that mediated or moderated this relationship (see page 135 et seq. for further discussion).	Both structural complexity and organisational size are positively related to organisational innovation and explain, about 15% and 12%, respectively, of variation in it. Contingency factors common to both indicators were: environmental uncertainty; use of service organisations; focus on technical innovations; and focus on product innovations.	Again, the demonstrated impact of organisational factors on innovativeness appears stable and challenges previously held views that the empirical literature is inconsistent.

[a]The reviews were: Daft,[494] Damanpour,[495] Kimberly,[352] and Tornatzky and Klein.[62] Also included were Rogers *et al.*[496] and Glazer and Montgomery.[497]

Table A.14 Empirical studies of 'inner' context determinants of innovation in health care organisations and selected other examples.

Author/year	*Innovation and context*	*Study design and size*	*Factors hypothesised to affect innovativeness*	*Significant associations actually demonstrated*	*Comment*
Baldridge and Burnham 1975[63]	Organisational innovations in US schools in the late 1960s	Qualitative interviews and questionnaires; 271 school districts	(a) Proportion of innovative individuals; (b) size and complexity; (c) changing environment	Size and complexity only	'Landmark' study that challenged previous assumptions that innovative individuals can make their organisations more innovative
Kimberly and Evanisko 1981[59] [see Tables A.16 and A.18]	Technological and administrative innovations in US hospitals in late 1970	Mixed methodology with questionnaires, described in a separate article;[498] number of hospitals not given	(a) Characteristics of individuals in authority (b) organisational characteristics; (c) contextual factors	Size was most significantly and consistently associated with innovation; other organisational variables also impacted on technological, but not administrative, innovations	The variables tested were much better predictors of the adoption of new medical technologies than of administrative innovations
Meyer and Goes 1988[38] [see Tables A.8, A.12 and A.18]	12 organisation-level medical innovations introduced into US community hospitals in late 1970s	Comparative case study over 6 years with over 300 interviews, and observation and surveys	Assimilation of innovations by organisations is influenced by (a) environment, organisational context and leadership; (b) attributes of the innovation and (c) interaction between these	Contextual factors accounted for only about 11% of the observed variation; environmental variables had little demonstrable impact	Results closely resemble those of Kimberly and Evanisko[59]
Champagne *et al.* 1991[64] [see Tables A.8 and A.18]	Sessional fee remuneration for general practitioners in hospitals in Canada	Qualitative study of long-term care hospitals in Quebec, 1984–1985; 27 in main study	(a) Political factors including leaders' satisfaction with the organisation's performance; (b) organisational factors including size; (c) urbanisation	Political factors had a strong positive association, and size a small negative association, with implementation	The surprising negative association between size and implementation is discussed in the text (page 144)

Continued

Table A.14 continued: Empirical studies of 'inner' context determinants of innovation in health care organisations and selected other examples.

Author/year	*Innovation and context*	*Study design and size*	*Factors hypothesised to affect innovativeness*	*Significant associations actually demonstrated*	*Comment*
Burns and Wholey 1993[65] [see Table A.16]	Unit/matrix management in US general hospitals	Retrospective and longitudinal questionnaire surveys (study specific and national data)	Several measures of organisational structure plus embeddedness in external networks and normative institutional pressures	(a) Diversification and scale (a measure of size); (b) sociometric location in network; (c) dissemination of information; (d) interorganisational norms	Combination of 'inner context' and 'outer context' factors were both found to be significant; no overall effect of organisational size, but small hospitals excluded from sample
Goes and Park 1997[68] [see Table A.16]	15 innovations in Californian acute care hospitals including 6 technical and 11 administrative	Prospective longitudinal study over 10 years; tracked year-to-year changes on 135 items	(a) Size; (b) interorganisational links ('enduring transactions, flows and linkages that occur among or between an organisation, and one or more organisations in its environment')	Positive association was shown between (a) size and (b) interorganisational links and adoption of both technical and administrative innovations	Hospital exhibiting multiple and extensive interorganisational links were more likely to be large; large hospitals were consistently more innovative than small hospitals
Anderson and West 1998[69]	US hospitals; any product or process judged as an innovation by staff	Postal survey of management teams in 27 hospitals – total sample of 155 managers	An 'organisational climate' scale with 4 subscales: vision, participative safety, task orientation, and support for innovation	Support for innovation was predicted on overall innovation score; participative safety predicted number of innovations and self-reported innovativeness	See Section 7.7, page 150, for definitions and further discussion
Wilson *et al.* 1999[74]	Medical imaging diagnostic technologies in US hospitals	Postal survey of 70 hospitals	Organisations with a greater risk-oriented climate are likely to (a) adopt innovations that are more radical and (b) adopt innovations with higher relative advantage	Risk-oriented organisations tend to adopt more radical innovations ($r = 0.22$, $p < 0.06$) and innovations that provide greater relative advantage ($r = 0.23$, $p < 0.05$)	Related analysis to Nystrom *et al.* (see below)

Continued

Table A.14 continued: Empirical studies of 'inner' context determinants of innovation in health care organisations and selected other examples.

Author/year	*Innovation and context*	*Study design and size*	*Factors hypothesised to affect innovativeness*	*Significant associations actually demonstrated*	*Comment*
Castle 2001[73]	Special and subacute care units in nursing homes in USA (1992–1997)	Analysis of national data-set	Organisations with (a) larger size; (b) membership of a chain; (c) for-profit and (d) greater proportion of private patients will adopt the innovation more rapidly	Size, chain membership and proportion of private patients were all significantly associated with earlier adoption	Findings may not be generalisable beyond the US health care setting
Fitzgerald *et al.* 2002[32] [see Tables A.8, A.14, A.16 and A.19]	UK NHS (1995–1999): 8 case studies (5 technological and 3 organisational)	In-depth comparative case studies (4 in acute sector, 4 in primary care)	(a) Organisational context; (b) absorptive capacity (i.e. underlying capacity of organisations to absorb new knowledge)	Diffusion influenced by interplay of (a) credibility of evidence; (b) characteristics of the multiple groups of actors; (c) features of the organisation; (d) context	Various factors interact in a complex way to influence diffusion
Nystrom *et al.* 2002[76] [see Table A.18]	Medical imaging diagnostic technologies in US hospitals (same data-set as Wilson *et al.*)	Postal questionnaire survey of 70 hospitals	Organisational size and slack, moderated by aspects of organisational climate (risk orientation and external orientation)	Organisational size and slack promotes innovation, and does so more strongly in organisations with a climate favouring risk-taking	Good example of a more contemporary approach that attempted to measure interaction between multiple variables
Gosling *et al.* 2003[70]	Australian acute hospital care: an online evidence retrieval system	Survey of team climate in 18 teams in 3 hospitals	Team size (< 15 or >15); team climate by validated Team Climate Inventory	Positive team climate has no effect on initial adoption decision but is independently associated with effective and sustained use	Small teams had higher levels of system awareness than large teams
Newton *et al.* 2003[71]	UK primary health care: new models and approaches to delivery of primary care services	Case study of a single personal medical service pilot	That the 8 factors Pettigrew *et al.* identified (e.g. quality and coherence of policy; key people leading the change – see text for others) make up the receptive context for change	Most significant association was between quality and coherence of policy, key people leading the change, supportive organisational culture and effective managerial clinical relations	Highlights the temporal ordering of factors: e.g. as the salience of 'policy' (factor 1) receded, the salience of networks (factor 6) increased

Table A.15 Empirical studies from health care that looked at the organisational context for innovation from a knowledge utilisation perspective (discussed in Section 7.8, page 154).

Author/year	*Research context and focus*	*Design*	*Main research question*	*Factors shown to enhance or support knowledge utilisation*	*Factors shown to inhibit knowledge utilisation*
Barnsley *et al.* 1998[61]	Implementation of integrated care delivery system in US hospitals	Review; in-depth case study	What are the barriers and facilitators to effective utilisation and dissemination of knowledge in integrated delivery systems in the health care sector?	(a) Shared vision of organisational goals and contribution of learning to these; (b) facilitative leadership (provides opportunities, resources, incentives, and rewards for learning); (c) diverse, 'organic' communication channels Consider predisposing, enabling and reinforcing activities under these headings (Table 7.6, page 156)	(a) Organisational instability; (b) unclear change process; (c) lack of middle managers to lead cross-organisational teams; (d) inappropriate budget practices that do not support systemwide learning; (e) information overload
Patel 1996[67]	Canadian public health	Editorial review	How can knowledge be used for health education? What are the barriers to knowledge use? What is the role of cognition in bridging some of these impediments?	(a) Proper communication between the 'designers' of the message and the 'users'; (b) understanding of the culture of end-users	(a) Clash of conceptual models; (b) differences in sociocultural belief systems; (c) symbols and images are considered as having universal standards for interpretation
Dufault *et al.* 1995[66]	Improving nurses' pain assessment practice	Quasi-experimental design testing the collaborative research use model	Does the model change nurses' practice? Does it improve their competency in research utilisation?	(a) There exists a body of validated knowledge with a high degree of predictability; (b) user has ability to translate and use knowledge; (c) organisation promotes a 'research climate'	(a) Lack of trust between change agent and intended user; (b) knowledge offered was not based on the needs of the nurses – i.e. was insufficiently 'personalised'

Dopson *et al.* 2002[75]	Implementing evidence-based practice	Secondary analysis of data from 7 previously published in-depth case studies, involving around 1400 interviews	What are the barriers and facilitators to getting research evidence into practice in health care organisations	(a) Social construction of the meaning of evidence between different actors and groups; (b) interprofessional networks; (c) opinion leaders; (d) external incentives; (e) creation of receptive context for change – comprising leadership, clear goals, good relationships, and information sharing	(a) Professional boundaries; (b) access to knowledge (often different for different professional groups); (c) different groups' different 'hierarchies' of evidence; (d) multiple types of evidence; (e) external disincentives
Rashman and Hartley 2002[72]	Knowledge transfer in the UK Beacon Council Scheme	In-depth case study involving 59 in-depth interviews plus observation of learning events	How do 'Beacons' work? Specifically, how is knowledge transferred between organisations?	(a) Social interaction between actors from originating and recipient organisations; (b) conversion of tacit knowledge to explicit knowledge; (c) matching of learning and training to the needs of the actor and the nature of the knowledge; (d) capacity for knowledge transfer in receiving organisation – comprising facilitative leadership, shared vision, trust, problem setting, strong internal networks, and distributed decision-making	(a) Initiative fatigue and financial pressures; (b) insufficient attention to need of learners to apply their learning in the context of their own organisation

Table A.16 Empirical studies of informal interorganisational influence amongst health care organisations and selected other examples.

Author/year	*Innovation and context*	*Study design and size*	*Interorganisational factors hypothesised to affect innovativeness*	*Significant associations actually demonstrated*	*Comment*
Damanpour 1991[14] [see Table A.13]	Various	Meta-analysis of 23 studies published prior to 1988 (see Section 7.2, page 135)	External communication: the degree of organisation members' involvement and participation in extraorganisational professional activities	Positive significant relationship ($p = 0.055$) with the rate of adoption of multiple innovations (demonstrated through 14 correlations)	External communication' was one of the three strongest and most significant of 14 determinants of organisational innovativeness
Kimberly and Evanisko 1981[59]	Technological and administrative innovations in US hospitals in late 1970s	Mixed methodology (described in separate article[498]) with questionnaires; number of hospitals not given	'External integration': extensiveness of a variety of mechanisms that increase the probability that information about innovations will enter the organisational system	No significant association ($\beta = 0.06$)	Authors express some surprise at the dominance of internal organisational variables in this study and suggest some contextual explanations for this
Robertson and Wind 1983[80]	Radiology innovations in 182 US hospitals	Postal questionnaire survey	'Cosmopolitanism' as measured by external contacts and activities of (a) physicians and (b) administrators	Highly innovative hospitals are characterised by externally oriented physicians (i.e. those who have extensive professional and academic links) but 'local' administrators (i.e. those *without* such links)	Differences between hospitals with different cosmopolitanism scores were not impressive and level of statistical significance was not given; speculative discussion on physician–manager power balance
Fennell and Warnecke 1988[36] [see Tables A.9, A.10 and A.18]	Multi-disciplinary interventions and shared decision-making in head and neck cancer in 7 US networks involving 88 hospitals in late 1970s	Descriptive 6-year retrospective case study of each network and a comparative analysis based on in-depth interviews with a range of key informants	(a) Environment affects the extent of diffusion and the form of diffusion network, and (b) 'fit' between environmental contingencies and form of diffusion network will affect network performance	(a) Linkage (density and stability) combined with resource capacity and organisational compatibility to influence the network forms to emerge, (b) interpersonal networks left no discernible structure; interorganisational networks led to sustained innovations	Supports arguments for importance of organisational – as well as individual – homophily; relates form and performance of networks to environmental context (Section 8.3, page 170)

Burns and Wholey 1993[65] [see Table A.14]	Unit (matrix) management in 346 US general hospitals (and 901 'control' hospitals) over a 17-year period	Retrospective and longitudinal questionnaire surveys (study specific and national data)	Embeddedness in external networks and normative institutional pressures	The cumulative force of adoption in interorganisational networks was one of four factors that significantly influenced adoption	Effect of organisational characteristics on adoption depends on (a) stage of diffusion and (b) extent to which innovation has been adopted in local area
Goes and Park 1997[68] [see Table A.14]	15 innovations in Californian acute care hospitals (6 technical and 11 administrative)	Prospective longitudinal study over 10 years; tracked year-to-year changes on 135 items	Interorganisational links: enduring transactions, flows and linkages among or between an organisation and others in its environment	Positive association was shown between interorganisational links and adoption of both technical and administrative innovations ($r^2 = 0.19$)	Hospitals exhibiting multiple and extensive interorganisational links were more likely to be large (see Section 6.3, page 126)
Westphal *et al.* 1997[81]	Total quality management (TQM) programmes in US hospitals	5492 US general medical surgical hospitals (1985–1993)	Various network effects (e.g. the later the date of adoption the greater the degree of conformity to the normative pattern set by other organisations)	Institutional factors moderated the role of network membership in affecting the form of administrative innovations adopted; later adopters conformed more closely to the normative pattern set by others	Note again how the stage of the diffusion process influences reason for adoption decision
Johnson and Linton 2000[385]	Environmentally clean process technology	Network analysis of 83 firms throughout North America	(a) Social networks, (b) local networks, (c) complexity of the implementation; hypothesised that 3 different elements are important: frequency of contact, perceived importance of contact and perceived reciprocity of contact	Interfirm and public networks were significantly associated ($p < 0.05$) with successful implementation but public networks had a negative relationship to success; for complex innovations, reciprocity of contact had a hugely significant impact ($p < 0.01$)	Used non-standard network analysis approach focusing on the networks of an individual responsible for implementation of the innovation within an organisation; this non-service sector study was included for reasons discussed on page 162
Fitzgerald *et al.* 2002[32] [see Table A.8, A.14 and A.19]	UK NHS (1995–1999): 8 case studies of evidence into practice (see Section 5.3, page 111)	Comparative case studies (4 in acute sector; 4 in primary care) using qualitative methods	Pattern of interorganisational relationships among doctors and their professional bodies	Networks are one of the key determinants of whether an innovation is successfully diffused into use	Little discussion on interorganisational networks although mentioned as a key influence

Table A.17 Empirical studies on health care quality improvement collaboratives (discussed in Section 8.2, page 163).

Author/year	*Setting and topic*	*Research question*	*Study design*	*Main findings*	Comment
O'Connor *et al.* 1996[82]	US hospital care: initiatives to reduce in-hospital mortality from coronary artery bypass grafting (CABG)	What is the nature, extent and magnitude of quality improvement activities in hospitals that take part in a multi-organisational structured collaborative?	Descriptive multi-organisational case study with before-and-after measurements of coronary artery bypass grafting (CABG) by 23 surgeons in 5 cardiology units over 20 000 cases	Following the intervention period, the mean reduction in in-hospital mortality was 24% ($p < 0.001$)	Good descriptive detail on the IHI model but little detail in this early article on the process of learning or change
Flamm *et al.* 1998[83]	US hospital care: initiatives to reduce unnecessary Caesarean section rates	What is the nature, extent and magnitude of quality improvement activities in hospitals that take part in a multi-organisational structured collaborative?	Descriptive multi-organisational case study with before-and-after measurements of Caesarean section rates in 28 obstetric units over 12 months	Of 28 participating units, 15% achieved Caesarean delivery rate reductions of 30% or more during the 12-month period of active collaborative work	Little detail given on the process of learning or change
Leape *et al.* 2000[84]	US hospital care: initiatives to reduce adverse drug events	To what extent can adverse drug events be reduced through a multi-organisational structured collaborative?	Descriptive multi-organisational case study in 40 hospitals over 15 months in which participants were taught data gathering and analysis techniques and encouraged to use the rapid-cycle test-of-change approach	The 40 hospitals conducted a total of 739 tests of changes; 8 types of changes were implemented by 7 or more hospitals, with a success rate (measured against the hospitals' own local criteria) of 70%	Process of care changes included non-punitive reporting, ensuring documentation of information, standardising medication administration times, and implementing chemotherapy protocols

Horbar *et al.* 2001[86] and Rogowski *et al.* 2001[85]	US neonatal intensive care units (NICUs): initiatives to reduce mortality and morbidity in low birth weight infants	(a) What is the nature, extent and magnitude of quality improvement activities in NICUs that take part in a multi-organisational structured collaborative? (b) What is the cost of these improvements?	Descriptive multi-organisation case study with before-and-after measurements of quantitative data on predefined quality criteria (infection rates, use of supplemental oxygen) in 6 NICUs; 66 NICUs not in the study served as contemporaneous 'controls'	Significant improvements in predefined quality measures in the 6 intervention NICUs, with significant reductions in cost per case; control NICUs showed smaller improvements and an increase in cost per case	Not an RCT so differences between intervention and control groups should be interpreted with caution
Green and Plsek 2002[396]	US hospital care: variety of initiatives aimed at improving efficiency and cost-effectiveness	To what extent does the 'coaching and leadership' model of collaborative quality improvement lead to sustained changes in service organisations?	Descriptive multi-organisation case study with before-and-after measurements of quantitative data on a wide range of predefined quality criteria in 26 clinical and administrative teams	17 of the 26 teams made significant improvements in predefined areas	Emphasises the importance of a cyclical learning process in which 'Wave 1' teams mix informally with 'Wave 2' teams to transfer ideas and enthusiasm for the process

Note: Much work on the collaborative quality improvement model has been undertaken as evaluation rather than research and has been published as 'grey literature'. For practical reasons, we have confined our own analysis to papers published in peer-reviewed journals.

Table A.18 Empirical studies of impact of environmental factors on innovation in health care organisations and selected other examples.

Author/year	*Innovation and context*	*Study design and size*	*Environmental factors hypothesised to affect innovativeness*	*Significant associations actually demonstrated*	*Comment*
Damanpour 1996[16]	Various	Meta-analysis of 21 studies (described in detail on page 135)	'Environmental uncertainty' considered as a contingency factor that mediates the relationship between organisational complexity and innovativeness	Environmental uncertainty moderated the relationship between innovativeness and both (a) structural complexity and (b) organisational size	Explanation is in terms of varied external pressure on organisations leading to greater opportunities for innovation
Baldridge and Burnham 1975[63]	Organisational innovations in US schools in late 1960s	Qualitative interviews and questionnaires; 271 school districts	(a) Environmental heterogeneity will increase organisational innovativeness; (b) a rapidly changing environment will also increase it	Environmental heterogeneity was significantly associated with innovativeness; changing environment was not	Impact of environmental heterogeneity was small compared with size and complexity (see Sections 7.4–7.6, page 141 et seq.)
Kimberly and Evanisko 1981[59] [see Tables A.14 and A.16]	Technological and administrative innovations in US hospitals in late 1970s	Mixed methodology with questionnaires described in separate paper;[498] number of hospitals not given	3 'contextual' [environmental] variables – competition; size of city; age of hospital	Age of hospital showed small but significant association with adoption of technological innovation; competition and size of city not significant	In our own typology 'age of hospital' would be considered as part of the 'inner' context rather than as an environmental ('outer') context variable
Meyer and Goes 1988[38] [see Tables A.8, A.12 and A.14]	12 organisation-level medical innovations introduced into US community hospitals in late 1970s	Comparative case study for 6 years with over 300 interviews, and observation and surveys	3 environmental variables – urbanisation, affluence, federal health insurance	Environmental variables had little demonstrable impact	Again, intraorganisational variables were dominant

Fennell and Warnecke 1988[36] [see Tables A.9, A.10 and A.16]	(a) Multi-disciplinary interventions and shared decision-making in head and neck cancer, and (b) linking primary care physicians and community hospitals with research medicine in 7 US networks	Descriptive 6-year retrospective case study of each network and a comparative analysis based on in-depth interviews with a range of key informants	(a) Environmental factors affects the extent of diffusion and the form of diffusion channel through which the process occurs; and (b) 'fit' between environmental factors and the form of diffusion network will affect network performance	(a) Linkage history (density and stability) combined with resource capacity and organisational compatibility to influence the network forms to emerge; (b) interpersonal networks did not leave a discernible structure after their termination; the interorganisational networks did lead to sustained innovations	Combines environmental factors with form of diffusion channel (network) in health care system and assesses impact of network type on sustainability of organisational innovations
Champagne *et al.* 1991[64] [see Tables A.8 and A.14]	Sessional fee remuneration for general practitioners in long-term hospitals in Canada over a 15-month period	Multiple case studies with interviews and documentary analysis in 5 hospitals; data on the independent variables were collected by questionnaires sent to the 27 study hospitals and 72 control hospitals	Urbanisation (distance of the organisation from a large urban centre)	The level of implementation of the innovation was positively and moderately associated with the level of urbanisation ($\beta = 0.38$; $r^2 = 0.11$)	This study was of an atypical innovation (a change in how the doctors were paid), which may reduce the generalisability of the findings

Continued

Table A.18 continued: Empirical studies of impact of environmental factors on innovation in health care organisations and selected other examples.

Author/year	*Innovation and context*	*Study design and size*	*Environmental factors hypothesised to affect innovativeness*	*Significant associations actually demonstrated*	*Comment*
Castle 2001[73]	Special and subacute care units in nursing homes in USA (1992–1997)	Analysis of national data-set	7 environmental factors: (a) higher average income of residents; (b) beds per 100 000 population; (c) prospective reimbursement; (d) less competition; (e) state legislative policies with regard to building of new facilities; (f) age of population; and (g) availability of hospital-based services	Environmental variables positively associated with innovation were (a) and (b), plus membership of a chain of homes (see Table A.14); those negatively associated with innovation were (c) and (d); the last 3 showed no association with innovation	See further detail in Table A.14, page 271, in relation to organisation-level variables
Nystrom *et al.* 2002[76] [see Table A.14]	Medical imaging diagnostic technologies in US hospitals	Postal questionnaire survey of 70 hospitals	'External orientation': defined as those organisations with boundary spanning roles, focusing particularly on the nature of communication links between the organisation and its patients/community	External orientation interacted significantly but negatively with size ($p < 0.05$) to determine innovativeness; also a significant and positive relationship with organisational age ($p < 0.10$)	Surprising negative association between external orientation and size and combined effect on innovativeness

Table A.19 Empirical studies of impact of political and policymaking forces on organisational innovation (discussed in Section 8.4, page 172).

Author/year	*Innovation and context*	*Study design and size*	Research question	*Main findings*	*Comment*
Hughes *et al.* 2002[87]	UK NHS 1996–1999: 5 case studies of 'evidence into action'	In-depth comparative case studies in primary care (or at primary–secondary interface) in inner London	What is the nature of the process when a team decides to implement a particular evidence-based practice initiative? What are the common features of such implementation projects and what are the generalisable lessons for implementation of health care innovations?	Multiple local factors interacted with wider environmental forces to determine the success of the implementation effort; continuity of staff, good working relationships (especially across boundaries), alignment with national policy directives, adequate resources and effective involvement of users were all associated with project success	One recommendation from this study was 'acknowledge the limitations of short-term, single-worker, demonstration projects for initiatives that require sustained change in complex organisations and community settings'
Fitzgerald *et al.* 2002[32] [see Tables A.8, A.14 and A.16]	UK NHS 1995–1999: 8 case studies, 5 technological and 3 organisational innovations	In-depth comparative case studies (4 in acute sector; 4 in primary care) using qualitative methods	What is the nature of the process when a team decides to implement a particular evidence-based practice initiative? What are the facilitators and barriers to the success of such initiatives in the real world?	Both micro ('inner context') factors and macro ('outer context') factors were critical to implementation success; these interacted in complex and unpredictable ways	Authors concluded that the interplay of micro and macro contexts 'demonstrate the critical and variable influence of context on the diffusion process'
Exworthy *et al.* 2002[88]	UK health policy (1999–2001): policies aimed at reducing health inequalities	In-depth comparative case studies in 3 UK health authorities	What factors and forces influence the implementation of local policies to redress health inequalities?	National priorities (e.g. to reduce health inequalities) do shape local policy agendas but are mediated by central and local conditions and expectations	Authors draw on Kingdon's theory of policy streams (explained in Section 8.4, page 172)

Continued

Table A.19 continued: Empirical studies of impact of political and policymaking forces on organisational innovation (discussed in Section 8.4, page 172).

Author/year	*Innovation and context*	*Study design and size*	Research question	*Main findings*	*Comment*
Riley 2003[215] [see Table A.23]	Canadian public health (CHIOPP heart health programme)	In-depth case study analysis of the same programme	Explored the interaction of several determinants: (a) innovation attributes; (b) user system capacity (skills and resources, leadership and mandate); (c) external factors (interorganisational links; externally supported predisposing and capacity-building initiatives) and (d) contextual factors (local demographics and priorities)	Qualitative findings highlighted (a) the importance of synchronous interaction between external (national and regional) incentives and mandates and internal (organisational) activity; (b) the long lead time (around 15 years) for outcomes to appear in a complex programme such as this	This study is discussed in more detail in Section 9.7, page 195, in relation to whole-systems approaches to implementation

Table A.20 Systematic reviews relevant to the question of dissemination, implementation and sustainability of innovations in service delivery and organisation (discussed in Section 9.3, page 180).

Author/year	*Scope of review*	*Methodological approach*	*Number of studies reviewed*	*Main findings*	*Strengths in relation to our own research question*	*Limitations in relation to our own research question*
Granados *et al.* 1997[89]	Dissemination of health technology assessment (HTA) reports	Hierarchy of evidence with randomised trials seen as 'best evidence'; most studies considered by the authors were experimental or quasi-experimental	110 references	Couched in terms of 'behaviour change' (i.e. did a particular report change professional behaviour?); barriers divided into environmental (e.g. political), prevailing professional norms and social standards, and individual factors (perceptions, tolerance of risk)	Empirical studies are all from health care field	Did not focus on service delivery and organisation; hence of tangential relevance to our own review. Now fairly dated. See page 180 for further discussion and our comment in Table A.6, page 255.
Meyers *et al.* 1999[91] [see Table A.6]	Implementation of industrial process innovations	Narrative overview of a range of primary studies similar in breadth to that covered in this review	About 120 primary studies	Summarised in Box 9.2: various characteristics of the user system, resource system, interface between these and wider environment had an impact on implementation and sustainability	(a) Strong theoretical basis; (b) range of research questions covered similar to our own	Addressed commercial sector; hence questionable generalisability of findings to service sector. See page 181 for further discussion.

Continued

Table A.20 continued: Systematic reviews relevant to the question of dissemination, implementation and sustainability of innovations in service delivery and organisation (discussed in Section 9.3, page 180)

Author/year	*Scope of review*	*Methodological approach*	*Number of studies reviewed*	*Main findings*	*Strengths in relation to our own research question*	*Limitations in relation to our own research question*
Gustafson *et al.* 2003[79] [see Table A.6]	Implementation of organisational change; focuses specifically on implementing service initiatives in the health care field	Narrative review of change management literature plus 'Delphi' style survey of experts	96 books and papers referenced	Summarised in Box 9.4, page 185; various characteristics of the innovation, structural features of the organisation, leadership, resources, change skills, linkage; retrospective testing of these factors against 221 studies in the literature had impressive predictive value (area under ROC curve 0.84).	Also includes an empirical study of an expert panel of organisational theorists using a Delphi-type method, to develop a Bayesian model to predict the success of any implementation programme	Not a full systematic review. Model has face validity but has yet to be prospectively tested. See page 185 for further discussion.
Grimshaw *et al.* 2004[11]	Guideline dissemination and implementation strategies	Draws on Cochrane methodology and centres on controlled trials	235 primary studies; 309 separate comparisons	Methodological quality of many studies was judged poor. Very few had an explicit theoretical basis. Much 'received wisdom' challenged.	Focused, systematic and thorough approach to health service–related topic area	Little attention to process found in primary studies so few conclusions about how to go about implementation; authors recommended further process studies. See page 183 for further discussion.

Table A.21 Surveys of perceptions about capacity or of association between capacity and implementation in health care organisations (discussed in Section 9.4, page 186)

Author/year	*Context*	*Innovation*	*Study design, size and intervention*	*Factors hypothesised to influence implementation or sustainability*	*Factors confirmed as influencing implementation or sustainability*	*Comment*
Taylor *et al.* 1998[90]	Canadian public health	Heart health promotion programmes	Semi-structured interviews with staff members ($n = 56$) supplemented by wider staff questionnaire survey ($n = 262$)	No prior hypothesis in qualitative stage	Factors perceived to be facilitators of predisposition were mostly external to the organisation (e.g. national directive, coalitions with other agencies); those perceived to be facilitators of actual implementation were mostly internal (e.g. dedicated funding, trained staff)	Suggests that external directives can have a powerful impact on organisations' motivation to implement innovations
Elliott *et al.* 1998[96]	Canadian public health	Heart health promotion programmes	Questionnaire survey at 2 levels: organisational ($n = 42$) and staff members ($n = 262$)	(a) Organisational predisposition towards the innovation; (b) organisational capacity (measured as per capita funding, dedicated budget, and coalitions)	Predisposition strongly linked to capacity; capacity moderately linked to implementation; but predisposition not independently linked to implementation	Predisposition is a necessary but not sufficient condition for implementation

Continued

Table A.21 continued: Surveys of perceptions about capacity or of association between capacity and implementation in health care organisations (discussed in Section 9.4, page 186).

Author/year	*Context*	*Innovation*	*Study design, size and intervention*	*Factors hypothesised to influence implementation or sustainability*	*Factors confirmed as influencing implementation or sustainability*	*Comment*
O'Loughlin *et al.* 1998[349]	Canadian public health (CHIOPP programme)	Heart health promotion programmes	Telephone survey of programme leaders and stakeholders involved in 189 interventions; asked whether they thought their programme was successfully implemented and would be sustained	15 potential determinants of implementation success including characteristics of the intervention, frequency of intervention, staff capacity and training, and intervention–provider fit	'Intervention used no paid staff' (odds ratio 3.7), 'intervention was modified during implementation' (odds ratio 2.7), 'there was a good fit between the local provider and the intervention' (odds ratio 2.4), and 'program champion' (odds ratio 2.3)	Interesting negative correlation between presence of paid staff and implementation success
Riley *et al.* 2001[431]	Canadian public health (CHIOPP programme)	Heart health promotion programmes	Postal survey of 42 health departments or units involved in CHIOPP	4 sets of possible determinants: (a) the organisation's predisposition (motivation and commitment), (b) its capacity (skills and resources), (c) internal organisational (structural) factors and (d) external system factors (including interorganisational links and external facilitation)	Results summarised in Box 9.5, page 193; various perceived critical factors including aspects of the innovation, user system predisposition and capacity, linkage, and monitoring and evaluation	Somewhat deterministic design, which confirmed all main hypotheses

Note: as explained in the text, the survey is a relatively weak design so these studies should be interpreted with this in mind.

Table A.22 Empirical studies of interventions to enhance user system capacity in health care organisations (discussed in Section 9.4, page 186).

Author/year	*Context*	*Innovation*	*Study design, size and intervention*	*Factors hypothesised to influence implementation or sustainability*	*Factors confirmed as influencing implementation or sustainability*	*Comment*
Controlled trials of capacity-building interventions						
McCormick *et al.* 1995[94]	Canadian public health	School health education programmes	Randomised controlled trial in 22 school districts with survey of individual classroom teachers; intervention in the RCT was staff training	(a) Process consultation (in which individual schools had a say in which of 3 programmes to teach); (b) staff awareness, concern and interest; (c) staff training; (d) organisational antecedents (size and climate)	Staff training did not change initial implementation rate but significantly improved success of 'later implementation', defined as the programme still being in place 4 years on (62% vs 30% of districts implemented the programme)	This study provides moderate support for staff training having an impact on sustainability
In-depth qualitative studies						
Green 1998[92]	US Health Maintenance Organisation	Integrated care pathway	Case study in a single HMO; intervention was a conventional quality improvement model (plan-do-check act) plus dedicated multi-disciplinary teams	(a) Tools and artefacts (e.g. protocols); (b) multi-disciplinary implementation teams; (c) multi-disciplinary, interorganisational collaborative practice committees with oversight role	In-depth qualitative evaluation suggested 7 key elements of success including positive organisational culture, 'just-in-time' training, detailed feedback, and broad-based support	Overall, provides weak support for capacity building in terms of creation of multi-disciplinary teams

Continued

Table A.22 continued: Empirical studies of interventions to enhance user system capacity in health care organisations (discussed in Section 9.4, page 186).

Author/year	*Context*	*Innovation*	*Study design, size and intervention*	*Factors hypothesised to influence implementation or sustainability*	*Factors confirmed as influencing implementation or sustainability*	*Comment*
Edmondson *et al.* 2001[95]	US cardiac surgery	New technology for cardiac surgery	Qualitative case study of cardiac teams in 16 hospitals (164 interviews)	(a) Aspects of the team learning process; (b) leadership; (c) interorganisational networks	All the hypothesised determinants were found to influence the depth of learning about the innovation and its implementation success	Successful implementers underwent a 'qualitatively different team learning process' than those who were unsuccessful

Table A.23 'Whole-systems' approaches to implementation and sustainability of innovations in health care organisations and selected other examples (discussed in Section 9.7, page 195).

Author /year	*Context*	*Innovation*	*Study design, size and intervention*	*Factors hypothesised to influence implementation or sustainability*	*Factors confirmed as influencing implementation or sustainability*	*Comment*
O'Loughlin *et al.* 1998[349] [see Table A.21]	Canadian public health (CHIOPP programme)	Heart health promotion programmes	Telephone survey of programme leaders and stakeholders involved in 189 interventions	15 potential determinants of implementation success including characteristics of the intervention, frequency of intervention, staff capacity and training, and intervention–provider fit; respondents were asked whether they thought their programme was successfully implemented and would be sustained	'Intervention used no paid staff' (odds ratio 3.7), 'intervention was modified during implementation' (odds ratio 2.7), 'there was a good fit between the local provider and the intervention' (odds ratio 2.4), and 'there was a program champion' (odds ratio 2.3).	Interesting negative correlation between presence of paid staff and implementation success; survey methodology precludes definitive causal inferences, especially since the instrument included several leading questions; interaction between variables was not explored
Riley *et al.* 2001[431] [see Table A.21]	Canadian public health (CHIOPP programme)	Heart health promotion programmes	Postal survey of 42 health departments or units involved in CHIOPP	4 sets of possible determinants: (a) the organisation's predisposition (motivation and commitment), (b) its capacity (skills and resources), (c) internal organisational (structural) factors and (d) external system factors (including interorganisational links and external facilitation)	5 variables explained almost half the variance in implementation: organisational capacity, priority given to heart health, coordination of programmes, use of resource centres and participation in interorganisational networks; the other half of the variance remained unexplained by any factors	Supports the model shown in Fig. 9.1, page 187, in which key determinants of implementation success are predisposition, capacity, process of implementation, and reinforcement; other (unmeasured) factors are likely also to be important

Continued

Table A.23 continued: 'Whole-systems' approaches to implementation and sustainability of innovations in health care organisations and selected other examples (discussed in Section 9.7, page 195).

Author /year	*Context*	*Innovation*	*Study design, size and intervention*	*Factors hypothesised to influence implementation or sustainability*	*Factors confirmed as influencing implementation or sustainability*	*Comment*
Riley 2003[215] [see Table A.19]	Canadian public health (CHIOPP programme)	Heart health promotion programmes	In-depth case study analysis of the same programme	Explored interaction of innovation attributes; user system capacity (skills and resources, leadership and mandate); external factors (interorganisational links; externally supported predisposing and capacity-building initiatives), and contextual factors (demographics and priorities)	Findings summarised in Box 9.5, page 193; implementation is a lengthy, staged process that moves from defining problems to evaluating outcomes; prior predisposing activities and concurrent capacity-building activities are essential, as is synchrony between national and local policymaking streams	Rich picture of the programme difficult to glean from this succinctly written article
Ellsworth 2002[432] [see Table A.6]	US education system	New technologies in education (schools and universities)	Narrative overview of whole-systems approaches to introducing new technologies	Provides overview of the educational sociology literature on a range of whole-systems approaches with different linked interventions at different levels	(a) Linkage initiatives with potential users of the technologies; (b) strategies for gaining broad-based support across the organisation; (c) strategic changes in organisational structure; and (d) linked staff development initiatives	In-depth overview that covered a wealth of primary sources; we have only included brief details in this report

Glossary

Absorptive capacity
A dynamic capability pertaining to knowledge creation and utilisation that enhances an organisation's ability to gain and sustain a competitive advantage (Zahra and George[23]). Four dimensions: acquisition (the ability to find and prioritise new knowledge quickly and efficiently); assimilation (the ability to understand it and link it to existing knowledge); transformation (the ability to combine, convert and recodify it) and exploitation (the ability to put it to productive use). Discussed in Section 3.13 (page 70).

Adoption of innovations (individual)
The decision to make full use of the innovation as the best course of action available (Rogers[3]). Discussed in Sections 1.4 (page 26) and 5.2 (page 103).

Adoption of innovations (organisational)
An organisation's means to adapt to the environment, or to pre-empt a change in the environment, in order to increase or sustain its effectiveness or competitiveness. Managers may emphasise the rate or speed of adoption, or both, to close an actual or perceived performance gap (Damanpour and Gopalakrishnan[130]). Discussed in Section 5.3 (page 106).

Assimilation of innovations
Another term for the adoption of innovations by organisations, often used in the literature relating to service sector innovations. Assimilation is the preferred term for adoption in organisations, since it emphasises the long and complex processes involved, with multiple decisions made by multiple agents. Discussed in Section 5.3 (page 106).

Change agency
An organisation or other unit that promotes and supports adoption and implementation of innovations. Discussed in Section 9.5 (page 190).

Change agent
An individual who influences clients' innovation decisions in a direction deemed desirable by a change agency (Rogers[3]). Discussed in Section 6.5 (page 130).

Concerns
The composite representation of the feelings, preoccupation, thought and consideration given to a particular issue or task. Depending on their personal make-up, knowledge, and experience, each person perceives and mentally contends with a given issue differentially; thus there are different kinds of concerns (Hall and Hord[46]). Discussed in Section 5.2 (page 103).

Diffusion
The process by which an innovation is communicated through certain channels over time among the members of a social system (Rogers[3]). Discussed in Section 1.4 (page 26).

Dissemination
Actively spreading a message to defined target groups (Mowatt *et al.*[131]). Discussed in Section 1.4 (page 26).

Implementation
Dissemination plus action to actively encourage the adoption recommendations contained in a message (Mowatt *et al.*[131]). Discussed in Section 1.4 (page 26).

Inner context
In this book, inner context relates to the intraorganisational determinants of innovation, including structural determinants (size, maturity, functional differentiation and so on, discussed in Section 7.3 et seq., page 140), leadership and locus of decision-making (discussed in Section 7.6 et seq., page 148), receptive context for change (discussed in Section 7.7 et seq., page 150) and absorptive capacity for new knowledge (discussed in Section 7.8 et seq., page 154).

Innovation (individual)
An idea, practice or object that is perceived as new by an individual or other unit of adoption (Rogers[3]). Discussed in Section 1.4 (page 26).

Innovation (organisational; general)
The implementation of an internally generated or a borrowed idea – whether pertaining to a product, device, system, process, policy, program or service – that was new to the organisation at the time of adoption. Innovation is a practice, distinguished from invention by its readiness for mass consumption and from other practices by its novelty (Damanpour and Euan[125]). Discussed in Section 1.4 (page 26).

Innovation (relating to health service delivery and organisation)
A set of behaviours, routines and ways of working, along with any associated administrative technologies and systems, which are (a) perceived as new by a proportion of key stakeholders; (b) linked to the provision or support of health care; (c) discontinuous with previous practice; (d) directed at improving health outcomes, administrative efficiency, cost-effectiveness, or the user experience; (e) implemented by means of planned and coordinated action by individuals, teams or organisations. Such innovations may or may not be associated with a new health technology. Discussed in Section 1.3 (page 25) and Chapter 4 (page 83).

Institutionalisation
The process by which the innovation becomes part of business as usual (the 'common-sense' world of practice) and ceases to be considered new. Synonyms include 'frozen', 'stabilised', 'accepted', 'sustained', 'durable', 'persistent', and 'maintained', 'routinised', 'incorporated', 'continued', and 'built in-ness'.[403,404] Discussed in Section 9.2 (page 178).

Meta-narrative
The term 'meta-narrative' was introduced by Lyotard[160] to indicate the grand cosmological and ideological lens through which a group of people views the world. Lyotard's meta-narratives included Judao-Christianity, Marxism, feminism, modernist–rationalist science and psychoanalysis. We use the term in a slightly more prosaic sense to depict the overarching 'storyline' of a research tradition: where did it come from and why; what is its core business; and where is it headed? Discussed in Section 2.7 (page 42).

Opinion leader
Those perceived as having particular influence on the beliefs and actions of their colleagues in any direction, whether 'positive' (in the eyes of those trying to achieve change) or 'negative' (Locock *et al.* [53]). Discussed in Section 6.2 (page 118).

Outer context
In this book, outer context refers to extraorganisational determinants of innovativeness, including the extent and quality of informal interorganisational networks (discussed in Section 8.1, page 157); the nature and success of planned strategies to promote interorganisational collaboration (discussed in Section 8.2, page 163); the prevailing political, economic, sociological and technological environment (and whether it is static or changing; discussed in Section 8.3, page 170) and the nature and timing of particular policymaking streams and other political initiatives (discussed in Section 8.4, page 172).

Paradigm
Models from which spring particular coherent traditions of scientific research (Kuhn 1962[159]). According to Kuhn, a paradigm has four key dimensions – conceptual (what are considered the important objects of study – and, hence, what

counts as a legitimate problem to be solved by science), theoretical (how the objects of study are considered to relate to one another and to the world), methodological (the accepted ways in which problems might be investigated) and instrumental (the accepted tools and instruments to be used by scientists). Discussed in Section 2.7 (page 42).

Receptive context for change
A combination of factors from both the inner and the outer context that together determine an organisation's ability to respond effectively and purposively to change. Receptive context was developed by Pettigrew *et al.*,[78] and comprises eight dimensions: external environmental pressure; presence of visionary people in key roles; good managerial and clinical relations; a supportive organisational culture; quality and coherence of local policy; presence of an effective interorganisational network; clarity of goals and priorities and aspects of the local setting. Discussed in Section 7.7 (page 150).

Research tradition
A coherent theoretical discourse and a linked body of empirical research in which successive studies are influenced by preceding enquiries. This definition is derived (and slightly adapted) from Kuhn.[159] Discussed in Section 2.7 (page 42).

Resource system
An organisation (or other unit – e.g. a research institution) that develops innovations. Discussed in Section 9.5 (page 190).

Routinisation
When an innovation becomes an ongoing element in the organisation's activities and loses its distinct identity (van de Ven *et al.*[123]). Discussed in Section 9.2 (page 178).

Social network
The pattern of friendship, advice, communication and support that exists among members of a social system (Valente *et al.*[4]). Discussed in Section 3.2 (page 51).

Spread
Spread means that the learning that takes place in any part of an organisation is actively shared and acted upon by all parts of the organisation. Improvement knowledge generated anywhere in the health care system becomes common knowledge and practice across the health care system (NHS Modernisation Agency[133]). Discussed in Section 1.4 (page 26).

Sustainability
When new ways of working and improved outcomes become the norm. Not only have the process and outcome changed, but the thinking and attitudes behind them are fundamentally altered and the systems surrounding them are transformed in support (NHS Modernisation Agency[133]). Discussed in Section 1.4 (page 26).

User system
An organisation (or other unit of adoption) that considers the innovation for adoption. Discussed in Sections 9.3 (page 180) and 9.4 (page 186).

References

1. Department of Health. *The NHS Plan*. London: NHS Executive, 2001.
2. Dixon-Woods M, Agarwal S, Jones D, Young B, Sutton A. Synthesising qualitative and quantitative evidence: a review of methods. *Journal of Health Services Research and Policy* 2005; **10**:45–53.
3. Rogers EM. *Diffusion of Innovations*. New York: Free Press, 1995.
4. Valente TW. Social network thresholds in the diffusion of innovations. *Social Networks* 1996;**18**:69–89.
5. Coleman JS, Katz E, Menzel H. *Medical Innovations: A Diffusion Study*. New York: Bobbs-Merrill, 1966.
6. Burt RS. The differential impact of social integration on participation in the diffusion of innovations. *Social Science Research* 1973;**2**:125–44.
7. Rogers EM, Kincaid DL. *Communication Networks: Toward a New Paradigm for Research*. New York: Free Press, 1981.
8. Bass FM. A new product growth model for consumer durables. *Management Science* 1969;**13**:215–27.
9. Bourdenave JD. Communication of agricultural innovations in Latin America: the need for new models. *Communication Research* 1976;**3**:135–54.
10. Potvin L, Haddad S, Frohlich KL. Beyond process and outcome evaluation: a comprehensive approach for evaluating health promotion programmes. *WHO Regional Publications European Series* 2001;45–62.
11. Grimshaw JM, Thomas RE, MacLennan G, Fraser C, Ramsay CR, Vale L, *et al*. Effectiveness and efficiency of guideline dissemination and implementation strategies. *Health Technology Assessment Report* 2004; **8**:1–72.
12. Ferlie E, Gabbay J, Fitzgerald L, Locock L, Dopson S. Evidence-based medicine and organisational change: an overview of some recent qualitative research. In: Ashburner L, ed. *Organisational Behaviour and Organisational Studies in Health Care: Reflections on the Future*. Basingstoke: Palgrave, 2001.
13. Lomas J. Improving research dissemination and uptake in the health sector: beyond the sound of one hand clapping. *Policy Commentary C97-1*. Hamilton, Ontario: Centre for Health Economics and Policy Analysis, McMaster University, 1997.
14. Damanpour F. Organisational innovations: a meta-analysis of effects of determinants and moderators. *Academy of Management Journal* 1991;**34**:555–90.
15. Damanpour F. Organizational size and innovation. *Organization Studies* 1992;**13**:375–402.
16. Damanpour F. Organizational complexity and innovation: developing and testing multiple contingency models. *Management Science* 1996;**42**:693–716.
17. Kanter RM. When a thousand flowers bloom: structural, collective and social conditions for innovation in organisation. In: Staw BM, Cummings LL, eds. *Research in Organisational Behaviour*. Greenwich, Conn: JAI Press, 1988, pp. 169–211.
18. Van de Ven AH, Polley DE, Garud R, Venkataraman S. *The Innovation Journey*. Oxford: Oxford University Press, 1999.
19. Granovetter M, Soong R. Threshold models of diffusion and collective behavior. *Journal of Mathematical Sociology* 1983;**9**:165–79.
20. Abrahamson E, Fairchild G. Management fashion: lifecycles, triggers and collective learning processes. *Administrative Sciences Quarterly* 1999;**44**:708–40.
21. Abrahamson E. Managerial fads and fashions: the diffusion and rejection of innovation. *California Management Review* 1991;**16**:586–612.
22. Nonaka I, Takeuchi H. *The Knowledge Creation Company: How Japanese Companies Create the Dynamics of Innovation*. New York: Oxford University Press, 1995.
23. Zahra AS, George G. Absorptive capacity: a review, reconceptualization and extension. *Academy of Management Review* 2002;**27**:185–203.
24. Czarniawska B. A narrative approach to organization studies. *Qualitative Research Methods Series 43*. London: Sage, 1998.
25. Gabriel Y. *Storytelling in Organisations: Facts, Fictions and Fantasies*. Oxford: Oxford University Press, 2000.
26. Buckler SA, Zein C. The spirituality of innovation: learning from stories. *Journal of Product Innovation Management* 1996;September:391–405.
27. Fonseca J. *Complexity and Innovation in Organisations*. London: Routledge, 2001.
28. Plsek P. Complexity and the adoption of innovation in health care. Paper presented at Accelerating Quality

Improvement in Health Care: strategies to speed the diffusion of evidence-based innovations. Washington, DC: National Institute for Health Care Management Foundation and National Committee for Quality Health Care, 2003.

29. Dirksen CD, Ament AJ, Go PM. Diffusion of six surgical endoscopic procedures in the Netherlands: stimulating and restraining factors. *Health Policy* 1996;**37**:91–104.
30. Marshall JG. Diffusion of innovation theory and end-user searching. *Library and Information Science Research* 1990;**6**:55–69.
31. Meyer M, Johnson D, Ethington C. Contrasting attributes of preventive health innovations. *Journal of Communication* 1997;**47**:112–31.
32. Fitzgerald L, Ferlie E, Wood M, Hawkins C. Interlocking interactions: the diffusion of innovations in health care. *Human Relations* 2002;**55**:1429–49.
33. Denis JL, Hebert Y, Langley A, Lozeau D, Trottier LH. Explaining diffusion patterns for complex health care innovations. *Health Care Management Review* 2002;**27**:60–73.
34. Foy R, MacLennan G, Grimshaw J, Penney G, Campbell M, Grol R. Attributes of clinical recommendations that influence change in practice following audit and feedback. *Journal of Clinical Epidemiology* 2002;**55**:717–22.
35. Aubert BA, Hamel G. Adoption of smart cards in the medical sector: the Canadian experience. *Social Science and Medicine* 2001;**53**:879–94.
36. Fennell ML, Warnecke RB. *The Diffusion of Medical Innovations: an Applied Network Analysis*. New York: Plenum Publishing, 1988.
37. Grilli R, Lomas J. Evaluating the message: the relationship between compliance rate and the subject of a practice guideline. *Medical Care* 1994;**32**:202–13.
38. Meyer AD, Goes JB. Organisational assimilation of innovations: a multi-level contextual analysis. *Academy of Management Review* 1988;**31**:897–923.
39. Yetton P, Sharma R, Southon G. Successful IS innovation: the contingent contributions of innovation characteristics and implementation process. *Journal of Information Technology* 1999;**14**:53–68.
40. Øvretveit J, Bate P, Cleary P, Cretin S, Gustafson D, McInnes K, *et al.* Quality collaboratives: lessons from research. *Quality and Safety in Health Care* 2002;**11**:345–51.
41. Wejnert B. Integrating models of diffusion of innovations: a conceptual framework. *Annual Review of Sociology* 2002;**28**:297–326.
42. Dobbins M, Cockerill R, Barnsley J. Factors affecting the utilization of systematic reviews. *International Journal of Technology Assessment in Health Care* 2001;**17**:203–14.
43. Adler PS, Kwon S-W, Singer JMK. The 'Six-West' problem: professionals and the intraorganizational diffusion of innovations, with particular reference to the case of hospitals. Working paper 3–15, 2003. Los Angeles, Marshall School of Business, University of Southern California. *http://www.marshall.usc.edu/web/MOR.cfm?doc_id=5561*.
44. O'Neill HM, Pouder PW, Buchholtz AK. Patterns in the diffusion of strategies across organisations: insights from the innovation diffusion literature. *Academy of Management Review* 2002;**23**:98–114.
45. Gladwin J, Dixon RA, Wilson TD. Rejection of an innovation: health information management training materials in East Africa. *Health Policy and Planning* 2002;**17**:354–61.
46. Hall GE, Hord SM. *Change in Schools*. Albany, NY: State University of New York Press, 1987.
47. Lynn J, Arkes HR, Stevens M, Cohn F, Koenig B, Fox E, *et al.* Rethinking fundamental assumptions: SUPPORT's implications for future reform. Study to understand prognoses and preferences and risks of treatment. *Journal of the American Geriatrics Society* 2000;**48**:214–21.
48. Dearing JW, Meyer G, Kazmierczak J. Portraying the new: communication between university innovators and potential users. *Science Communication* 1994;**16**:11–42.
49. Timmons S. How does professional culture influence the success or failure of IT implementation in health services? In: Ashburner L, ed. *Organisational Behaviour and Organisational Studies in Health Care: Reflections on the Future–*. Basingstoke: Palgrave, 2001, pp.218–31.
50. Eveland JD. Diffusion, technology transfer and implementation. *Knowledge: Creation, Diffusion, Utilisation* 1986;8:303–22.
51. West E, Barron DN, Dowsett J, Newton JN. Hierarchies and cliques in the social networks of health care professionals: implications for the design of dissemination strategies. *Social Science and Medicine* 1999;**48**:633–46.
52. Becker MH. Factors affecting the diffusion of innovation among health professionals. *American Journal of Public Health* 1970;**60**:294–304.
53. Locock L, Dopson S, Chambers D, Gabbay J. Understanding the role of opinion leaders in improving clinical effectiveness. *Social Science and Medicine* 2001;**53**:745–57.
54. Thomson O'Brien MA, Oxman AD, Davis DA, Haynes RB, Freemantle N. Local opinion leaders. *Cochrane Database of Systematic Reviews* 2000;**2**:CD000125.
55. Markham SK. A longitudinal examination of how champions influence others to support their projects. *Journal of Product Innovation Management* 1998;**15**: 490–504.
56. Schon DA. Champions for radical new inventions. *Harvard Business Review* 1963;**41**:77–86.
57. Backer TE, Rogers EM. Diffusion of innovations theory and work-site AIDS programs. *Journal of Health Communication* 1998;**3**:17–28.
58. Shane S. Uncertainty avoidance and the preference for innovation championing roles. *Journal of International Business Studies* 1995;**26**:47–68.

59. Kimberly JR, Evanisko JM. Organisational innovation: the influence of individual, organisational and contextual factors on hospital adoption of technological and administrative innovation. *Academy of Management Journal* 1981;**24**:689–713.
60. Tushman M. Special boundary roles in the innovation process. *Administrative Sciences Quarterly* 1977; **22**:587–605.
61. Barnsley J, Lemieux-Charles L, McKinney MM. Integrating learning into integrated delivery systems. *Health Care Management Review* 1998;**23**:18–28.
62. Tornatsky LG, Klein KJ. Innovation characteristics and innovation-adoption-implementation: a meta-analysis of findings. *Transactions on Engineering Management* 1982;**29**:28–45.
63. Baldridge JV, Burnham RA. Organisational innovation: individual organisational and environmental impacts. *Administrative Sciences Quarterly* 1975;**20**:165–76.
64. Champagne F, Denis J-L, Pineault R, Contandriopoulos A. Structural and political models of analysis of the introduction of an innovation in organizations: the case of the change in the method of payment of physicians in long-term care hospitals. *Health Services Management Research* 1991;**4**:94–111.
65. Burns LR, Wholey DR. Adoption and abandonment of matrix management programs: effects of organizational characteristics and interorganizational networks. *Academy of Management Journal* 1993;**36**:106–38.
66. Dufault MA, Bielecki C, Collins E, Willey C. Changing nurses' pain assessment practice: a collaborative research utilization approach. *Journal of Advanced Nursing* 1995;**21**:634–45.
67. Patel V. Cognition and technology in health education research. *Canadian Journal of Public Health* 1996;**87(Suppl 2)**:S63–S67.
68. Goes JB, Park SH. Interorganisational links and innovation: the case of hospital services. *Academy of Management Journal* 1997;**40**:673–96.
69. Anderson NR, West NA. Measuring climate for work group innovation. *Journal of Organizational Behaviour* 1998;**19**:235–58.
70. Gosling AS, Westbrook JI, Braithwaite J. Clinical team functioning and IT innovation: a study of the diffusion of a point-of-care online evidence system. *Journal of American Medical Informatics Association.* 2003;**10**:244–51.
71. Newton J, Graham J, McLoughlin K, Moore A. Receptivity to change in a general medical practice. *British Journal of Management* 2003;**14**:143–53.
72. Rashman L, Hartley J. Leading and learning? Knowledge transfer in the Beacon Council Scheme. *Public Administration* 2002;**80**:523–42.
73. Castle NG. Innovation in nursing homes: which facilities are the early adopters? *Gerontologist* 2001;**41**:161–72.
74. Wilson AL, Ramamurthy K, Nystrom PC. A multi-attribute measure for innovation adoption: the context of imaging technology. *Transactions on Engineering Management* 1999;**46**:311–21.
75. Dopson S, Fitzgerald L, Ferlie E, Gabbay J, Locock L. No magic targets: changing clinical practice to become more evidence based. *Health Care Management Review* 2002;**37**:35–47.
76. Nystrom PC, Ramamurthy K, Wilson AL. Organizational context, climate and innovativeness: adoption of imaging technology. *Journal of Engineering and Technology Management* 2002;**19**:221–47.
77. House R, Rousseau DM, Thomas-Hunt M. The meso paradigm: a framework for the integration of micro and macro organisational behaviour. *Research in Organizational Behaviour* 1995;**17**:71–114.
78. Pettigrew AM, Ferlie E, McKee L. *Shaping Strategic Change: Making Change in Large Organisations*. London: Sage, 1992.
79. Gustafson DH, Sainfort F, Eichler M, Adams L, Bisognano M, Steudel H. Developing and testing a model to predict outcomes of organizational change. *Health Services Research* 2003;**38**:751–76.
80. Robertson T, Wind Y. Organisational cosmopolitanism and innovation. *Academy of Management Journal* 1983;**26**:332–8.
81. Westphal JD, Gulati R, Shortell SM. Customization or conformity? An institutional and network perspective on the content and consequences of total quality management adoption. *Administrative Sciences Quarterly* 1997;**42**:394.
82. O'Connor GT, Plume SK, Olmstead EM, Morton JR, Maloney CT, Nugent WC, *et al.* A regional intervention to improve the hospital mortality associated with coronary artery bypass graft surgery. The Northern New England Cardiovascular Disease Study Group. *Journal of the American Medical Association* 1996;**275**:841–6.
83. Flamm BL, Berwick DM, Kabcenell A. Reducing cesarean section rates safely: lessons from a 'breakthrough series' collaborative. *Birth* 1998;**25**:117–24.
84. Leape LL, Kabcenell AI, Gandhi TK, Carver P, Nolan TW, Berwick DM. Reducing adverse drug events: lessons from a breakthrough series collaborative. *Joint Commission Journal on Quality Improvement* 2000;**26**:321–31.
85. Rogowski JA, Horbar JD, Plsek PE, Schuurmann BL, Deterding J, Edwards WH, *et al.* Economic implications of neonatal intensive care unit collaborative quality improvement. *Pediatrics* 2001;**107**:23–9.
86. Horbar JD, Rogowski J, Plsek PE, Delmore P, Edwards WH, Hocker J, *et al.* Collaborative quality improvement for neonatal intensive care. *Pediatrics* 2001;**107**:14–22.
87. Hughes J, Humphrey C, Rogers S, Greenhalgh T. Evidence into action: changing practice in primary care. *Occasional Paper/Royal College of General Practitioners* 2002; 1–51.
88. Exworthy M, Berney L, Powell M. How great expectations in Westminster may be dashed locally: the local implementation of national policy on health inequalities. *Policy and Politics* 2002;**30**:79–96.

89. Granados A, Jonsson E, Banta HD, Bero L, Bonair A, Cochet C, *et al.* EUR-ASSESS project subgroup report on dissemination and impact. *International Journal of Technology Assessment in Health Care* 1997;**13**:220–86.
90. Taylor SM, Elliott S, Robinson K, Taylor S. Community-based heart health promotion: perceptions of facilitators and barriers. *Canadian Journal of Public Health* 1998;Revue Canadienne de Sante Publique. **89**:406–09.
91. Meyers PW, Sivakumar K, Nakata C. Implementation of industrial process innovations: factors, effects, and marketing implications. *Journal of Product Innovation Management* 1999;**16**:295–311.
92. Green PL. Improving clinical effectiveness in an integrated care delivery system. *Journal for Healthcare Quality* 1998;**20**:4–8.
93. Kitson A, Harney G, McCormack B. Enabling the implementation of evidence based practice: a conceptual framework. *Quality in Health Care* 1998;**7**:149–58.
94. McCormick LK, Steckler AB, Mcleroy KR. Diffusion of innovations in schools: a study of adoption and implementation of school-based tobacco prevention curricula. *American Journal of Health Promotion* 1995;**9**:210–19.
95. Edmondson AC, Bohmer RM, Pisano GP. Disrupted routines: team learning and new technology implementation in hospitals. *Administrative Sciences Quarterly* 2001;**46**:685–716.
96. Elliott SJ, Taylor SM, Cameron R, Schabas R. Assessing public health capacity to support community-based heart health promotion: the Canadian Heart Health Initiative Ontario Project (CHHIOP). *Health Education Research* 1998;**13**:607–22.
97. Bate SP. The role of stories and storytelling in organisational change efforts: a field study of an emerging 'community of practice' within the UK National Health Service. In: Hurwitz B, Greenhalgh T, Skultans V, eds. *Narrative Research in Health and Illness*. London: BMJ Publications, 2004.
98. Valente TW. *Network Models of the Diffusion of Innovations*. Cresskill, NJ: Hampton, 1995.
99. Lomas J. Using 'linkage and exchange' to move research into policy at a Canadian foundation. *Health Affairs* 2000;**19**:236–40.
100. Henrich J. Cultural transmission and the diffusion of innovations: adoption dynamics indicate that biased cultural transmission is the predominate force in behavioral change. *American Anthropologist* 2001; **103**:992–1013.
101. Bailey NTJ. *The Mathematical Theory of Infectious Diseases and its Applications*. London: Charles Griffin, 1957.
102. Green LW, Johnson JL. Dissemination and utilization of health promotion and disease prevention knowledge: theory, research and experience. *Canadian Journal of Public Health* 1996;**87**:11–17.
103. Robert G, McLeod H, and Ham C. Modernising cancer services: an evaluation of phase 1 of the cancer services collaborative. Birmingham: Health Services Management Centre, University of Birmingham,**43**: 2003.
104. Robert G, Hardacre J, Locock L, Bate SP. Evaluating the effectiveness of the mental health collaborative as an approach to bringing about improvements to admission, stay and discharge on acute wards in the Trent and Northern and Yorkshire regions. An action research project. Birmingham: Health Services Management Centre, University of Birmingham, 2002.
105. Bate SP, Robert G. Knowledge management and communities of practice in the private sector: lessons for modernizing the NHS in England and Wales. *Public Administration* 2002;**80**:643–63.
106. Ham C, Kipping R, Meredith P. *Capacity, Culture and Leadership: Lessons from Experience of Improving Access to Hospital Services*. Birmingham: Health Services Management Centre, University of Birmingham, 2002.
107. NHS Modernisation Agency. *Improvement in the NHS*. London: Department of Health, 2002.
108. NHS Modernisation Agency. *From scepticism to support – what are the influencing factors?* Research into practice summary report No. 1. London: Department of Health, 2002.
109. NHS Modernisation Agency. *Sustainability and spread in the National Booking Programme*. Research into practice summary report No. 2. London: Department of Health, 2002.
110. NHS Modernisation Agency. *Spreading and sustaining new practices: sharing and learning from the Cancer Services Collaborative*. Research into practice summary report No. 3. London: Department of Health, 2002.
111. NHS Modernisation Agency. *Spread and sustainability of service improvement: factors identified by staff leading modernisation programmes*. Research into practice Report No. 4: overview of early research findings. London: Department of Health, 2003.
112. NHS Modernisation Agency. *NHS modernisation: making it mainstream*. London: Department of Health, 2003.
113. Bate SP, Robert G. Where next for policy evaluation? Insights from researching NHS modernisation. *Politics and Policy* 2003;**31**:237–51.
114. Bate SP, Robert G, Bevan H. The next phase of health care improvement: what can we learn from social movements? *Quality and Safety in Health Care* 2004;**13**: 62–66.
115. Forbes A, Griffiths P. Methodological strategies for the identification and synthesis of 'evidence' to support decision-making in relation to complex healthcare systems and practices. *Nursing Inquiry* 2002; **9**:141–55.
116. Gomm R. Would it work here? In: Gomm R, ed. *Using Evidence in Health and Social Care*. London: Sage, 2000, pp. 171–91.

117. Martin S, Sanderson I. Evaluating public policy experiments: measuring outcomes, monitoring processesor managing pilots? *Evaluation* 1999;5:3–245.
118. Mays N, Roberts E, Popay J. Synthesizing research evidence. In: Fulop N, Allen P, Clarke A, Black N, eds. *Studying the Organization and the Delivery of the Health Services: Research Methods*. London: Routledge, 2001, pp. 188–220.
119. Paterson BL, Thorne SE, Canon C, Jillings J. Metatheory. *Meta-Study of Qualitative Health Research: A Practical Guide to Meta-Analysis and Meta-Synthesis*. Thousand Oaks, CA: Sage, 2001, pp. 91–108.
120. Pawson R, Tilley N. *Realistic Evaluation*. London: Sage, 1997.
121. Osborne SP. Naming the beast: delivering and classifying service innovations in social policy. *Human Relations* 1998;**51**:1133–54.
122. Tushman ML, Anderson P. Technological discontinuities and organizational environments. *Administrative Sciences Quarterly* 2003;**31**:439–65.
123. Van de Ven AH. Central problems in the management of innovation. *Management Science* 1986;**32**:590–607.
124. Strang D, Soule S. Diffusion in organizations and social movements: from hybrid corn to poison pills. *Annual Review of Sociology* 1998;**24**:265–90.
125. Damanpour F, Euan WM. Organisational innovation and performance: the problem of organisational lag. *Administrative Sciences Quarterly* 1984;**29**:392–409.
126. Osborne SP. Naming the beast: delivering and classifying service innovations in social policy. *Human Relations* 1998; **51**:1133–54
127. Zairi M, Whymark J. The transfer of best practice: how to build a culture of benchmarking and continuous learning – part 1. *Benchmarking: An International Journal* 2000;**7**:62–78.
128. Stone EG, Morton SC, Hulscher ME, Maglione MA, Roth EA, Grimshaw JM, *et al.* Interventions that increase use of adult immunization and cancer screening services: a meta-analysis. *Annals of Internal Medicine* 2002;**136**:641–51.
129. von Hippel E. *The Sources of Innovation*. New York: Oxford University Press, 1988.
130. Damanpour F, Gopalakrishnan S. Theories of organizational structure and innovation adoption: the role of environmental change. *Journal of Engineering and Technology Management* 1998;**15**:1–24.
131. Mowatt G, Thomson MA, Grimshaw J, Grant A. Implementing early warning messages on emerging health technologies. *International Journal of Technology Assessment in Health Care* 1998; **14**:663–70.
132. Berwick DM. Disseminating innovations in health care. *Journal of the American Medical Association* 2003;**289**:1969–75.
133. NHS Modernisation Agency. *The improvement leader's guide to spread and sustainability*. London: Department of Health, 2003.
134. Von Krogh G, Roos J. A perspective on knowledge, competence and strategy. *Personnel Review* 1995;**243**:56–77.
135. Coyne KP. Sustainable competitive advantage – what it is, what it isn't. *Business Horizons* 1986; 54–61.
136. Grant RM. *Contemporary Strategy Analysis*. Oxford: Blackwell, 2002.
137. Weick KE. *Sensemaking in Organizations*. Thousand Oaks, CA: Sage, 1995.
138. Zeitz G, Mittal V, McAuley B. Distinguishing adoption and entrenchment of management practices: a framework for analysis. *Organization Studies* 1999;**20**:741–76.
139. Greve HR, Taylor A. Innovations as catalysts for organizational change: shifts in organizational cognition and search. *Administrative Sciences Quarterly* 2000;**45**:54–80.
140. Pawson R. Evidence-based policy: the promise of 'realist synthesis'. *Evaluation* 2002;**8**:340–58.
141. Bero L, Grilli R, Grimshaw JM, Mowatt G, Oxman A, Zwarenstein M. Cochrane effective practice and organisation of care review group. In: Bero L, Grilli R, Grimshaw JM, Mowatt G, Oxman A, Zwarenstein M, eds. *The Cochrane Library, Issue 2*. Oxford: Update Software, 2003.
142. Popay J, Rogers A, Williams G. Rationale and standards for the systematic review of qualitative literature in health services research. *Qualitative Health Research* 1998;**8**:341–51.
143. Barbour RS. Checklists for improving rigour in qualitative research: a case of the tail wagging the dog? *British Medical Journal* 2001;**322**:1115–17.
144. Pawson R. Evidence-based policy: in search of a method. *Evaluation* 2002;**8**:157–81.
145. Jensen LA, Allen MN. Meta-synthesis of qualitative findings. *Qualitative Health Research* 1996; **6**:553–60.
146. Campbell R, Pound P, Pope C, Britten N, Pill R, Morgan M, *et al.* Evaluating meta-ethnography: a synthesis of qualitative research on lay experiences of diabetes and diabetes care. *Social Science and Medicine* 2003;**56**:671–84.
147. Kearney MH. Enduring love: a grounded formal theory of women's experience of domestic violence. *Research in Nursing and Health* 2001;**24**:270–82.
148. Øvretveit J. *Evaluating Health Interventions: an Introduction to Evaluation of Health Treatments, Services, Policies and Organizational Interventions*. Milton Keynes: Open University Press, 1998.
149. Greenhalgh T, Robert G, Macfarlane F, Bate P, Kyriakidou O, Peacock R. Storylines of research: a meta-narrative perspective on systematic review. *Social Science and Medicine* 2005 (in press).

150. Grimshaw JM, Shirran L, Thomas R, Mowatt G, Fraser C, Bero L, *et al.* Changing provider behavior: an overview of systematic reviews of interventions. *Medical Care* 2001;**39** (**8 Suppl** 2):112–45.
151. Robert G. Identifying new health care technologies. PhD thesis. Southampton: University of Southampton, 2000.
152. Rosenthal R. *Meta-Analytic Procedures for Social Research.* Newbury Park, CA: Sage, 1984.
153. Boynton P, Greenhalgh, T. Selecting and designing your questionnaire *British Medical Journal* 2004;**328**:1312–15.
154. Mays N, Pope C. Quality in qualitative health research. In: Pope C, Mays N, eds. *Qualitative Research in Health Care.* London: BMJ Books, 2000, pp. 89–110.
155. Blaxter M. Criteria for the evaluation of qualitative research. *Medical Sociology News* 1996;**22**:68–71.
156. Egger M, Schneider M, Davey SG. Spurious precision? Meta-analysis of observational studies. *British Medical Journal* 1998;**316**:140–44.
157. Denzin M, Lincoln P. *Handbook of Qualitative Research.* London: Sage, 1994.
158. Øvretveit J. Reviewing medical management research for decision-makers: methodological issues in carrying out systematic reviews of medical management research. Stockholm: Karolinska Institute (Medical Management Centre internal discussion document), 2003.
159. Kuhn TS. *The Structure of Scientific Revolutions.* Chicago: University of Chicago Press, 1962.
160. Lyotard J-F. *The Postmodern Condition: A Report on Knowledge.* Manchester: Manchester University Press, 1984.
161. Valente TW, Rogers EM. The origins and development of the diffusion of innovations paradigm as an example of scientific growth. *Science Communication* 1995;**16**:242–73.
162. Cochrane Reviewers' Handbook 4.2.0 (updated March 2003). *The Cochrane Library* 2003.
163. Dixon-Woods M, Agarwal S, Young B, Jones D, Sutton A. *Integrative Approaches to Qualitative and Quantitative Evidence.* London: Health Development Agency, 2004.
164. Miles MB, Huberman M. *Qualitative Data Analysis: An Expanded Sourcebook.* London: Sage, 1994.
165. Evans D, Fitzgerald M. Reasons for physically restraining patients and residents: a systematic review and content analysis. *International Journal of Nursing Studies* 2002;**39**:739–43.
166. Roberts KA, Dixon-Woods M, Fitzpatrick R, Abrams KR, Jones DR. Factors affecting the uptake of childhood immunisation: a Bayesian synthesis of qualitative and quantitative evidence. *Lancet* 2002; **360**:1596–9.
167. Tashakkori A, Teddi C. *Mixed Methodology: Combining Qualitative and Quantitative Approaches.* Thousand Oaks, CA: Sage, 1998.
168. Thomas J, Harden A, Oakley A, Oliver S, Sutcliffe K, Rees R, *et al.* Integrating qualitative research with trials in systematic reviews. *British Medical Journal* 2004;**328**:1010–12.
169. Mays N, Popay J, Pope C. *Review and Synthesis of Qualitative and Quantitative Research and Other Evidence.* London: Canadian Health Services Research Foundation and NHS SDO Programme, 2004.
170. Paterson BL, Thorne SE, Canon C, Jillings J. *Meta-Study of Qualitative Health Research: A Practical Guide to Meta-Analysis and Meta-Synthesis.* Thousand Oaks, CA: Sage, 2003.
171. Gomm R, Hammersley M, Foster P. *Case Study Method.* London: Sage, 2000.
172. Yin RK. *Case Study Research: Design and Methods.* London: Sage, 1994.
173. Pawson R, Greenhalgh T, Harvey G, Walshe K. *Using Realist Methods to Produce Syntheses of Evidence for Use by Managers and Policy Makers.* London: Canadian Health Services Research Foundation and NHS SDO Programme 2004.
174. Wolfe B. Organisational innovation: review, critique and suggested research directions. *Journal of Management Studies* 1994;**31**:405–31.
175. Fiol CM. Squeezing harder doesn't always work: continuing the search for consistency in innovation research. *Academy of Management Review* 1996; **21**:1012–21.
176. Rogers E. *The Diffusion of Innovations.* New York: Free Press, 1962.
177. Rogers EM, Shoemaker FF. *Communication of Innovations: A Cross-Cultural Approach.* New York: Free Press, 1972.
178. Rogers EM. *Diffusion of Innovations.* New York: Free Press, 1983.
179. Ferrence R. Diffusion theory and drug use. *Addiction* 2001;**96**:165–73.
180. Johnson JL, Green LW. A dissemination research agenda to strengthen health promotion and disease prevention. *Canadian Journal of Public Health* 1996;**87**:S5–11.
181. Oldenburg BF, Hardcastle DM, Kok G. Diffusion of innovations. In: Glanz K, Lewis FM, Rimer B, eds. *Health Behaviour and Health Education: Theory, Research and Practice.* San Francisco: Jossey-Bass, 1997, pp. 207–86.
182. Tarde G. *The Laws of Imitation.* New York: Henry, Holt & Co, 1903.
183. Ryan BF. *Social and Cultural Change.* New York: Ronald Press, 1969.
184. Hagerstrand T. *Innovation Diffusion as a Spatial Process.* Chicago: University of Chicago Press, 1967.
185. Bourdieu P. *Distinction: a Social Critique of the Judgement of Taste.* London: Routledge, 1986.
186. Brown JS, Duguid KP. *The Social Life of Information.* Boston, MA: Harvard University Press, 2000.

187. Mort PR. Educational adaptability. *The School Executive* 1953;**23**:199–200.
188. Ryan B, Gross N. The diffusion of hybrid seed corn in two Iowa communities. *Rural Sociology* 1943;**8**:15–24.
189. Ryan B, Gross N. Acceptance and diffusion of hybrid seed corn in two Iowa communities. *Ames, Iowa Agricultural Station Research Bulletin* 1950; **372**:665–79.
190. Hightower J. *Hard Tomatoes, Hard Times: the Failure of America's Land Grant Complex*. Cambridge, MA: Schenkman, 1972.
191. Rogers EM. *A History of Communication Study*. New York: Free Press, 1994.
192. Becker MH. Sociometric location and innovativeness: reformulation and extension of the diffusion model. *American Sociological Review* 1970;**35**:267–82.
193. Burt RS. *Structural Holes: the Social Structure of Competition*. Cambridge, MA: Harvard University Press, 1992.
194. Burt RS. Innovation as a structural interest: rethinking the impact of network position on innovation adoption. *Social Networks* 1980;**2**:327–55.
195. Burt RS. Social contagion and innovation, cohesion versus structural equivalence. *American Journal of Sociology* 1987;**92**:1287–335.
196. Granovetter M. The strength of weak ties. *American Journal of Sociology* 1973;**78**:1360–80.
197. Stocking B. *Initiatives and Inertia: case studies in the NHS*. London: Nuffield Provincial Hospitals Trust, 1985.
198. Van den Bulte C, Lillein GL. Medical innovation revisited: social contagion versus marketing effort. *American Journal of Sociology* 2001;**106**:1409–35.
199. DeFleur M. *Theories of Mass Communication*. New York: David McKay, 1966.
200. DeFleur M. The growth and decline of research on the diffusion of news, 1945–1985. *Communication Research* 1987;**14**:109–30.
201. Macdonald G. Communication theory and health promotion. In: Bunton R, Macdonald G, eds. *Health Promotion: Disciplines, Diversity and Developments*. London: Routledge, 2002, pp. 197–218.
202. McGuire W, Lipstein B. *Evaluating Advertising: a Bibliography of the Communications Process*. New York: Advertising Research Foundation, 1978.
203. Ashford J, Eccles M, Bond S, Hall LA, Bond J. Improving health care through professional behaviour change: introducing a framework for identifying behaviour change strategies. *British Journal of Clinical Governance* 1999;**4**:14–23.
204. Meadows D, Meadows D. *The Limits to Growth – A Report for the Club of Rome's Project on the Predicament of Mankind*. London: St Martin's Press, 1972.
205. Brown LA. *Innovation Diffusion: A New Perspective*. London: Methuen, 1981.
206. Rogers EM. *Communication Strategies for Family Planning*. New York: Free Press, 1970.
207. Roling N. Alternative approaches in extension. In: Jones GE, Roll M, eds. *Progress in Rural Extension and Community Development*. Chichester: John Wiley, 1981.
208. Shingi P. Agriculture technology and the issue of unequal distribution of rewards. *Rural Sociology* 1981;**46**:430–45.
209. Oldenburg BF, Sallis JF, Ffrench ML, Owen N. Health promotion research and the diffusion and institutionalization of interventions. *Health Education Research* 1999;**14**:121–30.
210. Kotler P, Zaltman G. Social marketing: an approach to planned social change. *Journal of Marketing* 1971;**35**:3–12.
211. Lefebvre C. Social marketing and health promotion. In: Bunton R, Macdonald G, eds. *Health Promotion: Disciplines, Diversity and Developments*. London and New York: Routledge, 2002, pp. 219–45.
212. Farquhar JW, Fortmann SP, Flora JA, Taylor CB, Haskell WL, Williams PT, *et al*. Effects of community wide education on cardiovascular disease risk factors. The Stanford Five-City Project. *Journal of the American Medical Association* 1990;**264**:359–65.
213. Robinson KL, Elliott SJ. Community development approaches to heart health promotion: a geographical perspective. *Professional Geographer* 1999;**51**:283–95.
214. Green LW, Kreuter MW. *Health Promotion Planning: an Educational and Environmental Approach*. Mountain View, CA: Mayfield, 1991.
215. Riley BL. Dissemination of heart health promotion in the Ontario Public Health System: 1989–1999. *Health Education Research* 2003;**18**:15–31.
216. Haines A, Jones R. Implementing findings of research. *British Medical Journal* 1994;**308**:1488–92.
217. Dawson S. Never mind solutions: what are the issues? Lessons of industrial technology transfer for quality in health care. *Quality in Health Care* 1995;**4**:197–203.
218. Grilli R, Freemantle N, Minozzi S, Domenighetti G, Finer D. Mass media interventions: effects on health services utilisation. *Cochrane Database of Systematic Reviews* 2000;CD000389.
219. Freemantle N, Harvey EL, Wolf F, Grimshaw JM, Grilli R, Bero LA. Printed educational materials: effects on professional practice and health care outcomes. *Cochrane Database of Systematic Reviews* 2003;CD000172.
220. Davis D, O'Brien MA, Freemantle N, Wolf FM, Mazmanian P, Taylor-Vaisey A. Impact of formal continuing medical education: do conferences, workshops, rounds, and other traditional continuing education activities change physician behavior or health care outcomes? *Journal of the American Medical Association* 1999;**282**:867–74.
221. Zwarenstein M, Reeves S, Barr H, Hammick M, Koppel I, Atkins J. Interprofessional education: effects on professional practice and health care outcomes.

Cochrane Database of Systematic Reviews 2001;CD002213.

222. Sibley JC, Sackett DL, Neufeld V, Gerrard B, Rudnick KV, Fraser W. A randomized trial of continuing medical education. *New England Journal of Medicine* 1982;**306**:511–15.
223. Grol R. Improving the quality of medical care: building bridges among professional pride, payer profit, and patient satisfaction. *Journal of the American Medical Association* 2001;**286**:2578–85.
224. Wolff N. Randomised trials of socially complex interventions: promise or peril? *Journal of Health Services and Research Policy* 2001;**6**:123–6.
225. Campbell M, Fitzpatrick R, Haines A, Kinmonth AL, Sandercock P, Spiegelhalter D, *et al.* Framework for design and evaluation of complex interventions to improve health. *British Medical Journal* 2000; **321**:694–6.
226. Nutley S, Davies TR. Making a reality of evidence-based practice: some lessons from the diffusion of innovations. *Public Money and Management* 2000;October–December:35–42.
227. Zaltman G, Duncan R, Holbeck J. *Innovations and Organisation*. New York: John Wiley, 1973.
228. Pierce JL, Delbecq AL. Organisational structure, individual attitudes and innovation. *Academy of Management Review* 1977;**2**:27–37.
229. Kervasdoue J, Kimberly JR. Are organisations culture free? In: England G, Neghandi A, Wilpert B, eds. *Organisational Functioning in a Cross-Cultural Perspective*. Kent, OH: Kent State University Press, 1979.
230. Walton RE. The diffusion of new work structures: explaining why success didn't take. *Organizational Dynamics* 1975;**3**:3–22.
231. Burns T, Stalker GM. *The Management of Innovation*. London: Tavistock, 1961.
232. Lawrence PR, Lorsch JW. *Organisation and Environment*. Boston, MA: Harvard University Press, 1967.
233. Duncan R. Multiple decision making structures in adapting to environmental uncertainty: the impact on organisational effectiveness. *Human Relations* 1973;**26**:273–92.
234. Fitzgerald L, Hawkins C, Ferlie E. *Achieving change within primary care: final report*. Warwick: University of Warwick, CCSC, 1999.
235. Harrison D, Laberge M. Innovation, identities and resistance: the social construction of an innovation network. *Journal of Management Studies* 2002;**41**:497–521.
236. Huy QN. Emotional capability, emotional intelligence and radical change. *Academy of Management Review* 1999;**24**:325–45.
237. Klein KJ, Sorra JS. The challenge of innovation implementation. *Academy of Management Review* 1996; **21**:1055–80.
238. Kanter RM. The middle manager as innovator. *Harvard Business Review* 1982;**61**:95–105.
239. Kanter RM. *When Giants Learn to Dance*. New York: Simon and Schuster, 1989.
240. Kanter RM. *The Change Masters: Innovation for Productivity in the American Corporation*. New York: Simon and Schuster, 1983.
241. Kling N, Anderson N. *Innovation and Change in Organisations*. London: Routledge, 1995.
242. Di Maggio PJ, Powell WW. The iron cage revisited: institutional isomorphism and collective rationality in organizational fields. *American Sociological Review* 1983;**48**:147–60.
243. Ahuja G. Collaboration networks, structural holes and innovation: a longitudinal study. *Administrative Sciences Quarterly* 2000;**45**:425–55.
244. Abrahamson E, Rosenkopf L. Social network effects on the extent of innovation diffusion: a computer simulation. *Organization Science* 1997;**8**:289–309.
245. Kogut B, Zander U. Knowledge of the firm: combinative capabilities and the replication of technology. *Organization Science* 1992;**3**:383–97.
246. Bartlett CA, Ghoshal S. *Managing Across Borders: the Transnational Solution*. Boston, MA: Harvard Business School Press, 1989.
247. Garvin DA. Building a learning organization. *Harvard Business Review* 1993;**71**:78–92.
248. Holsapple CW, Joshi KD. Knowledge manipulation activities: results of a Delphi study. *Information and Management* 2002;**39**:477–90.
249. Kelly P. *Technological Innovation: a Critical Review of Current Knowledge*. San Francisco: San Francisco Press, 1978.
250. Dunn WN, Holzner B. Anatomy of an emergent field. *Knowledge in Society* 1988;**1**:3–26.
251. Polanyi M. *The Tacit Dimension*. New York: Anchor Day, 1962.
252. Hippel EV. 'Sticky information' and the locus of problem solving. *Management Science* 1991; **44**:429–39.
253. Malhotra Y. From information management to knowledge management. In: Srikantaiah TK, Koenig MED, eds. *Knowledge Management for the Information Professional*. Medford, NJ: Information Today, 2000.
254. Prusak L. *Knowledge in Organizations*. Oxford: Butterworth-Heinemann, 1997.
255. Lave J, Wenger E. *Cognition in Practice: Mind, Mathematics and Culture in Everyday Life*. Cambridge: Cambridge University Press, 1988.
256. Tsoukas H, Vladimirou E. What is organizational knowledge? *Journal of Management Studies* 2001;**38**:973–94.
257. Osterloh M, Frey BS. Motivation, knowledge transfer and organizational forms. *Organization Science* 2000;**11**:538–50.
258. Choo CW. *The Knowing Organization*. New York: Oxford University Press, 1998.
259. Holsapple C, Winston A. Knowledge-based organizations. *The Information Society* 1987;**5**:77–90.

260. Leonard-Barton D. *Wellsprings of Knowledge*. Boston, MA: Harvard Business School Press, 1995.
261. Nonaka I. The knowledge creating company. *Harvard Business Review* 1991;November–December:96–104.
262. Szulanski G. Exploring internal stickiness: impediments to the transfer of best practice within the firm. *Strategic Management Journal* 1996;**17**:27–43.
263. van der Spek R, Spijkervet A. Knowledge management. In: Liebowitz J, Wilcox L, eds. *Knowledge Management and its Integrative Elements*. New York: CRC Press, 1997.
264. Wiig K. *Knowledge Management Foundations*. Arlington, TX: Schema Press, 1993.
265. Cohen WM, Levinthal DA. Absorptive capacity: a new perspective on learning and innovation. *Administrative Sciences Quarterly* 1990;**30**:560–85.
266. Hansen MT, Nohria N, Tierney T. What's your strategy for managing knowledge? *Harvard Business Review* 1999;March:106–16.
267. Senge PM. *The FifthDiscipline - the Art and Practice of the Learning Organisation*. New York: Random House, 1993.
268. Fiske ST, Neuberg SL. A continuum of impression formation from category-based to individuating processes. *Advances in Experimental Social Psychology* 1990;**23**:1–74.
269. Bartunek JM. Changing interpretative schemes and organizational restructuring: the example of a religious order. *Administrative Sciences Quarterly* 1984;**19**:372.
270. Boland RJ, Tenkasi RV, Te'eni D. Designing information technology to support distributed cognition. *Organization Science* 1994;**5**:456–75.
271. Bruner J. *Actual Minds, Possible Words*. Cambridge: Harvard University Press, 1986.
272. Polkinghorne DE. *Narrative Knowing and the Human Sciences*. Albany, NY: State University of New York Press, 1988.
273. Gardner H. *Leading Minds: an Anatomy of Leadership*. London: HarperCollins, 1997.
274. Denning S. *The Springboard: How Storytelling Ignites Action in Knowledge-Era Organisations*. New York: Butterworth-Heinemann, 2001.
275. Humphreys JM, Brown AD. Narratives of organisational identity and identification: a case study of hegemony and resistance. *Organization Studies* 2002;**23**:421–47.
276. Higgins JM, McAllaster C. Want innovation? Then use cultural artefacts that support it. *Organizational Dynamics* 2002;**31**:74–84.
277. Cooperrider D, Sorensen P, Yaeger TF, Whitney D. *Appreciative Enquiry an Emerging Direction for Organization Development*. Champaign, IL: Stipes Publishing, 2001.
278. Waterman H, Tillen D, Dickson R, de Koning K. Action research: a systematic review and guidance for assessment. *Health Technology Assessment* 2001;**5(23)**: iii–157.
279. Plsek PE, Greenhalgh T. Complexity science: the challenge of complexity in health care. *British Medical Journal* 2001;**323**:625–8.
280. Stacey RD. *Complexity and Creativity in Organisations*. San Francisco: Berrett-Koehler, 1996.
281. Alemi F, Safaie FK, Neuhauser D. A survey of 92 quality improvement projects. *Joint Commission Journal on Quality Improvement* 2001;**27**:619–32.
282. Hays SP. Influences on reinvention during the diffusion of innovations. *Political Research Quarterly* 1996;**49**:631–50.
283. Riemer-Reiss ML. Applying Rogers' diffusion of innovations theory to assistive technology discontinuance. *Journal of Applied Rehabilitation Counseling* 1999;**30**:16–21.
284. Moore GC, Benbasat I. Development of an instrument to measure the perceptions of adopting an information technology innovation. *Information Systems Research* 1991;**2**:192–222.
285. Azjen I, Fishbein M. *Understanding Attitudes and Predicting Social Behaviour*. Engelwood Cliffs, NJ: Prentice-Hall, 1980.
286. Davis FD. Perceived usefulness, perceived ease of use, and user acceptance of information technology. *MIS Quarterly* 1989;**13**:319–40.
287. Davis FD, Bagozzi RP, Warshaw PR. User acceptance of computer technology: a comparison of two theoretical models. *Management Science* 1989;**35**:982–1003.
288. Moore GC, Benbasat I. An examination of the adoption of information technology by end users: a diffusion of innovations perspective. Vancouver, Canada: Department of Commerce and Business Administration, University of British Colombia, 1990, Working Paper 90-MIS-012.
289. Mustonen-Ollila E, Lyytinen K. Why organizations adopt information process innovations: a longitudinal study using diffusion of innovations theory. *Information Systems Journal* 2003;**13**:275–97.
290. Weiss JA, Dale BC. Diffusing against mature technology: issues and strategy. *Industrial Marketing Management* 1998;**27**:293–304.
291. Rogers E, Adhikayra R. Diffusion of innovation: an up-to-date review and commentary. *Communication Yearbook* 1979;**3**:67–81.
292. Fidler LA, Johnson JD. Communication and innovation implementation. *Academy of Management Review* 1984;**9**:704–11.
293. Downs GW, Mohr LB. Conceptual issues in the study of innovations. *Administrative Sciences Quarterly* 1976;**21**:700–14.
294. Rothman R. *Planning and Organizing for Social Change: Action Principles from Social Science Research*. New York: Columbia University Press, 1974.

295. Havelock RG. *Planning for Innovation Through Dissemination and Utilization of Knowledge*. Ann Arbor: Center for Research on the Utilization of Scientific Knowledge, Institute of Social Research, University of Michigan, 1971.
296. Lee FW. Adoption of electronic medical records as a technology innovation for ambulatory care at the Medical University of South Carolina. *Topics in Health Information Management* 2000;**21**:1–20.
297. Lia-Hoagberg B, Schaffer M, Strohschein S. Public health nursing practice guidelines: an evaluation of dissemination and use. *Public Health Nursing* 1999;**16**:397–404.
298. Vollink T, Meertens R, Midden CJH. Innovating 'diffusion of innovation' theory: innovation characteristics and the intention of utility companies to adopt energy conservation interventions. *Journal of Environmental Psychology* 2002;**22**:333–44.
299. Cain M, Mittman R. *Diffusion of Innovation in Health Care*. San Francisco, CA: HealthCare Foundation, 2002.
300. Dewar RD, Dutton JE. The adoption of radical and incremental innovation: an empirical analysis. *Management Science* 1986;**32**:1422–33.
301. Agarwal R, Tanniru M, Wilemon D. Assimilating information technology innovations: strategies and moderating influences. *Transactions on Engineering Management* 1997;**44**:347–58.
302. Tornatsky LG, Fleischer M. *The Processes of Technological Innovation*. Lexington, MA: Lexington Books, 1990.
303. Leonard-Barton D, Sinha DK. Developer-user interaction and user satisfaction in internal technology transfer. *Academy of Management Journal* 1993; **36**:1125–39.
304. Kaluzny A. Innovation of health services: a comparative study of hospitals and health departments. *Milbank Memorial Fund Quarterly: Health and Society* 1974;**52**:51–82.
305. Mohr LB. Determinants of innovation in organisations. *American Political Science Review* 1969; **63**:111–26.
306. Gopalakrishnan S, Bierly P. Analyzing innovation adoption using a knowledge-based approach. *Journal of Engineering and Technology Management* 2001; **18**:107–30.
307. Plsek PE. Techniques for managing quality. *Hospital and Health Services Administration* 1995;**40**:50–79.
308. Moore G. *Crossing the Chasm: Marketing and Selling High-Tech Products to Mainstream Consumers*. New York: Harper Business, 1991.
309. Furnham A. *The Psychology of Behaviour at Work: the Individual in the Organisation*. London: Psychology Press, 1997.
310. Berggren AC. Swedish midwives' awareness of attitudes to and use of selected research findings. *Journal of Advanced Nursing* 1996;**23**:462–70.
311. Estabrooks CA. Modelling the individual determinants of research utilization. *Western Journal of Nursing Research* 1999;**21**:758–72.
312. Pearcey P, Draper P. Using the diffusion of innovation model to influence practice: a case study. *Journal of Advanced Nursing* 1996;**23**:714–21.
313. Frambach RT, Schillewaert N. Organizational innovation adoption – a multi-level framework of determinants and opportunities for future research. *Journal of Business Research* 2002;**55**:163–76.
314. Prochaska JO, DiClemente CC. *The Transtheoretical Approach: Crossing Traditional Boundaries of Therapy*. Malabar, Florida: Kreiger Publishing, 1992.
315. Hansen G, Salter G. The adoption and diffusion of web technologies into mainstream teaching. *Journal of Interactive Learning Research* 2001;**12**:281–99.
316. Signer B, Hall C, Upton J. *A study of faculty concerns and developmental use of web based course tools*. ERIC database. 2000.
317. Jacobsen, DM. *Adoption patterns of faculty who integrate computer technology for teaching and learning in higher education*. ERIC database. 1998.
318. Hall GE, Wallace RC, Dossett WA. *A Developmental Conceptualization of the Adoption Process within Educational Institutions*. Austin, TX: Research and Development Center for Teacher Education, University of Texas, 1973.
319. Connor D. *Managing at the Speed of Change*. New York: John Wiley, 2000.
320. The SUPPORT principal investigators. A controlled trial to improve care for seriously ill hospitalized patients: the study to understand prognoses and preferences for outcomes and risks of treatments. *Journal of the American Medical Association* 1995;**274**:1591–8.
321. Greer AL. Adoption of medical technology: the hospital's three decision systems. *International Journal of Technology Assessment in Health Care* 1985;**1**:669–90.
322. Greer AL. Medical technology: assessment, adoption and utilization. *Journal of Medical Systems* 1981; **5**:129–45.
323. Greer AL. The state of the art versus the state of the science: the diffusion of new medical technologies into practice. *International Journal of Technology Assessment in Health Care* 1988;**4**:5–26.
324. Sicotte C, Denis JL, Lehoux P, Champagne F. The computer-based patient record challenges towards timeless and spaceless medical practice. *Journal of Medical Systems* 1998;**22**:237–56.
325. Sicotte C, Denis JL, Lehoux P. The computer based patient record: a strategic issue in process innovation. *Journal of Medical Systems* 1998;**22**:431–43.
326. Bobrowski P, Bretschneider S. Internal and external interorganizational relationships and their impact on the adoption of new technology: an exploratory study. *Technological Forecasting and Social Change* 1994;**46**:197–211.

327. Chaves M. Ordaining women: the diffusion of an organizational innovation. *American Journal of Sociology* 1996;**101**:840–73.
328. Feder G, Umali DL. The adoption of agricultural innovations: a review. *Technological Forecasting and Social Change* 1993;**43**:215–39.
329. Hedstrom P. Contagious collectivities: on the spatial diffusion of Swedish trade unions, 1890–1940. *American Journal of Sociology* 1994;**99**:1157–79.
330. Galaskiewicz J, Burt RS. Interorganization contagion in corporate philanthropy. *Administrative Sciences Quarterly* 1991;**36**:88–105.
331. Glick HR, Hays SP. Innovation and reinvention in state policy making: theory and the evolution of living will laws. *Journal of Politics* 1991;**53**:835–50.
332. Holden RT. The contagiousness of aircraft hijacking. *American Journal of Sociology* 1986;**91**:874–904.
333. Land KC, Deane G, Blau JR. Religious pluralism and church membership: a spatial diffusion model. *American Sociological Review* 1991;**56**:237–49.
334. Chan KK, Misra S. Characteristics of the opinion leader: a new dimension. *Journal of Advertising* 1990;**19**:60.
335. Katz E, Lazarsfeld PF. *Personal Influence: the Part Played by People in the Flow of Mass Communication*. New York: Free Press, 1955.
336. Katz E. Diffusion: interpersonal influence. In: Sills D, ed. *International Encyclopedia of the Social Sciences*. New York: Macmillan/Free Press, 1968, pp. 178–84.
337. Hiss RG, MacDonald R, David WR. Identification of physician educational influentials in small community hospitals. *Research in Medical Education* 1978; **17**:283–8.
338. Lomas J, Enkin M, Anderson GM, Hannah WJ, Vayda E, Singer J. Opinion leaders vs audit and feedback to implement practice guidelines. Delivery after previous cesarean section. *Journal of the American Medical Association* 1991;**265**:2202–07.
339. Soumerai SB, McLaughlin TJ, Gurwitz JH, Guadagnoli E, Hauptman PJ, Borbas C, *et al.* Effect of local medical opinion leaders on quality of care for acute myocardial infarction: a randomised controlled trial. *Journal of the American Medical Association* 1998;**279**:1358–63.
340. Searle J, Grover S, Santin A, Weideman P. Randomised trial of an integrated educational strategy to reduce investigation rates in young women with dysfunctional uterine bleeding. *Australian and New Zealand Journal of Obstetrics & Gynaecology* 2002;**42**:395–400.
341. Berner ES, Baker CS, Funkhouser E, Heudebert GR, Allison JJ, Fargason CA, Jr, *et al.* Do local opinion leaders augment hospital quality improvement efforts? A randomized trial to promote adherence to unstable angina guidelines. *Medical Care* 2003; **41**:420–31.
342. Dopson S, Locock L, Chambers D, Gabbay J. Implementation of evidence-based medicine: evaluation of the promoting action on clinical effectiveness programme. *Journal of Health Services and Research Policy* 2001;**6**:23–31.
343. Locock L, Chambers D, Surender R, Dopson S, Gabbay J. *Evaluation of the Welsh Clinical Effectiveness Initiative National Demonstration Projects: Final Report*. Templeton College; University of Oxford and Wessex Institute for Health Research and Development, University of Southampton, 1999, pp.81.
344. Maidique MA. Entrepreneurs, champions and technological innovation. *Sloan Management Review* 1980; **21**:59–76.
345. Collins OF, Moore DG, Umwalla DB. *The Enterprising Man*. Michigan: Board of Trustees, Michigan State University, 1964.
346. Shane S, Venkataraman S, Macmillan I. Cultural-differences in innovation championing strategies. *Journal of Management* 1995;**21**:931–52.
347. Royer I. Why bad projects are so hard to kill. *Harvard Business Review* 2003;**81**:48–56.
348. Carter FJ, Jambulingam T, Gupta VK, Melone N. Technological innovations: a framework for communicating diffusion effects. *Information and Management* 2001;**38**:277–87.
349. O'Loughlin J, Renaud L, Richard L, Gomez LS, Paradis G. Correlates of the sustainability of community-based heart health promotion interventions. *Preventive Medicine* 1998;**27**:702–12.
350. Valois RF, Hoyle TB. Formative evaluation results from the Mariner Project: a coordinated school health pilot program. *Journal of School Health* 2000;**70**:95–103.
351. Rao N, Svenkerud PJ. Effective HIV/AIDS prevention communication strategies to reach culturally unique populations: lessons learned in San Francisco, USA and Bangkok, Thailand. *International Journal of Intercultural Relations* 1998;**22**:85–105.
352. Kimberly J. Managerial innovation. In: Nystrom PC, Starbuck WH, eds. *Handbook of Organisational Design*. New York: Oxford University Press, 1981, pp. 84–104.
353. Tolbert PS, Sucker LG. Institutional sources of change in the formal sector of organisations: the diffusion of civil service reform 1880–1935. *Administrative Sciences Quarterly* 1983;**28**:22–39.
354. Sharma S, Rai A. An assessment of the relationship between ISD leadership characteristics and IS innovation adoption in organizations. *Information and Management* 2003;**40**:391–401.
355. Hage J, Aiken M. Program change and organizational properties: a comparative analysis. *American Journal of Sociology* 1970;**72**:503–19.
356. Ferlie E, Fitzgerald L, Wood M. Getting evidence into clinical practice: an organisational behaviour

perspective. *Journal of Health Services and Research Policy* 2000;**5**:96–102.
357. Burns LR. The diffusion of unit management among US hospitals. *Hospital and Health Services Administration* 1982;**27**:43–57.
358. Quinn JB. Managing innovation: controlled chaos. *Harvard Business Review* 1985;May–June:75–84.
359. van Maurik J. *Writers on Leadership*. London: Penguin Books, 2001.
360. Hage J, Dewer R. Elite values versus organisational structure in predicting innovation. *Administrative Sciences Quarterly* 1973;**18**:279–90.
361. Perrin B. How to – and how not to – evaluate innovation. *Evaluation* 2002;**8**:13–28.
362. Schneider B, Reichers AE. On the etiology of climates. *Personnel Psychology* 1983;**36**:19–39.
363. Ashforth BE. Climate formation: issues and extensions. *Academy of Management Review* 1985;**4**:837–47.
364. Tushman M, Nadler D. Organising for innovation. *California Management Review* 1986;**28**:74–92.
365. Dopson S, Gabbay J. *Getting Research into Practice and Purchasing*. Oxford: Regional NHS Executive, 1995.
366. Wood M, Ferlie E, Fitzgerald L. *Achieving Change in Clinical Practice: Scientific, Organisational and Behavioural Processes*. Warwick: University of Warwick, CCSC, 1998.
367. Dawson S, Sutherland K, Dopson S, Miller R, Law S. *The Relationship Between R&D and Clinical Practice in Primary and Secondary Care*. Cambridge: Judge Institute of Management Studies, 1998.
368. Gabbay J. *Clinical Effectiveness*. London: Clinical Standards Advisory Group, 1998.
369. Dopson S, Gabbay J, Locock L, Chambers D. *Evaluation of the PACE Programme: Final Report*. Oxford: Oxford Healthcare Management Institute, Templeton College and Wessex Institute for Research and Development, University of Southampton, 1999.
370. Litwin GH, Stringer RA. *Motivation and Organizational Climate*. Boston, MA: Harvard University Press, 1968.
371. McGill ME, Slocum JW, Lei D. Management practices in learning organizations. *Organizational Dynamics* 1992;Summer:5–17.
372. Snyder-Halpern R. Assessing health care setting readiness for point of care computerized clinical decision support system innovations. *Outcomes Management for Nursing Practice* 1999;**3**:118–27.
373. Hansen MT. The search-transfer problem: the role of weak ties in sharing knowledge across organizational subunits. *Administrative Sciences Quarterly* 1999; **44**:82–111.
374. Hage J, Aiken M. Elite values vs organisational structure in predicting innovation. *American Journal of Sociology* 1967;**18**:279–90.
375. Mansfield E. Technical change and the rate of imitation. *Econometrica* 1961;**29**:741–66.
376. Abrahamson E, Fombrun CJ. Macrocultures: determinants and consequences. *Academy of Management Review* 1994;**19**:728–55.
377. Baron JP, Dobbin F, Jennings PD. War and peace: the evolution of modern personnel administration in US industry. *American Journal of Sociology* 1986;**92**:250–83.
378. Davis G. Agents without principles? The spread of the poison pill through the intercorporate network. *Administrative Sciences Quarterly* 1991;**36**:583–613.
379. Palmer DA, Jennings PD, Zhou X. Late adoption of the multidivisional form by large US corporations: institutional, political and economic accounts. *Administrative Sciences Quarterly* 1993;**38**:100–31.
380. Darr ED, Argote L, Epple D. The acquisition and appreciation of knowledge in service organisations: productivity in franchises. *Management Science* 1995;**41**:1750–62.
381. Shan W, Walker G, Kogut B. Interfirm cooperation and startup innovation in the biotechnology industry. *Strategic Management Journal* 1994;**15**:387–94.
382. Abrahamson E, Rosenkopf L. When do bandwagon diffusions roll? How far do they go? And when do they roll backwards: a computer simulation. *Academy of Management Best Paper Proceedings* 1990;155–9.
383. Abrahamson E, Rosenkopf L. Institutional and competitive bandwagons: using mathematical modelling as a tool to explore innovation diffusion. *Academy of Management Review* 1993;**18**:487–517.
384. Swan JA, Newell S. The role of professional associations in technology diffusion. *Organization Studies* 1995;**16**:847–74.
385. Johnston DA, Linton JD. Social networks and the implementation of environmental technology. *Transactions on Engineering Management* 2000;**47**:465–77.
386. Teo HH, Wei KK, Benbasat I. Predicting intention to adopt interorganizational linkages: an institutional perspective. *MIS Quarterly* 2003;**27**:19–49.
387. Kilo CM. A framework for collaborative improvement: lessons from the Institute for Healthcare Improvement's Breakthrough series. *Quality Management in Health Care* 1998;**6**:1–13.
388. Kilo CM. Improving care through collaboration. *Pediatrics* 1999;**103**:384–93.
389. Dewan NA, Daniels A, Zieman G, Kramer T. The national outcomes management project: a benchmarking collaborative. *Journal of Behavioral Health Services and Research* 2000;**27**:431–6.
390. Bate SP, Robert G, McLeod H. *Report on the 'Breakthrough' collaborative approach to quality and service improvement in four regions of the NHS: a research based evaluation of the Orthopaedic Services Collaborative within the Eastern, South and West, South East, and Trent Regions*. Birmingham: Health

Services Management Centre, University of Birmingham, 2002.

391. Leatherman S. Optimizing quality collaboratives. *Quality and Safety in Health Care* 2002;**11**:307.

392. Wilson T, Plsek P, Berwick D. *Learning from Around the World: Experiences and Thoughts of Collaborative Improvement from Seven Countries.* Boston: Institute for Healthcare Improvement, 2001.

393. Kerr CM, Bevan H, Gowland B, Penny J, Berwick D. Redesigning cancer care. *British Medical Journal* 2002;**324**:164–6.

394. Thompson M. Five giant leaps toward integrating health care delivery and ways to drive organizations to leap or get out of the way. *Journal of Ambulatory Care Management* 2000;**23**:1–18.

395. NHS Confederation. *Clinical Networks – a Discussion Paper.* London: NHS Confederation, 2001.

396. Green PL, Plsek PE. Coaching and leadership for the diffusion of innovation in health care: a different type of multi-organization improvement collaborative. *Joint Commission Journal on Quality Improvement* 2002;**28**:55–71.

397. Nonaka I. A dynamic theory of organizational knowledge creation. *Organization Science* 1994;**5**:14–37.

398. Hansen MT. Knowledge network: explaining effective knowledge in multiunit companies. *Organization Science* 2002;**13**:232–48.

399. Shediac-Rizkallah MC, Bone LR. Planning for the sustainability of community-based health programs: conceptual frameworks and future directions for research, practice and policy. *Health Education Research* 1998;**13**:87–108.

400. Marble RP. Operationalising the implementation puzzle: an argument for eclecticism in research and in practice. *European Journal of Information Systems* 2000;**9**:132–47.

401. Zmud RW. An examination of 'push-pull theory' applied to process innovation in knowledge work. *Management Science* 1984;**30**:727–38.

402. Attewell A. Technology diffusion and organizational learning: the case of business computing. *Organization Science* 1992;**3**:1–19.

403. Ledford GF. The persistence of planned organisational change: a process theory perspective. Ann Arbor, University of Michigan: Doctoral thesis, 1984.

404. Goodman RM, Mcleroy KR, Steckler AB, Hoyle RH. Development of level of institutionalization scales for health promotion programs. *Health Education Quarterly* 1993;**20**:161–78.

405. Leonard-Barton D, Deschamps I. Managerial influence in the implementation of new technology. *Management Science* 1988;**34**:1252–65.

406. Goodman RM, Steckler A. The life and death of a health promotion program – an institutionalization perspective. *International Quarterly of Community Health Education* 1988;**8**:5–19.

407. Kaluzny A, Hernandez JB. Organisational change and innovation. In: Shortell SM, Kaluzny A, eds. *Health Care Management: a Text in Organisational Theory and Behaviour.* New York: John Wiley, 1988.

408. Nutbeam D. Improving the fit between research and practice in health promotion: overcoming structural barriers. *Canadian Journal of Public Health* 1996;**87**:S18–23.

409. Jarrar YF, Zairi M. Internal transfer of best practice for performance excellence: a global survey. *Benchmarking: An International Journal* 2000;**7**:239–46.

410. Zairi M, Whymark J. The transfer of best practice: how to build a culture of benchmarking and continuous learning – Part 2. *Benchmarking: An International Journal* 2000;**7**:146–67.

411. Ossip-Klein DJ, Karusa J, Tweet A, Howard J, Obermiller-Powers M, Howard L, *et al.* Benchmarking implementation of a computerized system for long-term care. *American Journal of Medical Quality* 2002;**17**:94–101.

412. Goodman PS, Dean JW. Creating long term organizational change. In: Goodman PS, ed. *Change in Organizations.* San Francisco: Jossey-Bass, 1982.

413. Yin RK. *Changing Urban Bureaucracies: How New Practices Become Routinized.* Lexington, ML: Lexington Books, 1979.

414. Øvretveit J. *Making Temporary Quality Improvement Continuous: a Review of Research Relevant to the Sustainability of Quality Improvement in Health Care.* Stockholm: Karolinska Institute MMC, 2003.

415. Grimshaw J, Campbell M, Eccles M, Steen N. Experimental and quasi-experimental designs for evaluating guideline implementation strategies. *Family Practice* 2000;**17**:S11–18.

416. Eccles M, Grimshaw J, Campbell M, Ramsay C. Research designs for studies evaluating the effectiveness of change and improvement strategies. *Quality and Safety in Health Care* 2003;**12**:47–52.

417. Grol R, Grimshaw J. From best evidence to best practice: effective implementation of change in patients' care. *Lancet* 2003;**362**:1225–30.

418. Green LW, Kreuter MW, Deeds SG, Partridge KD. *Health Education Panning: a Diagnostic Approach.* Mountain View, CA: Mayfield, 1980.

419. Parcel GS, Perry CW, Taylor CW. Beyond demonstration: diffusion of health promotion innovations. In: Brach N, ed. *Health Promotion at the Community Level.* Newbury Park, CA: Sage, 1990.

420. Rycroft-Malone J, Kitson A, Harvey G, McCormack B, Seers K, Titchen A, *et al.* Ingredients for change: revisiting a conceptual framework. *Quality and Safety in Health Care* 2002;**11**:174–80.

421. Harvey G, Loftus-Hills A, Rycroft-Malone J, Titchen A, Kitson A, McCormack B, *et al.* Getting evidence into practice: the role and function of facilitation. *Journal of Advanced Nursing* 2002;**37**:577–88.

422. Nault BR, Wolfe RA, Dexter AS. Support strategies to foster adoption of interorganizational innovations. *Transactions on Engineering Management* 1997;**44**:378–89.
423. Orlandi MA. Health promotion technology transfer: organizational perspectives. *Canadian Journal of Public Health* 1996;**87** (**Suppl 2**):S28–33.
424. Stachenko S. The Canadian heart health initiative: dissemination perspectives. *Canadian Journal of Public Health* 1996;**87** (**Suppl 2**):S57–9.
425. Schabas R. Promoting heart health promotion. *Canadian Journal of Public Health* 1996;**87** (**Suppl 2**):S547.
426. Potvin L, Cargo M, McComber AM, Delormier T, Macaulay AC. Implementing participatory intervention and research in communities: lessons from the Kahnawake Schools Diabetes Prevention Project in Canada. *Social Science and Medicine* 2003;**56**:1295–305.
427. Macaulay AC, Commanda LE, Freeman WL, Gibson N, McCabe ML, Robbins CM, *et al.* Participatory research maximises community and lay involvement. North American Primary Care Research Group. *British Medical Journal* 1999;**319**:774–8.
428. Chen TF, Crampton M, Krass I, Benrimoj SI. Collaboration between community pharmacists and GPs in innovative clinical services: a conceptual model. *Journal of Social and Administrative Pharmacy* 1999;**16**:134–44.
429. Chen TF, Crampton M, Krass I, Benrimoj SI. *Interprofessional Collaboration Between Community Pharmacists and General Practitioners in Medication Regimen Review.* Sydney: University of Sydney, 2001.
430. Caldwell R. Models of change agents a fourfold classification. *British Journal of Management* 2003;**14**:131–42.
431. Riley BL, Taylor SM, Elliott SJ. Determinants of implementing heart health: promotion activities in Ontario public health units: a social ecological perspective. *Health Education Research* 2001; **16**:425–41.
432. Ellsworth JB. Technology and change for the information age. 2002 http://horizon.unc.edu/projects/monograph/CD/Change_Innovation/ Ellsworth.asp
433. Snyder-Halpern R. Health care system innovation: a model for practice. *Advanced Practice Nursing Quarterly* 1996;**1**:12–19.
434. Stake R. *The Art of Case Study Research.* London: Sage, 1995.
435. Renholm M, Leino-Kilpi H, Suominen T. Critical pathways: a systematic review. *Journal of Nursing Administration* 2002;**32**:196–202.
436. Campbell H, Hotchkiss R, Bradshaw N, Porteous M. Integrated care pathways. *British Medical Journal* 1998;**316**:133–7.
437. Harkleroad A, Schirf D, Volpe J, Holm MB. Critical pathway development: an integrative literature review. *American Journal of Occupational Therapy* 2000;**54**:148–54.
438. Pearson SD, Goulart-Fisher D, Lee TH. Critical pathways as a strategy for improving care: problems and potential. *Annals of Internal Medicine* 1995; **123**:941–8.
439. Benham AJ. Managed care and critical pathway development: the joint replacement experience. *Orthopaedic Nursing* 1999;**18**:71–5.
440. Brugh LA. Automated clinical pathways in the patient record legal implications. *Nursing Case Management* 1998;**3**:131–7.
441. Johnson S, Smith J. Factors influencing the success of ICP projects. *Professional Nurse* 2000;**15**:776–9.
442. Syed KA, Bogoch ER. Integrated care pathways in hip fracture management: demonstrated benefits are few. *Journal of Rheumatology* 2000;**27**:2071–3.
443. Naglie IG, Alibhai SM. Improving outcomes in hip fracture patients: are care pathways the answer? *Journal of Rheumatology* 2000;**27**:2068–70.
444. Beavis D, Simpson S, Graham I. A literature review of dementia care mapping: methodological considerations and efficacy. *Journal of Psychiatric and Mental Health Nursing* 2002;**9**:725–36.
445. Kwan J, Sandercock P. In-hospital care pathways for stroke. *Cochrane Database of Systematic Review* 2002;CD002924.
446. Cannon CP, Hand MH, Bahr R, Boden WE, Christenson R, Gibler WB, *et al.* Critical pathways for management of patients with acute coronary syndromes: an assessment by the National Heart Attack Alert Program. *American Heart Journal* 2002;**143**:777–89.
447. Currie L, Harvey G. Care pathways development and implementation. *Nursing Standard* 1998;**12**:35–8.
448. Oakley P, Greaves E. Process reengineering: from command to demand. *Health Service Journal* 1995;**23** February:32–3.
449. Harrison S, Choudhury N. General practice fund holding in the UK National Health Service: evidence to date. *Journal of Public Health Policy* 1996;**17**: 331–46.
450. Hausman D, Le Grand J. Incentives and health policy: primary and secondary care in the British National Health Service. *Social Science and Medicine* 1999;**49**:1299–307.
451. Wilkin D. Primary care budget holding in the United Kingdom National Health Service: learning from a decade of health service reform. *Medical Journal of Australia* 2002;**176**:539–42.
452. Milne RG, Torsney B. Financial incentives, competition and a two tier service: lessons from the UK National Health Service internal market. *Health Policy* 2003;**64**:1–12.
453. Whitten PS, Mair FS, Haycox A, May CR, Williams TL, Hellmich S. Systematic review of cost effectiveness studies of telemedicine interventions. *British Medical Journal* 2002;**324**:1434–7.

454. Department of Health. *The Patient's Charter*. London: Her Majesty's Stationery Office, 1992.

455. Appleby J. Fundholding databriefing. *Health Service Journal* 1994;**5415**:32–3.

456. Rivett G. *From Cradle to Grave: Fifty Years of the NHS*. London: Kings Fund, 1998.

457. Baines DL, Whynes DK. Selection bias in GP fundholding. *Health Economics* 1996;5:129–40.

458. Warwicker T. Managerialism and the British GP: the GP as manager and as managed. *Journal of Medical Management* 1998;**12**:331–48, 320.

459. Kay A. The abolition of the GP fundholding scheme: a lesson in evidence-based policy making. *British Journal of General Practice* 2002;**52**:141–4.

460. Currell R, Urquhart C, Wainwright P, Lewis R. Telemedicine versus face to face patient care: effects on professional practice and health care outcomes. *Cochrane Database of Systematic Review* 2000;CD002098.

461. Grigsby J, Rigby M, Hiemstra A, House M, Olsson S, Whitten P. Telemedicine/telehealth: an international perspective. The diffusion of telemedicine. *Telemedicine Journal and E-Health* 2002;8:79–94.

462. Cook D, Whitten P. Telemedicine in Kansas 1994–2001. *Journal of Healthcare Information Management* 2002;**16**:60–6.

463. Hu PJ, Chau PY. Physician acceptance of telemedicine technology: an empirical investigation. *Topics in Health Information Management* 1999;**19**:20–35.

464. Pelletier-Fleury N, Fargeon V, Lanoe JL, Fardeau M. Transaction costs economics as a conceptual framework for the analysis of barriers to the diffusion of telemedicine. *Health Policy* 1997;**42**:1–14.

465. Tanriverdi H, Iacono CS. Diffusion of telemedicine: a knowledge barrier perspective. *Telemedicine Journal* 1999;5:223–44.

466. Weinstein RS, Descour MR, Liang C, Bhattacharyya AK, Graham AR, Davis JR, *et al*. Telepathology overview: from concept to implementation. *Human Pathology* 2001;**32**:1283–99.

467. Mair F, Whitten P. Systematic review of studies of patient satisfaction with telemedicine. *British Medical Journal* 2000;**320**:1517–20.

468. Mairinger T. Acceptance of telepathology in daily practice. *Analytical Cellular Pathology* 2002;**21**:135–40.

469. Wootton R. Recent advances: telemedicine. *British Medical Journal* 2001;**323**:557–60.

470. Field MJ, Grigsby J. Telemedicine and remote patient monitoring. *Journal of the American Medical Association* 2002;**288**:423–5.

471. Sujansky WV. The benefits and challenges of an electronic medical record: much more than a "word-processed" patient chart. *Western Journal of Medicine* 1998;**169**:176–83.

472. Department of Health. *Information for Health: an Information Strategy for the Modern NHS 1998–2005*. London: NHS Executive, 1998.

473. Weir C, Lincoln M, Roscoe D, Turner C, Moreshead G. Dimensions associated with successful implementation of a hospital based integrated order entry system. *Proceedings – the Annual Symposium on Computer Applications in Medical Care* 1994;653–7.

474. Retchin SM, Wenzel RP. Electronic medical record systems at academic health centers: advantages and implementation issues. *Academic Medicine* 1999;**74**:493–8.

475. Thiru K, Hassey A, Sullivan F. Systematic review of scope and quality of electronic patient record data in primary care. *British Medical Journal* 2003;**326**:1070.

476. Veronesi JF. Ethical issues in computerized medical records. *Critical Care Nursing Quarterly* 1999;**22**:75–80.

477. Gaunt N, Roger-France F. Security of the electronic health care record – professional and ethical implications. *Studies in Health Technology and Informatics* 1996;**27**:10–22.

478. Chilton L, Berger JE, Melinkovich P, Nelson R, Rappo PD, Stoddard J, *et al*. American Academy of Pediatrics. Pediatric Practice Action Group and Task Force on Medical Informatics. Privacy protection and health information: patient rights and pediatrician responsibilities. *Pediatrics* 1999;**104**:973–7.

479. Loomis GA, Ries JS, Saywell RM Jr, Thakker NR. If electronic medical records are so great, why aren't family physicians using them? *Journal of Family Practice* 2002;**51**:636–41.

480. Grigsby WJ. Telehealth: an assessment of growth and distribution. *Journal of Rural Health* 2002;**18**:348–58.

481. Fleuren M, Wiefferink K, Paulussen T. Determinants of innovation within health care organizations: literature review and Delphi study. *International Journal of Quality in Health Care* 2004;**16**:107–23.

482. Potvin L. Methodological challenges in evaluation of dissemination programs. *Canadian Journal of Public Health* 1996;**87** (**Suppl 2**):S79–S83.

483. Green LW. From research to 'best practices" in other settings and populations. *American Journal of Health Behavior* 2001;**25**:165–78.

484. Rootman I, Goodstadt M, Potvin L, Springett J. A framework for health promotion evaluation. *WHO Regional Publications European Series* 2001;7–38.

485. Amidon DM. *The Innovation Superhighway: Sustaining Collaborative Advantage*. Butterworth-Heinemann, 2002.

486. Tushman M, Moore WL. *Readings in the Management of Innovation*. Marshfield, MA: Pitman, 1982.

487. Rothwell R, Gardener P. *Innovation*. London: Design Council, 1985.

488. Jones T. *Innovating at the Edge: How Organisations Evolve and Embed Innovation Capability.* New York: Butterworth-Heinemann, 2002.
489. Tushman ML, O'Reilly A. *Winning Through Innovation: a Practical Guide to Leading Organisational Change and Renewal.* New York: Harvard Business School Press, 2002.
490. Ellsworth JB. Surviving change: a survey of educational change models. Syracuse, NY: ERIC Clearinghouse on Information and Technology (ED 443 417), 2000.
491. Kraft JM, Mezoff JS, Sogolow ED, Neumann MS, Thomas PA. A technology transfer model for effective HIV/AIDS interventions: science and practice. *AIDS Education and Prevention* 2000;**12**:7–20.
492. Drummond M, Weatherly H. Implementing the findings of health technology assessments. If the CAT got out of the bag, can the TAIL wag the dog? *International Journal of Technology Assessment in Health Care* 2000;**16**:1–12.
493. Gladwin J, Wilson TD. Validation of a theoretical model linking organisational fit and diffusion of innovation in information systems development. *Health Informatics Journal* 2000;**6**:219–27.
494. Daft RL. Bureaucratic versus nonbureaucratic structure and the process of innovation and change. In: Bacarach SB, ed. *Research in the Sociology of Organisations*, Vol. 1. Greenwich, CT: JAI Press, 1982, pp. 129–66.
495. Damanpour F. Innovation type, radicalness, and the adoption process. *Communication Research* 1988;**15**:545–67.
496. Rogers EM, Williams L, West RB. *Bibliography of the Diffusion of Innovations.* Stanford, CA: Institute for Communications Research, Stanford University, 1977.
497. Glazer RH, Montgomery DB. New products and innovations: an annotated bibliography. Technical report no. 65. Stanford, CA: Graduate School of Business, Stanford University, 1980.
498. Moch MK, Morse EV. Size, centralization, and organizational adoption of innovations. *American Sociological Review* 1977;**42**:716–25.
499. Porter R. *From Cradle to Grave: 50 Years of the NHS.* London: Kings Fund, 1998.
500. Oakley A. *Ways of knowing: gender and method in the social sciences.* London: Sage, 2000.
501. Stross JK, Bole GG. Evaluation of a continuing education program in rheumatoid arthritis. *Arthritis and Rheumatism* 1980;**23**: 846–9.
502. Stross JK, Hiss RG, Wattts CM, Davis WK, MacDonald R. Continuing education in pulmonary disease for primary-care physicians. *American Review of Respiratory Diseases* 1983;**127**:739–46.
503. Stross JK, Bole GG. Evaluation of an educational program for primary care practitioners, on the management of osteoarthritis. *Arthritis and Rheumatism* 1985;**28**:108–11.
504. Hong SW, Ching TY, Fung JP, Seto WL. The employment of ward opinion leaders for continuing education in the hospital. *Medical Teacher* 1990;**12**: 209–17.
505. Hodnett ED, Kaufman K, O'Brien-Pallas L, Chipman M, Watson-MacDonell J, Hunsburger W. A strategy to promote research-based nursing care: effects on childbirth outcomes. *Research in Nursing and Health* 1996;**19**:13–20.

Index

Note: Page numbers in *italics* represent figures, those in **bold** represent tables.

Abrahamson, Eric 70, 158
absorptive capacity 72
adopter traits 67, 100–3, *101*, 220
adopters 100–13, *225*
adoption 28–9, 61, 92, 100–13, **211–12**, *225*
  as process 103–6, *104*, *105*
  psychological antecedents 103
  rate of *57*
  stages of 104
adoptive curve *see* S-shaped adoption curve
advertising *57*
advocates 126–9
agricultural extension model 52
anthropology 50
appraisal phase 33, 38–40
appreciative enquiry 79
assimilation of innovations 106–13, *112*
audience segmentation 90, 132, 133
augmented product 102

bandwagons 157–8
Bass Forecasting Model *57*
Beacon Council Scheme 169
Berwick, Don 25
best practice 27
  transfer of 168–70
Bevan, Anyerin 22
bias
  context-transferability 59–60
  individual blame 59
  linear relationship 59
boundary spanners 41, 129–30, 162
Breakthrough model 163–4, 165
Brown and Duguid, *The social life of information* 74

Canadian Heart Health Implementation Programme 188
capacity 186
capacity-building activities 186
case studies 199–218, **202**, *210*
  electronic health record 208–10, **211–18**
  GP fundholding 204–6, **211–18**
  integrated care pathways 202–4, **202**, **211–18**
  telemedicine 206–8, **211–18**
centralisation **135**
centralised networks **132**
certainty-agreement matrix *80*
champions 41, 126–9
  executive 128
  exit 128
  product 127
change agents 130
chief executives 127
citation tracking 35
client orientation 131, 132
cliques 117
Cochrane Effective Practice and Organisation of Care Group 39
collaboration 191–4
communicability 89, 98
communication **23**, 55–6, 130–1, **213–14**
  channels 154
  key variables 56
  prestige 120, 123
community development 64
compatibility 84, 86, 87, 89, 95, 131
complexity **24**, 79–80, *80*, 84, 89, 96, **135**
  structural 138–40, **140**, 146–8
concerns-based adoption model 105–6, *105*
confirmation 104
conflicting evidence 41
consequences of innovation 60
context 187
context-transferability bias 59–60
contingency factors 139, **140**
cosmopolitanism 159
cost 56–8, 63, 132
credibility 131
critical appraisal checklists 234–44
critical success factors 26

Damanpour, Fariborz 27, 28, 67, 96, 135–41, 146, 148, 157, 159,172, 246
data extraction form 232–3
decentralised networks **132**
decision processes 182
definitions 26–31
demonstrations 131
Department of Health 21, 25
  Service Delivery and Organisation Programme 25
descriptive models 58
developing world, innovations in 61–2
development studies **23**, 60–2
diffusion 29, 114–32
diffusion of innovations research 20–2, *21*, **23–4**, *44*
  criteria for developing world 62

diffusion of innovations research (*continued*)
  history and sociocultural context 58
  limitations of 58–60
  origins of conventional approaches to 49–51
discussion 107
dissemination 29, 114–32, 225–6
divisibility 98
domain consensus 171

early adopters 52, 59, 102, 113
early majority 101, 102
ease of use 86
economic profitability 94
education 51, 56, 57, **64**, 77, 105, 183–4
effort 131
egocentric mapping 162
electronic health records 208–10, **211–18**
electronic searching 35
empathy 131
environmental impact 170–2
EPPIcentre method 45
EUR-ASSESS systematic review 180–1
evidence-based medicine **23**, 64–6
exchange theory 62, 132
executive champions 128
exit champion 128
explanatory models 58
explicit knowledge 71
external agencies **217–18**
external communication 119, **135**, 159
external integration 159
external orientation 171

facilitation 187
failed innovations 61
Ferlie, Ewan 65, 125
Fitzgerald, Louise 65, 69, 111, 122, 125, 134, 147, 162, 173
fixed innovation 59
forecasting models 57
formalisation **135**
formative evaluation research 132
functional differentiation **135**

Gabriel, Yiannis 77, 78
general systems theory 79–80, *80*, **81**, *82*
generative relationships 79
GP fundholding 204–6, **211–18**
Green, Larry 228
Grimshaw *et al.*, review of dissemination and implementation of guidelines 183–5
Grimshaw, Jeremy 54, 175, 245
guidelines 64–6
Gustafson *et al.*, narrative review of change management in organisations 185–6

Health Action Zones 64
Health Development Agency 64
Health Education Authority 64
health promotion **23**, 62–4, **64**
health technology assessments 57–8
heterophily 124
heuristics 106
hierarchies 117
high-technology innovations 102
homophily 63, 114, 115, 131, 167
human resources 182

illusion of manageability 70
image 86
implementation 104, 175–98, **215–16**, 227
  complexity 98
  EUR-ASSESS systematic review 180–1
  failure 69
  Grimshaw *et al.* model 183–5
  Gustafson *et al.* model 185–6
  Meyers *et al.* model 181–3
  whole-systems approach 195–8
included studies 255–92
inclusion criteria 37
individual blame bias 59
influence prestige 120, 123
information and communications technology 85
inner context 107, 134–56, **213–14**
innovation gap 61, *65*
innovations 26–8, 83–99
  adoption of *see* adoption
  assimilation of 106–13, *112*
  background literature 83–7
  consequences of 60
  diffusion of *see* diffusion of innovations research
  empirical studies 90–4
  environmental impact 170–2
  failure of 61
  further research 225
  high-technology 102
  impact of 61
  organisational 26–8
  politics and policymaking 172–4
  as progress 54
  service delivery 26–8
  structural determinants of 66–8, *67*
innovativeness 119
  organisation determinants of 140–1
innovators 102
Institute for Healthcare Improvement (IHI) model 163, 164
institutionalisation 68, 175–98
  EUR-ASSESS systematic review 180–1
  Grimshaw *et al.* 183–5
  Gustafson *et al.* 185–6
  measurement of 178–80
  Meyers *et al.* 181–3
integrated care pathways 202–4, **211–18**
interactive initiatives 183
interconnectedness 54
intermediary agents 194–5
internal communication **135**
internalisation 72–4
interorganisational networks **24**, 70, 157–8, 160
interpersonal communication 52, 57
interpersonal networks 114–16, **115**, 160
  and diffusion of innovations 116–18
intervention models 58
intervention studies 188–90
Iowa hybrid corn study 51–3, *52*
irreversible action 30

key observations 113
Kingdon's model of policy streams 173
knowledge 104
knowledge creation cycle *74*
knowledge enactment 154
knowledge manipulation 72–4, **73**, *74*
knowledge purveyors 190, 194

knowledge readiness 156
knowledge transfer 191–4
knowledge utilisation **24**, 154–6, **155**, **156**
knowledge-based approaches to diffusion of innovations 70–7
Kuhn, Thomas 32, 37, 42

labour-saving technologies 61
laggards 52, *59*, 101, 102
late adopters *see* laggards
late majority 101, 102
laws of imitation 50
leadership 69–70
  empirical studies 148–50
  see also opinion leaders
learning organisation 74–5, **75**
Leonard-Barton, Dorothy 73, 97
Level of Institutionalisation (LoIn) Scale 179
limited evidence 42
linear relationship bias 59
linkage activities 191–5
low complexity 167
Lyotard, Jean-François 43

managerial attitude towards change **135**
managerial tenure **135**
mapping phase 33, 37–8
market potential 57
market research 57
market segmentation 62–3
marketing **23**, 56–8
  mix 63, 132
  strategies 102
mass media 57
medical sociology **23**, 53–5
Medline *44*
meta-analyses 135–40
meta-narrative review 42–7, *43*, *44*, **45**
method 32–47
  appraisal phase 33, 38–40
  inclusion criteria 37
  mapping phase 33, 37–8
  meta-narrative review 42–7, *43*, *44*, **45**
  planning phase 33, 34
  recommendations phase 33
  search phase 33, 35–7, *36*
  synthesis phase 40–2
Meyers *et al.*, review of industrial process implementation 181–3
middle management 129
mission statements 66
models
  application 220–5
  Bass Forecasting 57
  Breakthrough 163–4, 165
  concerns-based adoption 105–6, *105*
  Grimshaw *et al.* 183–5
  Gustafson *et al.* 185–6
  Institute for Healthcare Improvement 163, 164
  Kingdon's model of policy streams 173
  Meyers *et al.* 181–3
  NHS Beacon 168–70
  PRECEDE 186
  threshold 54–5
Moore and Benbasat Perceived Characteristics of Innovations scale 86, 90, 93
Moore's chasm 101
multi-organisational improvement collaboratives 163–8

narrative organisational studies 77–9
narrative studies **24**
narrative summary 40, 44
National Health Service 22, 25
natural growth *21*
network facilitator 128
networks 70
  centralised **132**
  decentralised 132
  interorganisational **24**, 70, 157–63
  interpersonal 114–18, **115**, 160
  social 162
NHS Beacon model 168–70
NHS Modernisation Agency 22, 25, 164, 168
  definition of sustainability 29–30
niche saturation 179
non-adoption 105, 112
normal science 42
Northern New England Cardiovascular Disease Study Group 165

observability 84, 96
Ontario Heart Health Promotion Project 195
operational attributes 97–9
operational feasibility 98
opinion leaders 41, 52, 55, 118–26, 167
  background literature 118–20
  characteristics of 120
  empirical studies 120–5
  expert **121**
  general characteristics 119
  measurement of leadership 119
  monomorphic leadership 118
  peer **121**
  polymorphic leadership 118
Organisation SCAN 186, 188, 196
organisational buffer 128
organisational centrality 70
organisational climate 150–3
organisational context 69, 226
organisational cosmopolitanism 159
organisational culture 69–70
organisational determinants 135–8, **136**, **138**
organisational fads and fashions 70
organisational innovativeness **24**, 26–8, 69
  structural determinants of 66–8, *67*
organisational learning 70, **156**
organisational maverick 128
organisational opinion leadership 70
organisational process 68–9
  context and culture **24**
organisational readiness 123
organisational sense-making 75–7
organisational size 138–40, **140**
  empirical studies 141–6, **142**
organisational structure 182
organisational ties 70
outer context **215–16**
overadoption 110
Øvretveit, John 42, 164, 166, 167, 180, 197

paradigm shift 64, 65
passages 179
peer review 37
Perceived Characteristics of Innovations Scale 85, 86
personal computers 76
persuasion 104

pharmaceutical industry 53–5
pharmaceutical sponsorship 54
planning phase 33, 34
Plsek, Paul 79, 80, **81**, 165, 186, 197
policymaking 172–4
politics 172–4
Potvin, Louise 193, 228, 229
PRECEDE model 186
predisposition 186
pro-innovation bias 58–9
process tracking 132
process-based research 68
product champions 127
professionalism **135**
Promoting Action on Clinical Effectiveness (PACE) Programme 123

quantitative approach 71

randomised controlled trials 39, 65–6, 189
rate of adoption 57
realist review 46–7
receptive context 150–1, 197
redundancy 70
reference scanning 35
reinforcement 187
reinvention 84, 96, 97, 167
relative advantage 84, 86, 89, 94, 111, 167
Research Into Practice Team 25
research traditions **23–4**, 48–82
resisting erosion 30
resource system and change agency 190–1
result demonstrability 86
risk orientation 149–50
riskiness 86
Rogers, Everett 3, 6, 20, 26, 28, 29, 38, 49, 50, 53, 58, 60, 61, 67, 83–4, 96, 101, 115, 119, 130–1, 162, 191, 193
routines 179
routinisation 30
rural sociology **23**, 51–3, *52*

S-shaped diffusion curve *21*, 58, 60, 64
Sackett, David 65
saturation 63
search phase 33, 35–7, *36*
  citation tracking 35
  electronic searching 35
  formal search methods 35
  informal methods 35
  reference scanning 35
search strings 35–6
service delivery, innovation in 26–8
single interventions 183–4
slack resources **135**
snowball sampling 53
social construction of meaning 191
social influence 225–6
social marketing 62, 131
social networks 162
socialisation 72
specialisation **135**
spread 29, 130–3
stages of adoption 104
statistics 245–54

sticky knowledge 71
storytelling 77–9
strength of evidence 123
structural complexity 138–40, **140**
structural equivalence 51
structural holes 70
surveys 187–8
susceptibility to new ideas 64
sustainability 29–31
synthesis of data 44–5, **45**
synthesis phase 40–2
system antecedents 186
system openness 67
system readiness 226–7
systematic browsing 35
systematic reviews 91

tacit knowledge 71
Tarde, *The Laws of Imitation* 49–50
task diversity 147
task relevance 98
task usefulness 98
Team Climate Inventory 153
technical innovators 127
technical knowledge resources **135**
technology fit 182
telemedicine 206–8, **211–18**
temporary learning organisation 163
The Limits to Growth 58
The NHS Plan 22, 163–4
theoretical papers 38
Thomson O'Brien, Mary Ann 122, 245
threshold models 54–5
top-down initiatives 183
Tornatzky and Klein meta-analysis of innovation attributes 87–9, **88**
total quality management 161
transfer of best practice 168–70
transferability 98
transformational leader 128
trend-setting 111
trial 107
trialability 84, 86, 96, 167

underadoption 110
urbanisation 171

Valente, Thomas 43, 54, 55, 114, 118
Van de Ven, Andrew 27, 69, 96, 113, 150, 170, 177
vertical differentiation **135**
viral marketing 64
visibility 86
voluntariness 86

weak ties 54, 55
Weick, Karl 30, 73, 76, 170
Welfare State 22
Welsh Clinical Effectiveness Initiative National Demonstration Projects 123
whole-systems research 195–8, 227–31
World Health Organisation Health Evidence Network 42

Yin, Robert 178